*The
Drinking
Man*

The Drinking Man

DAVID C. McCLELLAND

WILLIAM N. DAVIS

RUDOLF KALIN

ERIC WANNER

The Free Press, NEW YORK
Collier-Macmillan Ltd., LONDON

The Free Press
A DIVISION OF THE MACMILLAN COMPANY
866 Third Avenue, New York, New York 10022

Collier-Macmillan Canada Ltd., Toronto, Ontario

Library of Congress Catalog Card Number: 79–143504

Printing Number
3   4   5   6   7   8   9   10

Contents

Preface   vii

Authors and Contributors   xiii

I. Social Drinking   1

1. The Effects of Male Social Drinking on Fantasy   3
2. Social Drinking in Different Settings   21

II. Motives for Drinking   45

3. A Cross-Cultural Study of Folk-Tale Content and Drinking   48
4. Power and Inhibition: A Revision of the Magical Potency Theory   73
5. The Need for Power in College Men: Action Correlates and Relationship to Drinking   99

III. Drinking and the Need for Power   121

6. The Effects of Drinking on Thoughts About Power and Restraint   123
7. The Influence of Unrestrained Power Concerns on Drinking in Working-Class Men   142
8. Drinking in the Wider Context of Restrained and Unrestrained Assertive Thoughts and Acts   162
9. Drinking: A Search for Power or Nurturance?   198

v

IV. Explaining Alcoholism 215

10. Self-Descriptions of College Problem Drinkers   217

11. Alcoholism in a Mexican Village   232

12. The Sacred Water: The Quest for Personal Power Through Drinking Among the Teton Sioux   261

13. Examining the Research Basis for Alternative Explanations of Alcoholism   276

14. A Pilot Attempt To Help Alcoholics by Socializing Their Power Needs   316

15. Summary   332

Appendices 337

I. Description of Power Scoring Categories Used in Chapter 6   338

II. Activities Questions Asked in Bar Study II, with Variants Noted for Bar Study I, If Any   342

III. Are Sex and Aggression Power Concerns in Fantasy Alternative Manifestations of the Same Drive?   348

IV. Scoring Manual for Personal and Social Power Concerns   351

V. Correlations of Marital Problems with Power Concerns and Drinking in Two Bar Studies   357

VI. Correlations with Drinking of Self-Descriptive Statements Not Grouped in Three Factors   358

VII. Picture Reproductions   360

VIII. Detailed Codes for Social Variables Related to Drinking   368

IX. Motives for Drug Taking Among College Men   370

Bibliography   379

Index   387

Preface

The purpose of this book is to report the results of a ten-year-long program of psychological investigation of the role of alcohol in human life. Though varied in conception and approach, the investigations were all guided by a single premise—that drinking alcohol is essentially a psychologically motivated act. This assumption has shaped the research we have undertaken in several ways. First, we have studied drinking as it occurs in natural social settings where the subject may choose freely how much and how often he drinks. Second, we have tried to discover the psychological states which influence the subject's choice. In short, we have sought to determine how a subject thinks, feels and fantasizes before, during, and after taking a drink. We would not deny that alcohol has important physiological and behavioral effects which have been the subject of prolonged study; but the question we have asked is why men willingly partake of a substance which elicits these effects. It is a psychological question, and to it we have applied predominantly psychological methods. However, a glance over the Contents will show that this fact has not served as a limitation. It has encouraged a diversity unusual in studies of alcohol, which are customarily limited to one approach—a questionnaire survey, a series of case studies, or perhaps a laboratory investigation in which alcohol is administered intravenously in a double blind experiment.

The reporting of such a diverse series of studies carried out over a ten-year period presents problems. The model for scientific writing is basically deductive: theories are constructed in advance; hypotheses are derived and tested; and conclusions are drawn. Although we can only speculate about how others live with the prescriptions of this model, it was clear to us at the outset that we had very few strong theoretical notions. Rather we had many ideas as to how drinking might affect thinking or "expand consciousness." Then, on the basis of our first results, we began to reject some of those ideas and entertain others. As we designed experiments to test the new ideas, we continuously adjusted our theories of the psychological factors which motivate drinking. Now, nearly ten years later, our theory has become more firmly fixed, but the path by which we have arrived at that theory is neither straight nor narrow—which presents an expository problem. Even the most dedicated reader, we felt, could not be asked to retrace our tortuous process of theory construction. The dilemma was whether to rewrite our own history or to ignore it; to go back and shape up our earlier opinions o to present only our final conclusions. In the end we decided against both options.

We considered trying to re-work all of our investigations in the light of our final understandings, but decided that we could not and probably should not. We could not because it proved impossible to explain on the basis of the final theory why we had conducted certain experiments or decided to employ certain measures. For instance, for several years we were convinced that drinking affected primarily what we thought were feelings of sentience (physical sex, physical aggression, and meaning contrasts). The experiments reported in Chapter 2 were designed to test this theory. Although the results discouraged us in this interpretation a little at the time, it was only later, after we had begun to entertain the power theory of liquor drinking, that we went back and began to see the results of this experiment in quite a different light. But how should we report this series of events? Should we write up the experiment exactly as it was conceived and interpreted at the time, or should we reinterpret what happened in the light of hindsight? What we have done is something of a compromise. Several of the chapters report studies much as they were conceived of at the time, but with comments added in the discussion sections pointing forward to later results. Thus, the reader should be able both to get a look at the original findings and to understand what we think their implications are with respect to later work.

For we also feel that we should not distort earlier findings too much in the service of current theoretical orientation. Though we have been guided to our present convictions by our own results, those results are open to more than one interpretation. Several times in the past ten years we have been thoroughly convinced of a theoretical interpretation, which later proved to be at best only partially correct, and on the basis of that conviction have at particular moments gone back and re-interpreted and re-written earlier results, only to find that subsequent evidence required still another re-writing. So now, although we find our current theory reasonably convincing, given our past experience it would be foolish for us to expect no further modification of the theory in the future. Thus, the sensible procedure is to present all of our findings in a fairly straightforward fashion so that they may be taken into account in the light of future theoretical revisions.

Therefore, the reader will discover that there is a certain interpretive inelegance about the chapters in this book. They do not fit perfectly together in a well-integrated scheme. Interpretations from one chapter to another are not perfectly consistent with each other. If in the end they do add up to a general case, it is by no means so foolproof a case that the reader could not set off to develop an alternative interpretation from the same data. Hence we have tried to report those data straight-forwardly just as we obtained them in order to make possible the search for an alternative.

Diversity in the book is created not only by the progression in our ideas over time but also by the variety of methods that we employed. Some chapters deal with the effects of alcohol on fantasy, others with folk-tale themes associated cross-culturally with heavy drinking, still others with the attitudes and needs of men who habitually drink too much. Measures are based on content analyses of thought samples, adjective check lists, questionnaires, attitude scales or reports of characteristic actions taken. As far as the main findings are concerned, studies were replicated to make sure that the results obtained a first time were reliably as well as statistically significant. But replications never yield exactly the same results obtained originally, and so new findings have to be explained or explained away.

Why approach the same phenomenon in so many different ways so many different times if it only makes a consistent scientific explanation harder to arrive at? The essence of the problem lies in one's conception of the nature of psychological theories or explanation. The conventional model of a scientific theory dictates that it should lead to a crucial operational test which will confirm or reject it. If an investigator has such a model in mind, he will concentrate on trying to design the most precise test of the theory possible. He will not be particularly interested in alternative methods of confirming or denying it, using the whole gamut of measurement and analytic techniques available to the psychologist. Were he to be lured into employing other techniques, he might well find that some of them seem to support the theory and others reject it. He might wonder which methodological approach is the more "valid" and might even decide to limit himself to one approach in order to avoid confusion as to whether his theory was really correct. For instance, many students of alcoholism restrict themselves to the case study method because it regularly seems to confirm their hypothesis that alcoholics have dependency problems without yielding messy alternative findings that cast doubt on this theory. Other measurement techniques, such as those reported in Chapters 1–4 of this book, provide no direct evidence for the claim that dependency problems are associated with drinking.

Obviously the situation presents problems in interpretation. One has the choice of sticking to the dependency theory and arguing that some methods are simply inadequate for testing it, or of modifying it in some way so as to account for all the different phenomena associated with drinking, however measured. To us, the second alternative has seemed not only preferable, but also the only really viable one. For in our experience psychological theories are seldom expressed in precise enough terms to be proved or disproved. Certain of our findings, for example, have led us to be skeptical about the dependency theory of alcoholism, widely held at the present time. Yet at no time have we ever been convinced that we had clearly "disproved" the dependency hypothesis. In fact there is a suggestion in some of the discussion in Chapter 3 that all we may have done is to reinterpret the dependency hypothesis and state it in somewhat different terms in the light of further findings.

But we believe this is precisely what psychological theorizing is all about. Its purpose is to state some kind of generalization that will tie together or make sense out of a series of related phenomena. The more separate facts it will satisfactorily account for, the better it is as a generalization. It is such a view of theory that has led us to employ so many different methods. A satisfactory generalization about the motives underlying drinking ought to enable us to create situations in which men drink more, to predict which societies around the world drink heavily, to explain how heavy drinkers think and act, to design a therapeutic program with a better method of curing alcoholism. Only by testing the theory in all of these different ways, with a variety of different methods, we felt, could we gain some assurance that our explanation was tenable. But inevitably casting such a broad net does not lead always to nice, neat, coherent explanations.

Finally some inconsistencies in the book result from the fact that different investigators are responsible for different portions of it. Most of the work reported was supported by a grant to the senior author from the National Institute of Mental Health (MH02980), and it has been his practice to point to a problem needing study and then to leave it largely to the graduate student investigator to design, carry out, and write up his exploration of the problem. Within the limits of the broad guidelines stated at the outset, he has not tried to dictate exactly what should be done or how the results obtained should be interpreted. His role has been that of providing continuity in the interpretation of different studies conducted over a period of ten years. Some chapters, notably Chapters 10 (Kalin) and 11 (Maccoby), were scarcely influenced by his ideas at all. And, as already noted, since theories kept changing with time, it sometimes happened that by the time an experiment designed in terms of one set of ideas had been completed and written up, other findings were forcing a revision in the interpretation of what was going on. Often the original investigator would quite understandably resist changing his opinion of why and what he had done and wonder whether in fact the latter conceptualizations were so persuasively required by the new evidence.

So the general interpretations in this book have been the subject of much internal discussion. They are certainly not accepted in every particular by all of the people associated with this enterprise over the ten-year period. In individual chapters, statements can be found which are not perfectly consistent with our basic theory. This is a product of the autonomy given individual investigators, and we see no reason to apologize for the inconsistencies. Although we believe we have made an empirical and theoretical contribution to the understanding of the role of alcohol in human experience, we are all too well aware of the gaps that still exist in our knowledge and the room for alternative interpretations on particular points.

In every sense this has been a cooperative research enterprise, steered somewhat remotely by the senior author, with all the confusion and excitement that description implies. Many have made important contributions which we wish to acknowledge with gratitude. At the outset we would like to acknowledge the continuing support of the National Institute of Mental Health which provided the financial backing necessary to carry out the studies reported. Of particular value was its willingness to continue the support on a long-term basis, thus enabling us to revise continually and check our theories until we could arrive at an interpretation which we felt was reasonably grounded in a lot of empirical evidence. We hope that this book may be taken as a token that the NIMH policy of long-term support of basic research does pay off in accumulated knowledge.

It was difficult to know whom to acknowledge as authors of this report, since so many have been involved at various points in the total enterprise. In the end we have listed the four of us who have been associated with the project for the longest period of time. The names of others appear as authors or co-authors of individual chapters, and the assistance of many in various research capacities is acknowledged in connection with each chapter. Needless to say, we are tremendously grateful to those who spent hours and hours coding or otherwise tabulating and analyzing the figures which form the basis for the various chapters.

And finally we should like to express our thanks to those who typed and retyped the various chapters of this book as they were written and rewritten—particularly to Lynn Lundstrom and Beth Holden. We also owe a special debt to them and to Alice Thoren for keeping some semblance of order in the project over the years so that bills would be paid, materials filed, computer printouts stored, and personnel appointments made. A scientific report is just the tip of the iceberg in the extent to which it reflects the enormous amount of work that goes into a scientific enterprise, and we who are writing it are fully aware of how little we could have accomplished without the help of the many others who contributed to it.

> David C. McClelland, *Harvard University*
> William N. Davis, *Payne Whitney Clinic*
> Rudolph Kalin, *Queen's University*
> Eric Wanner, *Harvard University*

Postscript: After the manuscript was completed and in the process of being published, some data became available showing how the use of newer mind-altering substances—pot, speed, and acid (LSD)—was related in a college population to the motivational syndromes discussed in this book. In view of the great popular interest in motives for drug-taking among the young, we have added an appendix describing these preliminary findings.

Authors and Contributors

Dr. William N. Davis is Assistant Professor of Psychology in Psychiatry at the Cornell University Medical College and Attending Psychologist at the Payne Whitney Psychiatric Clinic of The New York Hospital. Dr. Davis divides his time between direct clinical services and clinical consultation at several New York City schools. In addition, he is both clinical and research consultant at the Addiction Research and Treatment Corporation, located in Brooklyn, New York.

Michael Kahn is Associate Professor of Psychology at University of California, Santa Cruz, where he is teaching and helping launch the newest college there, Kresge College.

Rudolf Kalin is Assistant Professor of Psychology at Queen's University in Kingston, Ontario, where he is teaching personality and social psychology and doing research on personal and social correlates of deviant behavior.

Michael Maccoby is a psychoanalyst and social psychologist who is currently a visiting fellow at the Institute for Policy Studies in Washington, D.C. In 1960, after receiving a Ph.D. from the Department of Social Relations at Harvard, he went to Mexico to investigate with Erich Fromm the social character of the peasant and to study at the Mexican Institute of Psychoanalysis. Dr. Maccoby is now directing a study of Technology and Character sponsored by the Harvard Program on Technology and Society.

David C. McClelland is Professor of Psychology in the Department of Social Relations at Harvard University. With support from the National Institute of Mental Health, he has been studying empirically for over ten years the causes and action consequences of variations in thought content.

Gerald Mohatt, a School and Community Psychologist, has worked on a school dropout prevention program for the United Sioux Tribes and an alcoholism program for the Rosebud Tribe.

Reeve Vanneman is a graduate student in the Department of Social Relations at Harvard. His major interests are in the social psychological aspects of modernization. He is currently doing research on the relationship between relative deprivation and social change and the development of formal organizations in modernizing societies.

Eric Wanner is an Assistant Professor in the Department of Psychology at Harvard University and the director of the Computer Based Psychological Laboratory. His current research is in the area of psycholinguistics.

Sharon Carlson Wilsnack is a candidate for the Ph.D. degree in clinical psychology at Harvard University. She received her M.A. from Harvard in 1968 and served a clinical psychology internship at the Massachusetts Mental Health Center, Boston. She is currently completing her doctoral thesis, a study of psychological factors in female social drinking and female alcoholism.

David G. Winter is Assistant Professor of Psychology at Wesleyan University, Middletown, Connecticut. A former Rhodes Scholar, he received a Ph.D. degree in Social Psychology from Harvard University in 1967. Currently he is writing a book on the need for Power, and is studying the psychological significance of the Don Juan legend.

I
SOCIAL DRINKING

The initial studies reported in this section are basically exploratory. They were undertaken on the simple assumption that men drink alcohol because they enjoy the experiences it produces. One distinct possibility is that it produces different types of pleasant experiences for different people, depending on their personal characteristics and expectations about its effects. So our first objective was to determine whether drinking had any general or average mental effects that could be identified reliably, at least among men, in a variety of situations in which drinking normally occurs.

We turned to fantasy as our indicator of what men experience while drinking rather than to self-reports because people have learned from their culture—from reading popular magazines, listening to stories from their friends and to psychiatrists—what effects alcohol is *supposed* to have. Thus we were afraid that people would simply report experiences that they had been told they should have while drinking. Since different cultures and even different sub-groups within a culture create different expectations about the psychological effects of alcohol, self-reports may provide useful information about the social psychology of drinking;

but if alcohol does have a common effect on all men, it is likely to be obscured in self-reports by the embroideries of time, place, individual expectations, or culture. So we tried to minimize expectations as to what responses should be given by not calling particular attention to the fact that we were studying the effects of alcohol, but rather by asking for spontaneously created stories which are less easily shaped by conscious beliefs, attitudes or sets. That is, we tried to get the "raw stuff" of experience so that we could code it in ways to show the common effects of drinking across men rather than let our subjects code their own experience for us in self-reports.

Trying to find the right way to code the raw stuff of experience so as to capture the effects of alcohol is an extremely difficult task. There are literally thousands of possible ways of coding the differences in "dry" and "wet" fantasies, and we tried out dozens of them. These chapters reflect some of the resulting coding sprawl, as we attempted to refine our categories and establish the consistency of the obtained differences in a variety of social drinking situations. All along the way, we were trying to group our codes under some generic heading— searching for some common denominator in the various apparently unrelated mental effects of drinking we were finding.

This was not just a matter of creating some order out of miscellaneous empirically discerned differences. Previous experience has shown that the mental effects of an "arousal experience" like drinking, may also serve as an advance indicator of who is most likely to perform the act that will produce these effects. For instance, an achievement arousal experience leads to clearly identifiable mental effects, which, if found in abundance in the fantasies of a person not in an achievement situation, will predict that he is more likely to perform acts which will produce those effects (McClelland *et al.*, 1953). This phenomenon is usually conceptualized in motivational terms: the unique mental effects of an arousal experience become a good way of measuring individual differences in the motive to have that experience. So we were proceeding along a familiar path in trying to classify the experienced affects of drinking under some motivational heading which would give us a clue as to why some people drink more than others.

Our initial attempt to conceptualize alcoholic experiences under the heading of sentience was not very successful. But the chapters still provide clear evidence of several interesting phenomena: that drinking has a number of common effects on fantasy across individuals, at least among young American males; that these effects persist in a variety of settings though they are also influenced by those settings; and that some combination of the mental effects, measured in advance, might serve to predict who would be most likely to drink more and who less.

Chapter 1

The Effects of Male Social Drinking on Fantasy

by Rudolf Kalin, David C. McClelland, and Michael Kahn[1]

The research literature on the psychological effects of alcohol consumption is singularly unenlightening as to why so many people drink small amounts of alcohol, often daily, in social settings. What it reveals primarily is that alcohol impairs functioning at all levels—starting with blurring the higher mental processes and ending with psychomotor inefficiency. Yet it is hard to believe that people drink in order to think, talk, or act in an uncoordinated, inefficient way (Takala *et al.*, 1957; Frankenhaeuser *et al.*, 1962). On the contrary, such confusion should theoretically create anxiety, if anything, because the individual would find himself unable to control his behavior. Yet a common explanation for social drinking is the precise opposite: people drink to reduce anxiety, tension or conflict. "Alcohol solves the problem of anxiety reduction" (Horton, 1943). "As complex society generates increasingly greater tension, the alcoholic means of solving it becomes more prominent" (Jellinek, 1945, p. 27).

Without even reviewing the criticisms that have been made of the

[1]This chapter is a slightly revised version of an article with the same title which appeared in the *Journal of Personality and Social Psychology*, 1965, 1, 441-452.

cross cultural (cf. Field, 1962) or animal studies (Weiss, 1958) on which this conclusion is based, one may question whether the average person who has a drink or two before dinner in the evening is doing so in order to reduce his anxiety. At least this is not what people say universally when asked why they drink. College students, as reported by Straus and Bacon (1953), either gave positive reasons for drinking ("to get high," "for a sense of well-being") or the traditional ones involving reduction of conflict ("not to be shy," "to meet crises"). Is it possible that the American puritan tradition has led even scientists to overlook some of the "positive" effects of social drinking and to stress that its only value is to deaden the individual to real life, to anesthetize him a little to the stresses of anxiety?

The present investigation was undertaken to discover empirically why people drink in normal amounts in natural social settings. It differs from much previous alcohol research in several respects:

1. It is designed to cover what happens psychologically after two or three drinks; that is, it deals neither with the physiological effects of alcohol nor with the gross disturbances in psychological functions that occur after heavy drinking.

2. It focuses on the effects of drinking on fantasy, because fantasy has been shown to respond sensitively to changes in psychological states (McClelland *et al.*, 1953; Winter, Chapter 5 in this volume) and because fantasy provides important clues as to what actions men will take in a wide variety of circumstances (McClelland, 1961, 1966). Thus, we felt it might be possible to discover empirically a type of fantasy effect which, if it occurred even when the person was not drinking, would predict who would drink heavily.

3. Our research also differs from others in that it studies people when they are drinking as they normally do—in normal amounts, in a natural social setting, in the mixtures and at the rate to which they are individually accustomed. Most studies in this field have a physiological orientation; predetermined amounts of alcohol (by body weight) are administered according to a fixed time schedule, perhaps even by a continuous intravenous drip (cf. Frankenhaeuser *et al.*, 1962), so that the person will not know whether he is getting alcohol or a placebo solution. The purpose of such studies is to determine the effects of alcohol *per se* (i.e., apart from "suggestion") in psychological functioning. But it is impossible to *eliminate* suggestion from psychological research. One can only work with different settings that influence the subject in different ways. Certainly strapping the subject down and administering an unknown substance to him (maybe alcohol) intravenously while his every reaction is being checked must have a powerful effect on him: very probably it makes him anxious at this strange, threatening procedure taking place in a laboratory or hospital, with all its concomitant negative

associations in our culture. Thus the results obtained are obviously a product of the interaction of the set and setting with alcohol.

The expectation is, of course, that the effects of alcohol can be *isolated* because the same set and setting operate on the subjects who receive only a placebo. But a little reflection will show how unwarranted such an expectation may be, particularly if the effects are slight and require an anxiety-free atmosphere to develop. Suppose, for the sake of argument, that alcohol consumption in interaction with settings B, C, and D gives rise to feelings of good cheer. Is it surprising that in interaction with setting A (anxiety-arousing intravenous administration) the investigators found (Frankenhaeuser *et al.*, 1962) no increase in the frequency with which the subjects who had had alcohol said they felt "happy" or "carefree" as compared with control subjects? It was a totally "cheerless" experience for all subjects: to expect a little alcohol to overcome this massive effect of the set and setting is unreasonable.

Obviously, what is needed is a series of studies in which alcohol is taken in a variety of settings where the range of interaction effects can be studied. It makes no methodological sense to assume that one type of set and setting (no knowledge of what is being ingested: laboratory conditions) is somehow better or "purer" for studying the effects of alcohol than another. After all, the results are only generalizable to that particular condition, and who ingests alcohol in that way? If one were to pick a set or setting as "best," it would seem most logical to pick the one that is modal for the culture. Hence we have decided to study the effects of social drinking, without any illusions that we (or anyone else) can study the effects of alcohol apart from the conditions under which it is consumed.

PROCEDURE

Young male subjects were recruited from two different educational institutions ostensibly to take part in psychological research "on the effects of various social atmospheres on people's imaginativeness or fantasy." Alcohol was not mentioned as the focus of interest because it was felt that subjects might be set to react in certain ways by this information. Instead social settings were chosen in which either alcoholic or non-alcoholic beverages could be served without being considered unusual.

Subjects in the first study were first- and second-year male students in a graduate school of business administration, averaging about 25 years of age. They were invited to attend a discussion in the living room of an apartment in groups of three to six at four o'clock in the afternoon or at eight o'clock in the evening. Alcoholic beverages were served to nine such groups (totaling 39 subjects) chosen at random, and non-alcoholic beverages to five other groups (totaling 24 subjects). The former will be referred to as the *wet* condition and the latter as the *dry* condition.

Subjects in the second study were male undergraduates belonging to two fraternities (average age = 19.5 years) at a liberal arts college for men. They were invited to attend one of two parties being given at four o'clock on a Friday afternoon by the researchers "to study the effects of a party atmosphere on fantasy." At both parties there was food (snacks) and music, but one served alcoholic (wet condition) and the other soft drinks (dry condition). Half of the men in each fraternity were randomly assigned to the wet ($N = 35$) and half to the dry ($N = 38$) parties. Unfortunately, since most subjects had expected alcohol to be served at both parties—which was normal on such occasions—the subjects in the dry condition were angry when they discovered no liquor available. To keep their cooperation, the experimenter had to promise them a keg of beer after the party was over, but obviously their mood meanwhile was not ideal for a control or "neutral" condition.

A few men in each study did not drink any alcohol in the wet condition. They were classified as dry subjects.[2]

When the subjects arrived, it was explained that they were going to be given a test of imagination, since the experimenters were interested in discovering the effects of various social situations on imagination. This was simply one type of social situation that was being studied (that is, a living room discussion or a fraternity party, depending on the study), and, they were told, other situations were also being investigated. After some further introduction to the Thematic Apperception Test (TAT) as a measure of imaginativeness, they wrote a set of stories to four different pictures (TAT I). The social interaction was then set in motion for about 25 minutes, during which alcoholic or non-alcoholic beverages were served as naturally as possible. Next, the subjects wrote stories to four new pictures (TAT II), conversed again socially for another 25 minutes, and finally wrote four more stories to a new set of pictures. During the 25-minute periods of social interaction, subjects in the first study were engaged by the experimenter in a discussion of what it means to be a businessman—why had they come to the business school? what was their attitude toward making money? what is the businessman's place in society? etc. In the second study, the periods of social interaction proceeded without much help from the experimenters in the context of a stag party, complete with a jazz combo and bar.

---

[2]It could be argued that abstainers are probably different from subjects who are not offered alcoholic beverages. However, the fact that only two subjects in Experiment I and three in Experiment II were so classified makes it unlikely that the decision could have affected the results in any significant way.

In both studies, alcohol was served in the form of the usual drinks: scotch and soda, martinis, etc. In the living room discussions, the men were encouraged simply to serve themselves whenever they felt like it. One experimenter was present in the room, ostensibly taking notes on the conversation, though actually he had trained himself to estimate and record accurately the amount of alcohol consumed from various-sized glasses, with and without ice cubes. In the fraternity party, participants could go to a bar for drinks, each of which contained two shots (3 oz. 86-proof beverage). In order to get the drink, they had to sign a slip, so that a record of the amount of alcohol obtained by each subject was available after the experiment. It should be noted that the alcohol estimates are only approximate in both studies; in the first one, there was undoubtedly some observer error; and in the second, the record was for the amount *obtained* (say before TAT II), not for the amount *consumed* (as in the first study). Often the subjects would be sipping a drink while writing their stories.

The instructions for taking the TAT were the standard ones used for experimental purposes (Atkinson, 1958). Subjects were allowed about five minutes for each story. Twelve pictures were specifically chosen for the present study, so that three sets of four different pictures could be available for each man. The themes suggested by the pictures were chosen to represent areas of thought which alcohol might be expected to affect—namely, sex (S), aggression (A), elation (E), conflict (C), and "mysteries of life" (M). Since there were 12 pictures and three TAT administrations, three pictures were chosen to represent two themes each. A short description of the pictures and the themes which they were meant to elicit follows:[3]

1. Young couple walking on a sidewalk. (S)
2. Couple crossing the street in a snowstorm. (S)
3. Blonde model sitting pensively on a rotten, decaying boat. (S)
4. Boss leaning back in a desk chair looking at blonde secretary who is taking dictation. Picture of wife and children on the desk. (C)
5. Hoodlum in leather jacket leaning against a lamp post. Young college couple walking by, young man turned around toward the "hood." (C) (A)
6. Boxer in gym, looking pensive. In background someone shadow-boxing. (E) (A)
7. Negro in a race riot, taunted by a number of white fellows. (C) (A)
8. Two racing cars cutting a corner. (E)
9. Ski jumper in midair. (E)

[3]See Appendix VII for picture reproductions.

10. Man looking into a tent. (M)
11. Man looking into a tunnel. (M)
12. Boatman rowing on a lake on moonlit night. (M)

The order of pictures was arranged so that (1) each of four themes (S, E, C, M) occurred in each four-picture-TAT; (2) each four-picture-TAT also contained one aggression picture; (3) the order of appearance of the four thematic categories was random in each four-picture-TAT; (4) the order of the three pictures constituting a category was random across the different four-picture TATs.

CODING SCHEME

Categories for coding the imaginative stories written were chosen partly on theoretical and partly on empirical grounds, and underwent several revisions. A number of categories thought to be of theoretical importance were dropped because of (1) infrequent occurrence, (2) low inter-scorer reliability, or (3) no changes in frequency of occurrence as a function of social drinking. Among the categories extensively tested and discarded were: *provoking press* (e.g., temptation to sex or challenge to aggression), *conflict* (in particular, approach and avoidance conflicts over sex or aggression), *impulsive conflict resolution* (impulsive, unplanned action, without response-produced guilt), *elation* (including all words connoting positive affect), *pleasant physical impulses*, *deception* (e.g., villainy, immorality, illicit love), and *poetic usage* (e.g., metaphors, similes, hyperbole, etc.). The coding scheme reported here developed out of some of these categories, but it is worth recording as a guide to future research what types of "associative chains" proved unreliable or invalid in this study.

The scoring scheme which finally evolved included one set of categories which generally increased with drinking and another set which decreased.[4] The former we will refer to for convenience as *sentience* thoughts, the latter as *restraint* thoughts. The sentience categories were "sex," "aggression" and "meaning contrasts."

Sex was defined as any reference to sex, love, or romance. Such references were classified as physical and non-physical. *Physical sex* included any reference containing a physical or body image; for example, "beautiful knees," "he wants to sleep with her." *Non-physical*

[4]Only a brief indication of coding definitions can be included here. The complete set of scoring instructions is on file with the American Documentation Institute. Order Document No. 8302 from ADI Auxiliary Publications Project, Photoduplication Service, Library of Congress, Washington, D.C. 20540. Remit in advance $1.75 for microfilm or $2.50 for photocopies and make checks payable to: Chief, Photoduplication Service, Library of Congress.

sex included all such references not classified as physical; for example, "he asks her for a date," "they are in love."

Aggression was defined as any reference to human aggressive thought, emotion, or action. As with sex, such references were classified as physical or non-physical. Examples of *physical aggression* are: "his face is red with anger," "he slapped him." Examples of *non-physical aggression* are: "he is angry," "he insulted him."

Meaning contrasts were themes of sharply contrasting ideas where the contrast is immediate (in the same or adjacent sentences) and involves the meaning of life or some similar major experience. For example, "death provides meaning to life"; "do you take the easy road in life or get caught up in society's rat-race?"; "he placed 23rd, but he is happy."

Properly speaking, the term sentience applies to these categories only by expansion of the definition given by Murray (1938) referring to the desire to seek and enjoy sensuous impressions, e.g., through tactile sensations (as in erotic pleasure), or pleasurable muscular movements as in dancing, driving, or, by extension, smashing someone in the face (as in physical aggression). "Meaning contrasts" comes under this heading only in the sense that the primary process type of thinking involved might suggest a kind of pleasure in the release of id impulses.

The class of restraining thoughts included "sex and aggression restraints," "fear," and "time concern." A *restraint* is anything that involves an avoidance reaction to sex or aggression. Restraints may be objective frustrations, subjective fears, regret, guilt, or punishment for sexual or aggressive activities.

The *fear* category to some extent includes references also coded under the previous two categories, although it is broader in the sense that it includes all references to anxiety of any sort.

Time concern we defined as references to waiting, having enough time, etc.; for example, "He is almost late now," "It seems an interminable time to the tournament."

These categories were worked out using a small number of the protocols from the first study to test for coder reliability and validity in discriminating between "wets" and "drys." They were then applied to the remainder of the stories from this study and to all those from the second study. The stories were detached from the test booklets and randomly mixed together so that the coders could not be biased in their judgments. In the end, the results from the forty-odd stories used to develop the code were included in calculating means, since they differed in no way from scores on the remaining stories and since belief in the dependability of the results rests largely on cross-validation anyway. Two coders were trained in the use of the coding scheme, and each scored half the stories. Inter-coder reliability checks were made at the beginning and at the end of the coding. Agreement coefficients were computed by the formula:

$$\frac{2 \times \text{number of agreement}}{\text{total number scored by both judges}}$$

The respective median coding reliabilities were .94 and .96, when agreements on *absence* of a category were included. However, as will appear later, agreement on *presence* of "meaning contrasts" was considerably lower and ultimately required a revision in its scoring definition.

RESULTS AND DISCUSSION

Table 1.1 summarizes the mean levels of various sentient thoughts for "wet" and "dry" groups for the three different TAT administrations. So far as the relaxed discussion groups are concerned, most of the categories showed no significant shifts, despite their initial promise based on scoring the trial protocols. No significant shifts appear in the inhibitory thoughts either, the findings on which are summarized in Table 1.2. In a negative sense this result is very important, since it casts doubt on the most widely held theory as to why people drink. Certainly there is no evidence here of a *decrease* in inhibitory or anxious thoughts after one or two drinks in a normal living room discussion. Nor is there any evidence of a release of id-thoughts dealing with sex and aggression (which might be attributable to a decrease in inhibitions not reflected in the protocols).

"Meaning Contrast" is the one category which showed a marked, regular and significant increase in the wet condition (TAT II > TAT I, $p < .05$, TAT III > TAT II, $p < .05$, TAT III > TAT I, $p < .001$) and not in the dry condition. A newcomer to theories about the effects of alcohol, it contains the first hint as to why people indulge in drinking small amounts of alcohol in social settings of this kind. Apparently it acts to allow or encourage them to think in contrasting terms about large or existential life issues. Many of the themes have a meditative and ironic twist to them, as in such poetic statements as "Paths of glory lead but to the grave," or "To be or not to be, that is the question." One can think of these contrasts as involving primary process thinking—that is, entertaining contradictory thoughts or feelings at the same time—or as indicating a yearning for reflecting on some of life's basic issues (success-failure, life-death, pleasure-unpleasure, etc.) which is encouraged or released by alcohol in small quantities under social conditions.

It should be recalled, however, that the living-room discussions had focused around such "existential issues" as why they had come to the business school, the meaning of business in national life, etc. Perhaps

Table 1.1—Average frequency of various sentient thoughts in four-story protocols obtained at intervals during male social interaction

CONDITION	EXPERIMENT I (Relaxed discussion)					EXPERIMENT II (Fraternity party)				
	N	TAT I M	TAT II M	TAT III M	Difference TAT III −TAT I	N	TAT I M	TAT II M	TAT III M	Difference TAT III −TAT I
Meaning Contrast										
Wet	39	.46[a]	.85	1.33	+.87**	35	.69	1.26[b]	1.06	+.37
Dry	24	.75	.54	.79	+.04	38	.97	.92	.63	−.34
Physical Sex										
Wet	39	.64	.51	.36	−.28	35	.80	2.54	2.91	+2.11**
Dry	24	.17	.38	.29	+.12	38	1.45	2.00	2.37	+.92*
Non-physical Sex										
Wet	39	2.26	2.72	2.08	−.18	35	3.20	3.60	3.00	−.20
Dry	24	1.96	2.08	1.54	−.42	38	3.39	2.76	2.68	−.61
Physical Aggression										
Wet	39	.69	.74	.69	.00	35	.83[c]	1.40[b]	1.20	+.37
Dry	24	.50	.63	.75	+.15	38	1.71	1.34	1.39	−.32
Non-physical Aggression										
Wet	39	2.38	2.26	2.51	+.13	35	2.17	1.80	1.60	−.57[d]
Dry	24	2.46	2.08	2.58	+.12	38	1.96	1.66	2.42	.46
Cumulative average alcohol consumed (ounces, 86-proof beverage)[e]		1.61		4.07			7.2		14.1	

[a]Standard deviations range from .8 for means around .5 to 2.3 for means around 2.00.
[b]Difference TAT II—TAT I is significant at $p < .05$ in the predicted direction.
[c]Difference between means of Dry and Wet conditions significant at $p < .05$.
[d]A Physical-Nonphysical Aggression score for each subject shows a significant average increase from TAT I to TAT III ($p < .05$ in the predicted direction).
[e]For the Wet conditions only.
*$p < .05$ by t tests for differences between correlated means.
**$p < .001$ by t tests for differences between correlated means.

Table 1.2—Average frequency of various inhibiting thoughts in four-story protocols obtained at intervals during male social interaction

CONDITION	EXPERIMENT I (Relaxed discussion)					EXPERIMENT II (Fraternity party)				
	N	TATi M	TATii M	TATiii M	Difference TATiii −TATi	N	TATi M	TATii M	TATiii M	Difference TATiii −TATi
Sex Restraints										
Wet	39	.46	.59	.36	−.10	35	.23	.43	.49	+.26
Dry	24	.08	.46	.38	+.30	38	.84ª	.74	.68	−.16
Aggression Restraints										
Wet	39	.56	.49	.72	+.16	35	.41	.31	.11	−.30*
Dry	24	.58	.54	.54	−.04	38	.53	.31	.40	−.13
Fear-Anxiety										
Wet	39	.46	.49	.54	+.08	35	.69	.37	.17	−.52*
Dry	24	.54	.42	.21	−.33	38	.61	.66	.76	+.15
Time Concern										
Wet	39	1.21	.82	.95	−.26	35	2.14	2.40	.97	−1.17*
Dry	24	1.25	.92	1.04	−.21	38	1.82	1.63	1.53	−.29
Cumulative average alcohol consumed (ounces, 86-proof beverage)ᵇ		1.61		4.07			7.2		14.1	

aThe number of Sex Restraints in the Dry condition is significantly higher than in the Wet condition, but so is the number of sex-related stories in which such imagery could occur; see Table 1.1.
bFor the Wet conditions only.
*p < .01.

this line of thinking was just picked up more easily by the wets because they were in a more suggestible state. Yet, the findings for the cocktail party, where there was no organized discussion, do not support this view. There too stories showed a significant increase in Meaning Contrast from TAT I to TAT II after an average consumption of 7.2 oz., 86-proof beverage, followed by a slight decrease from TAT II to TAT III. The increase in Meaning Contrast as a result of social drinking is cross-validated.

Unfortunately, in view of the importance and novelty of this finding, real difficulties were encountered in maintaining high inter-judge agreement for the Meaning Contrast category, particularly for the fraternity party protocols. Judge B (a woman) found very few instances of Meaning Contrast in Study 2—less than one-third the number coded by Judge A (a man)—which produced low inter-scorer agreement. It was therefore decided to have Judge A score all the protocols in Study 2, so that the means in Table 1.1 represent his judgments exclusively. A year later two new judges, C and D, recoded all these protocols to check the result. Again Judge D (a woman) did not recognize as many instances of Meaning Contrast, making agreement with Judge C (a man) low. The results obtained by Judge C, however, were very similar to those obtained by Judge A. Even when the means per subject are based only on the half of the stories scored by Judge C, the increase in Meaning Contrast thoughts from TAT I to TAT II is highly significant ($t = 3.91$, $p < .0001$) leaving little doubt as to the "reality" of the increase shown in Table 1.1. This experience convinced us, nevertheless, that the coding definition had to be revised since, while two male judges had obtained the result, two female judges had not.

Other changes in fantasy in the second study are marked and in line with general expectations based on pilot studies. After moderate to heavy drinking (up to nine drinks containing 1.5 oz. shots), there is a marked increase in references to Physical Sex and a not quite so marked increase in references to Physical Aggression, among young college males at a stag party. The increase in physical sex references also occurs in the dry condition, although the increase in the wet condition is at a higher level of significance. Unfortunately this finding is marred by the fact that the drys also started out higher in physical sex and perhaps could not show as great an increase. Even so, evidence presented below in Experiment III and in Chapter 2 serves to strengthen the case that drinking does indeed increase themes of physical sex as compared to a control group.

Some confusion is introduced into the comparisons of aggression by the fact that the irritation of the dry subjects at not being served liquor, showed up in their first TAT, producing a significantly higher mean on physical (but not non-physical) aggression. Thus while the wet subjects showed a significant increase in physical aggression from TAT I to TAT II, they could not really be compared with the dry subjects who started at a significantly higher level. What seems more appropriate and less influenced by initial level is the ratio of physical to non-physical aggression. Physical aggression starts out low (mean of .83 to 2.17) and increases significantly in the wet condition (1.20 to 1.60), whereas it decreases in the dry condition—perhaps as the subjects' anger wore off. What is interesting both for sex and aggression is that the key changes occurred not in *any* reference to sex and aggression, but only in those references having a *physical* aspect—using body, sensory, or feeling imagery.

Table 1.2 shows a significant decrease in Aggression Restraints in the protocols written in the wet condition in Experiment II. The slight increase in Sex Restraints is only apparent, since a glance at Table 1.1 shows that the increase could easily be due to the much larger number of sex-related stories in the wet condition for TATs II and III. The significant reduction in Fear-Anxiety is direct confirmation of the most prevalent theory as to the psychological effects of alcohol. Finally Time Concern also shows a big drop after the heaviest drinking, suggesting that a key type of "reality constraint" drops out with heavy consumption of alcohol—a constraint which also interferes with many other ego functions like writing or speaking clearly, problem-solving, etc. (cf. Takala *et al.*, 1957).

EXPERIMENT III

We decided to check the results for the fraternity cocktail party, since, unlike the subjects in the discussion groups, these subjects were all exposed to a single social atmosphere which may have been unique in some way. Additional subjects would also provide data for a more detailed analysis of the effects on fantasy of different levels of alcohol consumption.

Protocols were therefore obtained from 50 more male undergraduates at another college as they took part in cocktail parties normal for that institution—12, 17, 8, and 13 subjects (*S*s) from each of four different parties. Conditions differed from those reported for Experiment II in the following respects: (1) A faculty member was not present, nor was either of the two experimenters used in the other two studies. A naive undergraduate experimenter was used to eliminate any possible effects of experimenter bias (Rosenthal, 1963) or of the presence of an "authority figure." (2) For this and other reasons the parties were less under experimental control. In two cases less than half of the protocols were available, either because the subjects had been drinking before they arrived or because they failed to write enough on one or more of the TATs. At one party, many other guests were also present who were not participating in the experiment. We did not look upon these variations as unfortunate because our goal was to see whether the effects held up despite such changes in conditions. (3) The advance announcements of the experiment probably suggested more definitely that alcohol was the subject of study. (4) Alcohol was provided by the bartender in 1 oz. shots to cut down on the amount of drinking and to provide a condition in which average consumption was between that of Experiment I and Experiment II. (5) A number of new pictures were used (cf. Kalin, 1964) to eliminate those that had low "drawing power" for the categories used. And (6) the coding definition for Meaning Contrast was revised to cover instances in which contrasting (positive and negative) *emotions* occurred in immediate succession over some meaningful life event. Inter-scorer reliability under this new definition was 82 per cent.

Table 1.3 presents the results for the six categories that showed some significant change in Tables 1.1 and 1.2. The findings are similar for these subjects despite the many variations in procedure. There is

Table 1.3—Average frequency of various thoughts in four-story protocols obtained during male undergraduate social drinking

	TAT I	TAT II	TAT III	Difference TAT III −TAT I
Meaning Contrast	.82	1.04	.78	−.04
Physical Sex	.96	2.56	3.04	+2.08*
Physical Aggression	.94	1.10	1.00	+.06
Aggression Restraints	2.24	.96	.72	−1.52*
Fear-Anxiety	.90	.38	.22	−.68
Time Concern	1.02	.68	.50	−.52*
Cumulative average alcohol consumed (ounces, 86-proof beverage)	4.42	8.84		

Note.—$N = 50$.
* $p < .0001$.

a marked and significant increase in references to Physical Sex (but not Non-physical Sex) and marked decreases in references to Aggression Restraints, Fear-Anxiety, and Time Concern, just as in Experiment II. It should be noted, however, that there are marked differences between the living room discussions and these cocktail parties. Consumption of two to three drinks (a little over 4 oz., 86-proof alcoholic beverage) had *none* of these effects on TAT III in the living-room discussions, but *all* of them on TAT II in the setting of the cocktail party.

The results for Meaning Contrast and Physical Aggression suggest curvilinearity, as they do in Table 1.1. The effect for Meaning Contrast shows up clearly in Figure 1.1, which was constructed in the following way: First, an attempt was made to establish a baseline for appearance of the category without ingestion of alcohol by averaging the frequency of its occurrence for TATs II and III under the dry condition (available only in Experiments I and II) and TAT I under the wet condition (to include the same subjects whose later protocols contribute to other points on the curve). Then the number of Meaning Contrasts in TAT II or TAT III were classified according to how much alcohol the person had consumed prior to writing the stories. Four levels of consumption were established across the three experiments—.1 to 3.99 oz.; 4–6 oz.; 6.1–12 oz.; and over 12 oz. of 86-proof alcoholic beverage—and each wet subject contributed two values to this part of the curve depending on how much he had drunk prior to TAT II and prior to TAT III.

Obviously there are flaws in this procedure: more subjects in Experiment I drank lightly (less than 4 oz., 86-proof) and more in Experiments II and III drank heavily; also those who drank heavily

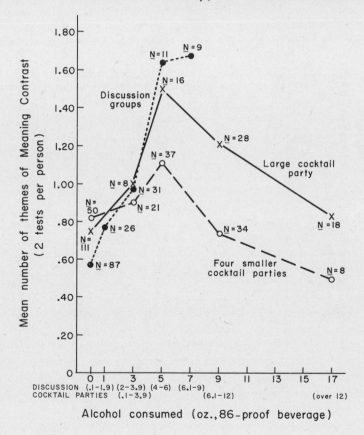

Figure 1.1   Average frequency of Meaning Contrast themes in TATs as a function of alcohol consumed in discussion groups and cocktail parties.

in the first experiment or lightly in the cocktail party probably differed in some key respects from the other subjects. Nevertheless, the results are instructive; in all three experiments there is a sharp increase in the number of Meaning Contrast images to a maximum after ingestion of 4–6 oz. (3–4 drinks) followed by a regular decrease in the two experiments in which drinking continued beyond this point. The increase after two drinks is not significant ($t = 1.47$, $p < .10$, in the predicted direction for all results combined), but it is very significant after three to four drinks ($t = 3.42$, $p < .01$). The finding is not so marked in Tables 1.1 and 1.3 because at any given TAT administration, individuals are writing who have consumed different amounts of alcohol.

The results for images of Physical Aggression, when plotted in the same way in Figure 1.2, are not so easily understood. Although there are no significant changes by amount of alcohol consumed for the discussion groups, several changes occur in the cocktail parties. The

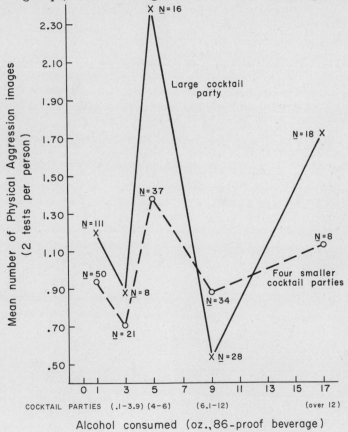

Figure 1.2 Average frequency of Physical Aggression images in TATs as a function of alcohol consumed in cocktail parties.

pattern is so irregular, one would be inclined to dismiss it as due to chance fluctuations except that it is identical in shape for the two experiments, and when the results are combined, nearly all the shifts are significant. First, with small amounts of drinking, there seems to be a decrease in Physical Aggression images ($t = 1.46$, $p < .20$), followed by a sharp increase ($t = 3.19$, $p < .01$), then a decrease ($t = 4.13$, $p < .01$), followed again by a final increase ($t = 2.03$, $p < .05$) with very heavy drinking. The first increase is significantly above the base line ($t = 2.43$, $p < .02$), just as the decrease at an average 9 oz., 86-proof consumption is significantly below the baseline, ($t = 2.26$, $p < .05$). These changes cannot readily be explained by reference to alternating patterns in writing about aggression, as they do not occur markedly in Tables 1.1 and 1.3. The pattern of changes in images of Non-physical Aggression is both irregular and dissimilar for the two groups, as is the pattern of changes in differences or sums of Physical vs. Non-physical Aggression images. So one must apparently accept the results in Figure 1.2 at face value: in cocktail parties with increasing consumption of alcohol, images of Physical Aggression first increase in young males (when they are "high" or excited), then decrease (when they are "sodden"), and finally increase again (when they are really "drunk"). These findings need to be checked in other settings.

The curves for the other variables when plotted in this way show more or less linear changes in the cocktail parties and no significant changes in the discussion groups. Of considerable interest is the point in the course of drinking at which the trends really begin to be marked. So far as Physical Sex images are concerned, the increase appears immediately, at the lowest levels of drinking recorded in the cocktail parties; but it rises significantly above the high baseline that exists in the dry party of Experiment II only after about five to six drinks containing 1.5 oz. shots of 86-proof beverage. Although no such increase appears in the discussion groups, perhaps it would have if alcohol consumption had been continued to higher levels.

There is some evidence for a decrease in images of Aggression Restraint in Experiments II and III at moderate levels of drinking, but the decrease becomes marked and significant in both cases only at around a consumption of 9 oz. and up (six drinks or more)—a level not reached by anyone in the discussion groups. The same can be said for Fear-Anxiety and Time Concern images, though a really good case for a decrease in the latter can be made only at even higher levels of consumption (15 oz. and up, or 10 drinks or more).

To summarize, at the level of consumption of a single drink (a 1.5 oz. shot of 86-proof beverage), no changes in fantasy are detected. At two drinks, themes of Meaning Contrast appear more often, both in the discussion groups and in the cocktail parties. At three to four drinks, the subjects appear to be "high" in the sense that their thoughts deal most often in Meaning Contrast and with Physical Aggression. At five to six drinks, they think more about Physical Sex even than usual, and Physical Aggression drops out. At seven drinks or more, Meaning Contrast also begins to disappear, and the decrease in inhibitory thoughts become *clearly* apparent for the first time—i.e., Aggression Restraint, Fear-Anxiety, and Time Concern—and there may be a final increase in Physical Aggression, this time combined with fewer thoughts about Aggression Restraint. The results match fairly well the stages of alcoholic intoxication as commonly understood or described in the clinical literature. What has not been previously stressed is the early "positive" stage in which subjects think more often in emotionally contrasting terms about the meaning of life. If this type of thinking is regarded as pleasurable, its appearance may help to explain why so many people drink small amounts of alcohol socially. The anxiety reduction hypothesis, on the other hand, is supported by these data only for heavy drinking.

One final note: in previous research of this kind, it has been found useful to compute scores for individuals consisting of the frequency with which they normally inject images into their stories of the type associated with changes in the experimental variable. It turned out here that the tendency to use these images in TAT I, before drinking started, is associated with the amount of subsequent drinking. This is particularly true of the images that *increase* with alcohol consumption—i.e., Meaning Contrast, Physical Sex, and Physical Aggression. Subjects whose initial protocols contained only two or fewer of these images less often drank heavily in all three experiments—42 per cent above the median in the discussion groups ($\chi^2 = 2.92$), 38 per cent in the large cocktail party ($\chi^2 = 2.30$), and 31 per cent in the smaller cocktail parties ($\chi^2 = 1.92$). The combined chi-square is significant in the predicted direction ($\chi^2 = 7.14$, $df = 3$, $p < .05$).

Or, to put it the other way, those who had more "sentient" thoughts to start with drank more subsequently. There was also a tendency for those who had more inhibitory thoughts to start with to drink less. This was particularly true in the cocktail parties for the categories of Aggression Restraint and Time Concern. The Fear Category was inconsistently related to subsequent drinking in the two cocktail party experiments. So a total "sentience" score (cf. Murray, 1938) was computed for TAT I by adding the number of instances of Meaning Contrast, Physical Sex, and Physical Aggression, and subtracting the number of instances of Aggression Restraint and Time Concern. This score was significantly related to subsequent drinking in Experiments II and III. In the large cocktail party, of those who scored high in sentience (+1 or more), 80 per cent drank more than average, as compared with only 25 per cent of those who scored low in sentience ($\chi^2 = 10.3, p < .01$). In the smaller parties of Experiment III, the same comparison yielded a 75 per cent vs. 35 per cent split ($\chi^2 = 12.3, p < .01$), although the proportion of people scoring $+1$ or more was considerably smaller (32 per cent vs. 43 per cent). In short, in these parties if the sentience-inhibition ratio is positive to start with, the person is likely to drink more. The same tendency exists in the discussion groups (64 per cent vs. 44 per cent), but at an insignificant level, perhaps because not enough drinking occurred to sharpen up the difference.

The interpretation of this finding is uncertain; it may be a kind of conditioned response evoked in anticipation of drinking, since the initial testing is done in a party setting. That is, subjects may anticipate the effects of drinking from past experience and project into their initial TATs the thoughts it will produce. Those who project more such thoughts are those who are more in a "party mood"—readier to drink more at the moment. On the other hand, a high sentience score may represent a more stable personality characteristic signifying an individual who is more open to sentient experience and likely to drink more. If so, it may provide a clue to why some people drink heavily and perhaps even become alcoholics.

An obvious way to check such an hypothesis is to get a measure of it away from the party setting and correlate that measure with drinking behavior. We ultimately report such a test in Chapter 7 (Bar II), but only after we had reconceptualized the meaning of some of the variables here grouped under the heading of sentience.

Chapter **2**

Social Drinking in Different Settings

by Rudolf Kalin

T he experiments reported in Chapter 1 have all the earmarks of pilot research. Interesting possibilities are raised, but many questions are left open. The results move towards the conclusion that a concern with sentient experience motivates the use of alcohol and that restraining thoughts inhibit such behavior. However, it is evident that these results by no means force such a conclusion. There are several reasons.

First, there are the puzzling problems caused by the outlying results of Experiment I. In this experiment only the category of meaning contrasts appeared to be affected by drinking. The remaining sentient themes (Physical Sex, Physical Aggression) showed no significant increases after drinking, and the restraint cluster (time concern, aggression restraints, and fear) gave no evidence of decreasing.

Second, there is the matter of control groups. Of the two experiment (II and III) in which interesting thematic changes arise, only one had a dry control group. And that control group was not entirely satisfactory because subjects had expected liquor to be served and were obviously disturbed when it was not served. Thus it is possible to argue that the fantasy changes observed in Experiments II and III are due solely to repeated administrations of the TAT in a relaxed social atmosphere and that they have little to do with alcohol. By this line of reasoning, the results of Experiment I are not outliers at all, but are the only fantasy changes which can be definitely attributed to drinking.

The third problem concerns the definition of sentience and its relation to the thematic categories which increase after drinking in Experiments II and III. As noted in Chapter 1, the themes of physical sex, physical aggression, and meaning contrasts were grouped together under the general notion of sentience, after it was discovered that they increased with drinking. But they may be three quite unrelated themes all affected by drinking, or they may be components of some other general state of mind besides sentience. In order to verify the sentience grouping, it would be necessary to find that drinking affects at least one other thematic category that bears a clear relation to sensuous experience and is not explicitly connected with physical sex, physical aggression, or meaning contrasts. Without such evidence the use of the term sentience is little more than a convenience—a kind of shorthand for referring to the three thematic categories which increase with drinking.

Finally, there is the difficult question of determining whether sentience may be properly understood as a motive which leads to heavier drinking. A direct way to get at this question is to arouse the "sentience motive" situationally and see if it leads to more drinking. An indirect way is to examine the correlation between the predrinking sentience score and subsequent alcohol consumption. As noted in Chapter 1, one interpretation of this finding is that the score reflects a sentience motive which leads people to drink more subsequently. But another is that the score is simply a product of the same situationally aroused cues (party atmosphere) which lead some student also to drink more. It seemed possible to shed some further light on this question by examining what happened to the correlation under a variety of situational conditions. For instance, if the correlation remains more or less constant regardless of the number of sentience cues in the situation, one might argue that the sentience score is an indicator of a general sentience motive.

The study reported in this chapter was designed to deal with each of the problems raised by the experiments in Chapter 1. Its first purpose was simply to replicate the original work with appropriate control groups. The basic procedures of the earlier studies were maintained. Young males attended cocktail parties and wrote TATs, once before and two times after drinking alcohol or non-alcoholic beverages. This time, however, precautions were taken to insure that the dry groups would not have reason to assume that they would be served liquor.

The second purpose was to get at the apparent anomalies of Experiment I. The difference between the results of Experiment I and those of the other two experiments suggests the interesting possibility that the effects of alcohol may vary according to the drinking context. Experiment I differed in several respects from the other experiments. In Experiment I the setting was quite "reality oriented." Subjects, who were students in a course in "Creative Marketing Strategy" at a Graduate Business School, were asked to take a "test of imagination." At the experimental sessions they also talked about the life of a businessman, a topic of vital importance to them. It may have been the case that the "reality cues" in the setting of Experiment I induced a state of inhibition in the experimental subjects. This inhibition may have acted to suppress the fantasy effects normally generated by alcohol in more relaxed settings.

To test this possibility, we ran cocktail parties in two different settings: a classroom and a private apartment. It seemed reasonable to suppose that a classroom would be rich in reality cues while an apartment would provide a more relaxed atmosphere. Thus, we expected that the classroom would provide an inhibiting situation which would raise restraining thoughts, lower sentient feelings, and reduce alcoholic consumption, as compared to the apartment. Thus, we would be checking the effects of drinking in an inhibiting setting directly against those in a relaxing setting, to confirm our impression from Experiment I, Chapter 1, that the setting can suppress the "normal" experiential effects that drinking produces.

To get at the question of whether sentience might be considered a motive responsible for drinking, we also attempted to arouse it directly. Because physical sex was one of the components of the sentience syndrome, situational sentience was created by adding sexual cues, in the form of an attractive female folksinger, to some of the parties. In control parties, neutral recorded music provided the entertainment. It was expected that sentience arousal would increase drinking and maximize its sentient effects on fantasy, just as situational restraints (classroom setting) would minimize both.

This design also permitted testing the correlation of the predrinking sentience score with subsequent drinking under conditions of sentience arousal and restraint. By examining the size of the correlation under varying conditions, it was hoped that some insight could be obtained on the question of whether the sentience score is an index of a stable personality characteristic or in some way a response to situational cues. Thus if the correlation remains high under all conditions, one might suppose that the score is an index of something like a motive to have fun regardless of the situation.

Finally we developed a new coding category, "Sensuous Physical Pleasure," to check on the appropriateness of applying the concept of sentience to the fantasy changes we had so far observed. That is, if their common characteristic was really sentience, then a category more definitely and explicitly in the sentience domain ought also to increase with consumption of alcohol.

The three independent variables, alcohol, situational inhibition and situational sentience, could be combined to yield a $2 \times 2 \times 2$ factorial design, that is, eight different experimental conditions. In fact only six of the eight conditions were run, for reasons of economy and because these conditions were sufficient to test the major hypotheses of the study. The six conditions were run as two partly overlapping experiments.

The first of these, hereafter called the Alcohol Experiment, was for the purpose of examining the effects of alcohol on fantasy in conditions differing in situational sentience. It follows a 2×2 factorial design, the two factors being alcohol (presence of alcoholic *vs.* nonalcoholic beverages at the parties, or, in short, Wet *vs.* Dry parties) and situational sentience (presence or absence of an attractive female folksinger).

The second experiment, hereafter called the Setting Experiment, also followed a 2×2 design, with the factors of situational inhibition (classroom *vs.* private apartment) and situational sentience (presence or absence of the folksinger). The purpose of this experiment was to study the effects of situational sentience and inhibition on fantasy and on alcohol consumption. The Alcohol and the Setting Experiments were overlapping in that two conditions (Wet parties in the apartment with and without the folksinger) were common to both experiments. It should be noted that alcohol consumption was an independent variable in the Alcohol Experiment and a dependent variable in the Setting Experiment.

METHOD

Experimental Conditions

Young males wrote TAT stories at cocktail parties, once before drinking (TAT I), a second time after a drinking period of 45 minutes (TAT II), and a third time after another drinking period of 30 minutes (TAT III). The nature of these parties was varied through the experimental manipulation of the setting.

In order to create situational sentience, the subjects at some parties were entertained by a female folksinger with distinctly feminine physical attributes. The selection of the girl as sexually attractive was later validated by her appearance as the playmate of the month in *Playboy* magazine. It was anticipated that there might be problems with having a live sex stimulus. As Clark (1952) found, the presence of a girl can inhibit rather than stimulate the expression of sexual fantasies. It was also feared that the girl might inhibit the consumption of alcohol. Although every attempt was made to present the girl in a way that would not have these undesirable effects (presenting her as an entertainer rather than as an accomplice in a scientific venture, etc.), it was decided that the girl should exit at TAT II. Therefore only men were present in the second drinking period.

At parties without situational sentience, a record player was playing neutral, unarousing music. The selections were from modern jazz and included Dave Brubeck, Gerry Mulligan and Ahmad Jamal.

Situational inhibition was varied by having the parties in two different settings. One set of parties was held in an academic building, in a room that is normally used for classes. It was reasoned that such academic paraphernalia as school chairs, blackboard, etc. would serve as "reality" cues. In order to create disinhibition, parties were held in a nice looking, private bachelor apartment. Also, in the apartment the experimenters appeared in casual clothes (sportshirt) whereas in the classroom they wore jackets and ties.

Alcohol was an independent variable in that subjects in some conditions (Wet) could drink alcoholic beverages while in other conditions (Dry), only soft drinks were served. The amount of alcohol consumed in the Wet conditions was recorded to give information about alcohol as a dependent variable.

The six experimental conditions were run as a series of parties, with two or three parties per condition. Ideally the sequence of the conditions should have been randomized in order to eliminate series effects. Because of the possibility of rumors developing that alcohol was served at all parties, and because such rumors might induce inappropriate expectancies in potentially Dry Subjects, a different procedure was followed. In order to avoid subjects' disappointment at finding no alcohol at parties where they expected it, the conditions were run in order of increasing pleasantness. The sequence is given below:

1. Apartment, No Singer, Dry
2. Apartment, Singer, Dry
3. Classroom, No Singer, Wet
4. Apartment, No Singer, Wet
5. Classroom, Singer, Wet
6. Apartment, Singer, Wet

Possible sequence effects, however, were still a serious difficulty in this procedure. As a partial solution the following steps were taken. The conditions were run in the above listed order, with two parties for each condition. After 12 parties had been run, two more were given, one for condition four and one for condition five. When the results were checked for sequence effects, no systematic pattern in the dependent variables emerged. That is, dependent variables such as alcohol consumption, thematic sex, etc. sometimes had higher means in later parties, and sometimes in early parties. It was therefore decided that if sequence effects did occur, they were not strong enough to warrant serious consideration.

Selection and Arrangement of TAT Pictures

Some of the pictures used in the present study had been used in the earlier experiments; others were selected specifically for the present study. The goal was to construct sets of TAT pictures to pull those themes that were positively affected by alcohol in the previous experiments, that is sex, aggression and meaning contrast. In addition, the thematic category of Pleasant Physical Impulses was reintroduced as Sensuous Physical Pleasure because it seemed theoretically important for the concept of sentience. A short description of the pictures and the themes which they were meant to elicit follows. (An asterisk in the list refers to a picture that was new in this study.)

1.* Horse-drawn wagon in moonlight (Sensuous Physical Pleasure)
2.* Small boy in cemetery (Meaning Contrast)
3. Negro in a race riot, taunted by a number of white fellows (Aggression)
4. Boss leaning back in a desk chair looking at blond secretary who is taking dictation. Picture of wife and children on the desk (Sex)
5.* Swimmer in pool (Sensuous Physical Pleasure)
6.* Mad scientist looking at a test tube (Meaning Contrast)
7. Hoodlum in leather jacket leaning against a lamp post. Young college couple walking by, young man turned around toward the "hood" (Aggression)
8. Young couple walking on a sidewalk (Sex)
9.* Trumpet player under a blooming cherry tree (Sensuous Physical Pleasure)
10. Boatman rowing on a lake on moonlit night (Meaning Contrast)
11.* Accident scene. Young man in sportscar has apparently just hit a car coming out of a parking space (Aggression)
12.* Young couple lying on the grass on a riverbank (Sex)

The pictures were arranged into sets of three, for three different

TAT administrations. Each set contained a picture for sensuous physical pleasure, and one for sex. As a third picture, one half of the sets contained an aggression picture while the other half contained one for meaning contrast. Thus there were three sets with two alternate forms each. Set I contained pictures 1–4, Form A with picture 2 and Form B with picture 3; Set II pictures 5–8, Form A having picture 6 and Form B picture 7; Set III pictures 9–12, Form A picture 10, Form B picture 11. The pictures were always presented in the same sequence, namely, sensuous physical pleasure, meaning contrast, or aggression, sex.

The reason for giving only half the subjects an aggression or meaning contrast picture was that it was felt that too much writing would interfere with a party mood.

Subjects

One hundred sixty-three subjects from 16 different fraternities at the Massachusetts Institute of Technology were recruited to participate in a "study of sociability." It was not mentioned that alcohol was a major focus of the investigation. Members from two to four different fraternities were present at each party. A given fraternity was represented by one to eight members at any one party. Some fraternities appeared in successive parties and some had as many as seven parties between the first and the last appearance. The subjects were from all four college years and their average age was 19.55 years.

Several subjects were eliminated from the analysis for the following reasons. Nine did not consume any alcohol. Four subjects left the parties early. Finally, the TAT protocols of one subject were missing at the time of analysis. There was a total of 149 usable subjects.

Procedure

The groups were run at four in the afternoon, i.e., at a time close to the usual cocktail hour. Weekend afternoons (Friday, Saturday, and Sunday) were chosen as the culturally natural times to drink. They were also unlikely to interfere with school work. Drinking just before a meal insured the maximum physiological effects of alcohol.

When a group of subjects appeared at the appropriate locale, they were met by two experimenters. The author was the major experimenter and gave all the instructions. The second experimenter was introduced as a "friend who is helping out." As an introduction, the experimenter revealed the purpose and plan of the study as being "to learn something about situations where people socialize." They were further told to relax and behave as they would at an ordinary party. The same initial introduction was given to subjects in all experimental conditions. The experimenter then introduced the folksinger or the records, depending on the conditions.

> I am convinced the "atmosphere" is very important for people to have a good time. I thought that a little music would help to get people in the right mood.

To introduce the folksinger he went on:

> So I asked Sally to come over and provide some entertainment. Sally is a folksinger, and because of the recent popularity of folksinging, we felt that most people would enjoy this. So why don't you settle back and see for yourselves.

To introduce the recorded music he continued:

> So I decided to put on some music. I think the selections are pretty good to put you in a party mood.

The initial concert went on for 15 minutes. During this time subjects sat around in chairs or on the floor. Some conversations were carried on. Where the folksinger was present, however, most subjects just sat and listened. With the recorded music, discussions were started, some in sub-groups, some among all subjects. The two experimenters tried to be as nondirective as was possible without at the same time being unnatural. After this initial exposure to a concert, the experimenter went on:

> I am now ready to ask you to do one of the things I mentioned before. People seem to like to tell stories when they socialize, like for example, at parties. One of the things that I'm interested in is story-telling. So, I'm going to ask you to tell some stories. In order to standardize the results and to help you in your storytelling, we have made up a little booklet with some pictures about which I'd like you to write the stories. You will find a more detailed description of what you are to do on the first page of the booklet.

The instructions for the TAT were adapted from the standard ones used in experimental research (see Atkinson, 1958). However, an effort was made to rid the instructions of anything which might induce a "testing set." Subjects were told that the five minutes they were allowed per story was not a strict time limit but that in order to provide some guide lines about how long the stories should be, the experimenter would announce when five minutes were up.

At the completion of the TAT, the experimenter introduced the drinks. In both the Wet and Dry conditions he said:

> Parties usually don't last too long without refreshments. So I have some refreshments for you here. Take whatever you like and as much as you like. Don't worry, the money for the drinks doesn't come out of my pocket.
> The only thing I have to ask you is to sign your name on a little slip of paper

each time you get a drink. Also put down what you would like to drink. The reason for this is that I have to turn in some sort of receipt in order to get my money back.

The real purpose of the slips was to obtain a record of alcohol consumption. In the Wet conditions a bar was set up with scotch, bourbon, rye, sherry, and various mixes available. The second experimenter acted as bartender and handled the distribution of liquor.

After subjects had been encouraged to drink as much as they liked, the concert was resumed for drinking period 1. In parties with the folksinger a short intermission occurred after the first three songs. Although subjects could go to the bar throughout the concert, the intermissions were used primarily for the purpose of obtaining drinks. For the rest of the drinking period there were two more songs, another short intermission, two further songs. This first drinking period lasted 45 minutes.

The first drinking period at parties without the folksinger proceeded similarly except that there was more conversation and spontaneous activity among the subjects.

After the first drinking period, subjects were asked to write TAT II. Upon completion of these stories the folksinger officially left the parties and socializing resumed among the subjects for drinking period 2. During this time a record player was turned on in all conditions. After 30 minutes of socializing and social drinking, subjects wrote TAT III. The total procedure lasted about two and one-half hours.

Coding of Stories and Intercoder Reliability

The coding scheme was basically the one described in the previous chapter, although the coding definitions of some categories—for example, sex restraints—were expanded and elaborated. In order to measure sentience independently of sex and aggression, the new category of Sensuous Physical Pleasure was defined to cover themes that contain both pleasure and sensuous physicality. The scorer first locates something indicating physical activity ("diving"), a sensory experience ("wind in the face"), or certain physical objects ("a warm fire"), then he looks for pleasure in it as indicated by statements of positive affect ("enjoying diving") or desire ("wanting to feel the wind in his face"). In a few obvious cases ("a blossoming cherry tree"), it was assumed that the sensory experience was pleasurable. Other examples are "a warm fire," "a pleasure boat," "he relaxed in the cool caressingness of the summer water."

For the purpose of coding, the stories were given an identification code (subject, ID; picture, TAT) on the back. The story booklets were then disassembled and mixed together, so that stories from all conditions and all TAT administrations would follow each other in random order.

Two coders who had already scored the protocols of the third experiment reported in the previous chapter, but who did not know the purpose and design of the present experiment, coded the stories. Each scored about half the protocols. Reliability checks were made three times: at the beginning, in the middle, and at the end of coding all the protocols. Reliability was defined as:

$$\frac{2 \times \text{number of agreements}}{\text{total number scored by both scorers}}$$

The median reliability without counting agreement on absence of a category was .82; with counting absence it was .95.

Data Analysis

It will be recalled that the present study consisted of two partially overlapping experiments, each with a 2×2 design. The use of two TAT forms extended the designs to $2 \times 2 \times 2$. Thus in the Alcohol Experiment we had Alcohol $\times$ Singer $\times$ Form, and in the Setting Experiment there was Setting $\times$ Singer $\times$ Form. The effects of TAT form were of peripheral interest except for the aggression and meaning contrast variables. But Form was made part of the design anyway, since it represented a known source of variance which could be eliminated. Three-way analyses of variance were carried out on the two designs. In order to overcome the problem of unequal subjects in the various cells an approximation method to estimate the error variance (Walker & Lev, 1953, p. 381) was used. This method has disadvantages because it evaluates effects using the complete design, whereas we might have predictions that pertain only to parts. Also, because the method is approximate, it may not be able to detect real effects. For these reasons, *t*-tests were performed, for relationships hypothesized in advance, even though the main effects in the analysis of variance were not significant.

The thematic scores were added through the three stories constituting a TAT for each subject. To test the effects of alcohol, the folksinger, and the setting on fantasy, TAT II and III were combined in order to obtain a more stable measure.

RESULTS AND DISCUSSION

The effects of the setting and the singer on the predrinking TAT are not a major concern in this report and are therefore only briefly described. More detail can be found in Kalin (1964). The experimental manipulation of situational sentience and inhibition had no clear effects at TAT I. There was some indication that the folksinger lowered thematic sexual responses and raised thematic sexual restraints when the level of sexual imagery was controlled. These results, which are similar to those obtained by Clark (1952), suggest that sexual arousal in certain settings leads to conflict over sex. The setting had no discernible effects at TAT I and none of the other thematic variables was affected by the folksinger.

Effects of Situational and Personal Sentience and Inhibition on Alcohol Consumption

The average amounts of alcohol consumed in the four Wet conditions are presented in Table 2.1. The results show that less alcohol was consumed in the classroom than in the apartment. After pooling the conditions with and without the singer, a t-test showed that the difference between the means of the classroom and the apartment was significant at the .05 level. The effects of the singer were not consistent; statistical tests showed no reliable differences between conditions with and without the singer. Of the two predictions concerning alcohol consumption, therefore, only the one involving the setting was confirmed.

Table 2.1—Means of average amount of alcohol consumed (*Total of two drinking periods in oz., 86-proof beverage*)

	No Singer	Singer	S—NoS[a]
1. Apartment	7.29 (28)	7.75 (26)	.46
2. Classroom	6.45 (20)	6.06 (32)	−.39
Setting Effect, difference 1–2	−.84	−1.69[b]	

Note.—Numbers in parentheses = number of subjects per condition. The subject whose TAT was missing was included in this analysis.
[a]Difference Singer—No Singer conditions.
[b]Combining Singer and No Singer conditions, difference Classroom-Apartment, $t = 1.70$, $p < .05$ (one-tailed).

An inhibiting, as compared with a relaxed, setting can lower the consumption of alcohol. It seems therefore reasonable to interpret the lower alcohol consumption in Experiment I, as compared with Experiments II and III, reported in the previous chapter, as having been partly determined by the more inhibiting setting of that experiment. This is not to say, however, that the differences among the consumption levels of the previous experiments have been totally accounted for by the present results. Comparing the various experiments we see that the average consumption level of the present experiment (6.88 oz.) is on the lower end of the range obtained in the earlier studies (4.07 oz. to 14.1 oz.). Also, the range among the four conditions of this experiment (6.06–7.75 oz.) is much smaller than that previously obtained. In retrospect it appears that all of the present conditions were relatively inhibiting. Among the likely reasons for this situation are the facts that subjects in the present experiment attended parties away from home with people they didn't know whereas in Experiments II and III parties took place in the fraternity houses among brothers.

In the previous chapter it was shown that the Sentience score from TAT I (consisting of the sum of physical sex, physical aggression and meaning contrast minus time concern and aggression restraints) was positively associated with subsequent drinking in all three experiments. In the current study, two questions were asked. One, does the relationship between predrinking Sentience and subsequent alcohol consumption hold? Two, is the relationship similar in the different experimental conditions? Results relevant to these questions are presented in Table 2.2.

**Table 2.2—Correlations between predrinking TAT sentience[a]
and subsequent alcohol consumption[b]**

	No Singer	Singer
1. Apartment	.14 (27)	.15 (26)
2. Classroom	−.10 (20)	.39** (32)
All Conditions	.16* (105)	

Note.—Numbers in parentheses = number of subjects per condition.
[a]Sentience = Physical Sex +Physical Aggression+Meaning Contrast—Time Concern.
[b]Total from both drinking perods.
*$p < .05$, **$p < .01$.

It should be noted that the present Sentience score differs slightly from the earlier one. In this study, as in Chapter 1, those subjects whose initial TATs contained more instances (here at least two) of physical sex, physical aggression, or meaning contrast, later drank significantly ($p < .05$) more than those whose initial TATs contained fewer instances of any of these thematic categories. Those whose initial TATs contained more time concern (two or more instances) drank less subsequently ($p < .06$). (See Kalin, 1964.) The presence of more aggression restraints, however, did not predict less drinking, probably because restraints are highly correlated with aggression imagery, which is positively associated with later drinking. Since there is no simple way to correct for this correlation, aggression restraints are not included here in the total Sentience score.

Table 2.2 shows that the correlations between the Sentience score and alcohol consumption was positive in three of the four conditions. Combining all four conditions yields a correlation that is low but statistically significant. The condition where the relationship is reversed was the one in the classroom, without the singer—in other words, the condition least like a natural party. Overall, then, the relationship between Sentience and drinking was very similar to that found in the earlier experiments. In situations that contain some party cues (the fraternity settings of Experiments II and III in Chapter 1, or a private apartment and/or the presence of a female singer) the dry Sentience score is positively related to drinking. This relationship does not obtain, or may even be reversed, when the setting contains no party cues (Experiment I above and the present classroom setting with no singer present).

Unfortunately these results are not decisive as to whether the Sentience score represents a stable personality characteristic or a situational response. Obviously there is considerable variation in the size of the relationship across situations, a variation which suggests at the very least that if a stable motive is involved, it is differently tapped by a TAT administered in different settings. On the other hand, one might well expect, according to the interpretation by situational response, that the correlation would be highest in the condition of maximum sentience arousal (apartment, folksinger—which is not the case. It seems best to conclude modestly that some relation may exist between the components of the predrinking Sentience score and subsequent alcohol consumption, but that we have not yet succeeded in clarifying the nature of the relationship.

Effects of Alcohol, the Female Folksinger, and the Setting on Fantasy

The presentation of the effects of the three independent variables on post-drinking fantasy is arranged by dependent variable. A descrip-

Table 2.3—Mean frequencies of thematic physical sex in six conditions (TAT$_{II}$ + TAT$_{III}$)

	No Singer	Singer	S–NS[a]
1. Apartment, Dry	1.18 (17)	.70 (27)	−.48
2. Apartment, Wet	2.48 (27)	4.39 (26)	1.91[b]
3. Classroom, Wet	1.80 (20)	1.31 (32)	−.49
Drinking Effect, difference 2–1	1.30[c]	3.69[c]	
Setting Effect, difference 3–2	−.68[d]	−3.08[d]	

Note.—Numbers in parentheses = number of subjects per condition.
[a]Difference Singer—No Singer conditions.
[b]In Apartment, Wet conditions, difference No Singer—Singer $t = 1.96$, $p < .05$ (in the predicted direction.)
[c]In alcohol experiment, main effect, alcohol, $F = 11.69$, $p < .01$.
[d]In setting experiment, main effect, setting, $F = 7.57$, $p < .01$.

tion and discussion of these results in terms of each independent variable appears below. Rows 1 and 2 in each Table contain the results of the Alcohol Experiment; the Setting Experiment is presented in rows 2 and 3. Although Form effects were used in the analyses, results were pooled across Form to achieve a simpler presentation.

Physical Sex. Table 2.3 shows that alcohol significantly raised the frequency of Physical Sex imagery. The female folksinger had the same effect but only in the apartment, wet condition. In the Setting Experiment, we can see that Physical Sex was significantly lower in the classroom than in the apartment.

Nonphysical Sex. It was not expected that nonphysical sex would be affected by any of the independent variables, and the results bore this out.

Sex Restraints. The outcome of sex restraints proved to be complex and unclear. Some detailed analyses are presented in Kalin (1964). For present purposes it suffices to say that no definite conclusions can be drawn about the effects of alcohol or the setting on thematic sex restraints.

Table 2.4—Mean frequencies of thematic physical aggression in six conditions ($TAT_{II} + TAT_{III}$)

	No Singer	Singer	S—NS[a]
1. Apartment, Dry	.47 (17)	.93 (27)	.46
2. Apartment, Wet	1.22 (27)	.88 (26)	−.34
3. Classroom, Wet	1.40 (20)	.81 (32)	−.59
Drinking Effect, difference 2–1	.75[b]	−.05	
Setting Effect, difference 3–2	.18	−.07	

Note.—Numbers in parentheses = number of subjects per condition.
[a]Difference Singer—No Singer conditions.
[b]In Apartment No Singer conditions, difference Dry—West $t = 1.70$, $p < .05$ (one-tailed).

Physical Aggression. The only variable significantly affecting physical aggression was alcohol. This effect was, however, apparent only in the condition without the folksinger, that is, in the condition most similar to the settings of Experiments II and III reported in the previous chapter. It appears, therefore, that the effects of alcohol on physical aggression are complex. They can be obscured by the presence of a female, and we remember from the earlier experiments, that physical aggression is related to the amount of alcohol consumed in a nonmonotonic fashion. In order to replicate the earlier relationships the following steps were taken. Each Wet subject was categorized according to how much alcohol he had obtained just before writing a set of stories. The cutting points to establish consumption intervals were identical to those employed in the previous chapter with the following exceptions: (a) Intervals were chosen that gave the most even distribution of subjects among the intervals. (b) Subjects who did not drink alcoholic beverages at all, but who were in Wet parties, were eliminated. (c) Three subjects at TAT II and two subjects at TAT III were eliminated because they fell in the .1–1.9 oz. range, and the number of subjects in that interval would have been so small that no reliable estimate of the amount of imagery could have been made. (d) Only subjects with Form B (containing the aggression picture) were included.

Figure 2.1 shows an increase of physical aggression thoughts from a dry control level among subjects who had consumed up to 9 oz., followed by a sharp decrease among subjects who had consumed 9.1 oz. or more. The similarity between the curves from TAT II and TAT III is striking. In order to evaluate the significance of the shifts, *t*-tests were

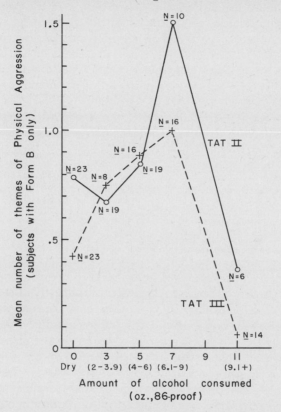

Figure 2.1 Average frequency of thematic Physical Aggression as a function of amount of alcohol consumed.

performed.[1] Comparison of the consumption group (6.1–9 oz.) at TAT II and TAT III with the Dry control level, yielded differences which could have arisen by chance fairly often (about 1 in 5 times). Subjects who consumed 9.1 oz. and over did not differ significantly from the Dry group either at TAT II nor at TAT III. Comparing the consumption

[1] A *t*-test is a measure of how often a difference might be expected to arise by chance. The probability (p) that a difference might arise by chance is stated in terms of how many times out of 100 it could arise by chance alone. Thus $p < .20$ is to be read, the probability that this difference could arise by chance is less than 20 in 100 (or 1 in 5). Ordinarily in psychology differences are not thought to be significant unless they could have arisen by chance rarely— e.g., less than 5 times in 100 opportunities.

groups of 9.1 and over with those of 6.1–9, *t*s of 1.50, *p* < .10, (TAT II) and 2.81, *p* < .01, (TAT III) were obtained.

Nonphysical Aggression. From Table 2.5 we can see that alcohol significantly lowered thoughts of nonphysical aggression. Combining the results of Tables 2.4 and 2.5, we see that images of aggression become increasingly physical after drinking. The same result was obtained in Experiment II of Chapter 1. There is also a suggestion in Table 2.5 that thoughts of nonphysical aggression were decreased by the singer.

Aggression Restraints. None of the independent variables significantly affected aggression restraints.

Table 2.5—Mean frequencies of thematic nonphysical aggression in six conditions (*TAT*$_{II}$ + *TAT*$_{III}$)

	No Singer	Singer	S−NS[a]
1. Apartment, Dry	3.18 (17)	2.07 (27)	−1.11[b]
2. Apartment, Wet	1.93 (27)	1.38 (26)	−.55[b]
3. Classroom, Wet	1.90 (20)	2.03 (32)	.13
Drinking Effect, difference 2–1	−1.25[c]	−.69[c]	
Setting Effect, difference 3–2	−.03	−.65	

Note.—Numbers in parentheses = number of subjects per condition.
[a]Difference Singer−No Singer conditions.
[b]In Alcohol Experiment, main effect Singer $F = 3.87$, $.10 > p > .05$.
[c]In Alcohol Experiment, main effect Alcohol $F = 6.67$, $p < .05$.

Meaning Contrast. The category of meaning contrast presented unsatisfactory results in several respects. The frequencies of such imagery obtained in the present study were so low as to make statistical treatment almost impossible. Even though half the subjects had in each of their TAT forms a picture that was meant to elicit meaning contrast, very few such themes appeared. In fact only two of the three pictures specifically included for meaning contrast ("Mad scientist" and "Boatman rowing on a moonlit night") reliably elicited a greater frequency of this theme. None of the other effects was significant.

An attempt was then made to relate meaning contrast to amount of alcohol consumption, as was done with physical aggression; in the earlier studies a curvilinear relationship between this variable and amount of alcohol consumed had been discovered. When subjects from all four Wet conditions were included in this analysis, the pattern that emerged was quite irregular. It was noticed, however, that the two conditions most like the experiments run earlier presented similar results and that the irregularities occurred in the two conditions with the folksinger. Only the results of the two Wet conditions without the folksinger were consequently plotted, these being presented in Figure 2.2.

Figure 2.2 shows that the peak of meaning contrast occurs at both TATs among subjects who had consumed between 4–6 oz. of alcoholic beverages. Among subjects who consumed more alcohol the average

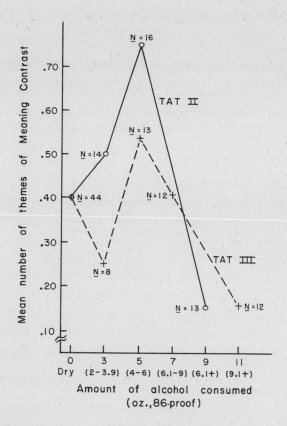

Figure 2.2 Average frequency of thematic Meaning Contrast as a function of amount of alcohol consumed.

frequencies dropped to a level below that of the Dry control subjects. *t*-tests run to evaluate the significance of the shifts gave the following results. At TAT II the difference between the group of subjects who consumed between 4–6 oz. and the Dry control group yielded a *t* of 1.84 (*p* < .10, two-tailed). The group which consumed 6.1 oz. and more was significantly lower than the 4–6 oz. group (*t* = 2.84, *p* < .01, two-tailed). At TAT III the difference between the 4–6 oz. group and the Dry control group yielded a *t* of less than 1. The difference between the 4–6 oz. group and the 9.1 oz. and more group resulted in *t* = 1.74 (*p* < .10, two-tailed.

Sensuous physical pleasure is an important thematic category in view of the concept of sentience. It will be remembered that in the present study the old category of pleasant physical impulses was conceptually elaborated and renamed, and that pictures were specifically included to pull this theme. Despite these efforts, the category did not behave as expected. None of the experimental manipulations had a significant effect on this variable.

Time Concern. The means of Time Concern for the six conditions are presented in Table 2.6. Alcohol decreased the number of references indicating Time Concern. Time Concern was also lower in all conditions

Table 2.6—Mean frequencies of thematic time concern in six conditions (TAT_{II} + TAT_{III})

	No Singer	Singer	S−NS[a]
1. Apartment, Dry	1.65 (17)	.67 (27)	−.98[c]
2. Apartment, Wet	.85 (27)	.58 (26)	−.27[c]
3. Classroom, Wet	1.60 (20)	1.31 (32)	−.29
Drinking Effect, difference 2–1	−.80[b]	−.09[b]	
Setting Effect, difference 3–2	.75[d]	.73[d]	

Note.—Numbers in parentheses = number of subjects per condition.
[a]Difference Singer—No Singer conditions.
[b]In Alcohol Experiment, main effect Alcohol F = 3.86, p < .05 (one-tailed).
[c]In Alcohol Experiment, main effect Singer F = 8.51, p < .005 (one-tailed).
[d]In Setting Experiment, main effect Setting F = 4.72, p < .025 (one-tailed).

with the singer, although the effect of the singer was significant only in the Alcohol Experiment. The setting had a clear effect on Time Concern. As anticipated, the level of Time Concern was higher in the classroom than in the apartment conditions.

Fear. The results of thematic fear appear in Table 2.7. Only alcohol had a significant main effect on fear. Fear references were fewer among Wet than Dry subjects.

Table 2.7—Mean frequencies of thematic fear in six conditions (TAT_{II} + TAT_{III})

	No Singer	Singer	S−NS[a]
1. Apartment, Dry	.71 (17)	.85 (27)	.14
2. Apartment, Wet	.59 (27)	.27 (26)	−.32
3. Classroom, Wet	.40 (20)	.69 (32)	.29
Drinking Effect, difference 2–1	−.12[b]	−.58[b]	
Setting Effect, difference 3–2	−.19	.42	

Note.—Numbers in parentheses = number of subjects per condition.
[a]Difference Singer—No Singer conditions.
[b]In Alcohol Experiment, main effect Alcohol F = 4.53, p < .025 (one-tailed).

In the following section, the results are summarized and discussed according to the three independent variables. The main questions asked in the present investigation can be more easily answered with the results in this form.

Effects of Alcohol on Fantasy. A major purpose of the present study was to replicate the findings on the effects of alcohol reported in the previous chapter; in general, this replication was successful. Alcohol increased physical sex images. Alcohol also raised references to physical aggression but only when the conditions without the folksinger were compared. References to nonphysical aggression were lowered by alcohol, so that we can say that thematic aggression becomes increasingly physical with drinking. As in the earlier investigations, however, the increase in images of physical aggression was not monotonically related to the amount of alcohol consumed. The present curves were partially similar to those obtained earlier. In the earlier experiments a slight initial drop (statistically not significant) of physical aggression thoughts from a Dry control level to consumption up to 3.9 oz. was observed. In the interval 4–6 oz. a sharp increase was observed, followed by a drop at 6.1–12 oz., followed again by an increase among subjects who consumed over 12 oz. The present study showed an initial increase, followed by a decrease.

But a slight shift in the peak of physical aggression imagery occurred. Whereas in the earlier investigation the highest point was for the group that consumed between 4–6 oz., the present curves continued to rise up to the consumption interval of 6.1–9 oz. The other major discrepancy between the present results and the earlier ones, was an absence of the increase with high consumption (over 12 oz.). Several points should be kept in mind, however, when making such comparisons. (a) The lower overall alcohol consumption in the present study necessitated slightly different groupings into consumption groups. Thus, it was considered more appropriate in this study to split the interval of 6.1–12 oz. used earlier into half and create two intervals. (b) The small numbers of subjects in the present study, especially at the upper end of consumption, should be taken into account when considering the failure of very high consumers to show an increase in physical aggression. There were very few subjects who consumed more than 12 oz. The present study therefore does not give adequate evidence concerning the relationship between high levels of alcohol consumption and the appearance of physical aggression imagery.

In view of the partial correspondence of the results obtained in this study with those obtained earlier, it still seems warranted to conclude that with increasing consumption of alcohol, images of physical aggression first increase when subjects are "high or excited," then decrease when they are "sodden." Whether or not they increase again when subjects really are "drunk" is not ascertainable from the present results.

Further support was provided for the relationship between alcohol consumption and the occurrence of meaning contrast. Even though the initial increase with moderate amounts of alcohol (up to 6 oz.) among subjects in parties without the folksinger did not reach very high levels of significance, the following points should be noted. The peak of thematic meaning contrast was in the consumption group of 4–6 oz. both at TAT II and at TAT III. This finding parallels the peaks found among groups with identical alcohol consumption scores in all three previous experiments. The decrease in the occurrence of this theme among subjects who consumed more than 6 oz. of alcohol was also similar at TAT II and III, replicating a similar decrease in the three previous experiments. Thus the conclusion still seems warranted that among young males, at stag cocktail parties, themes of meaning contrast first increase with consumption of alcohol up to 6 oz. With higher consumption of alcoholic beverages, the frequency of such themes decreases. The phrase 'at stag cocktail parties' is a necessary qualification of this conclusion as quite an irregular relationship between amount of alcohol consumed and the occurrence of meaning contrast was observed among subjects entertained by a female folksinger.

Of the restraint categories, time concern and fear were reliably reduced by alcohol, paralleling earlier findings.

The only results not replicated in the present study were the earlier findings that aggression restraints are decreased by alcohol. Among the possible reasons for this discrepancy is the fact that less alcohol was consumed in the present study.

Of the thematic categories not affected by alcohol, sensuous physical pleasure deserves special mention because of its theoretical relevance to the concept of sentience. The implications of this fact are taken up in the general discussion below.

Effects of the Inhibition Setting on Fantasy

The second major goal of this experiment was to investigate the invariance of alcohol effects across different settings; or, to put it differently, whether the drinking context can modify the effect of alcohol. More specifically, the question was asked whether an inhibiting setting can reduce those fantasies usually generated by alcohol, and raise fantasies typically reduced by alcohol. The results showed that with regard to physical sex and time concern, this was the case. Among subjects who had been drinking alcohol, the average level of physical sex expressed in the classroom was less than half as high as that in the apartment, and time concern was greater in the classroom as compared with the apartment. The question arises whether the effect of the setting on fantasy was a direct or an indirect result of the fact that less alcohol was consumed in the classroom. It seems likely that the setting had, at least in part, a direct influence on fantasy, for two reasons. One, the difference in the average levels of physical sex between the two settings was much larger than the difference between the levels of alcohol consumption. Two, in a later study (Kalin, 1966) run only under dry conditions, it was shown that an inhibiting, as compared with a relaxed setting, greatly decreases physical sex and increases time concern.

Inhibition inherent in experimental settings seems to have obscured the effects of alcohol in other studies. Frankenhaeuser, Myrsten and Järpe (1962) found that subjects did not report increases in mood variables like "friendly" and "happy" under alcohol, but did report that they were less clearheaded and able to concentrate. On the other hand, in a study by Ekman, Frankenhaeuser, Goldbert, Bjerver and Myrsten (1962) subjects' self-ratings of mood were *more* affected by alcohol than ratings on intellectual functions like ability to concentrate. This contradiction can be explained by taking note of the difference in purpose and procedure of the two studies.

The major purpose of Frankenhaeuser *et al.* was to investigate intellectual functioning under alcohol. The subjects had to perform a number of complex tasks, and self-ratings were only an incidental part of the procedure. Furthermore, a first dose of alcohol was given in the form of pure alcohol. To keep blood alcohol level constant, alcohol was subsequently administered by intravenous drip. Accordingly, a "scientific" atmosphere must have prevailed in the experimental setting which may well have inhibited the "normal" sentient fantasies associated with drinking and focussed the attention of the subjects on their lack of clearheadedness. In the study by Ekman *et al.*, however, subjects drank whiskey and a much greater emphasis was placed on ratings of intoxication and mood. In short, the setting in the first study was inhibiting because of the "scientific" and "intellectual" atmosphere, whereas in the second study it was less inhibiting and permitted normal mood changes to appear.

Effects of the Female Folksinger on Fantasy

The effects of the attractive female folksinger were far from clear. Two types of effects were observed. (a) Direct effects were those where a thematic variable was either raised or lowered by the presence of the folksinger. (b) Indirect effects occurred when the presence of the singer obscured a relationship between alcohol and fantasy that obtained under nonsinger conditions. Of the direct effects, only the one showing that the folksinger raised Physical Sex in the setting of the apartment, under Wet conditions, was expected. No definitive conclusions concerning the effects of an attractive female on sexual imagery can be drawn on the basis of this result, however, when we consider that the same effects did not occur in the Classroom setting, nor in the Dry conditions. Based on the present results, we can only conclude that the extent to which sexual arousal leads to increased expression of thematic physical sex, depends on alcohol consumption *and* the setting in which the arousal takes place.

The other direct effects were not expected, and it is not immediately clear why the folksinger lowered Nonphysical Aggression and Time

Concern in the Alcohol Experiment. A possible interpretation, that the folksinger simply relaxed subjects as did alcohol, does not seem warranted. The strongest effects of the Singer on Nonphysical Aggression and Time Concern occurred in the Dry conditions, that is, in those conditions where the folksinger aroused conflict over sex and not relaxation (cf. Kalin, 1964). A more likely interpretation seems to be that the Singer channeled the subjects' concern into the sexual sphere, and consequently caused a decrease in other imagery.

Even harder to understand are the indirect effects of the folksinger. Alcohol raised Physical Aggression in the condition of no singer present (and in the earlier Experiment II), but not in the condition of the Singer present; and the functional relationship between alcohol and Meaning Contrast established in the earlier experiments was only replicated in the conditions without the Singer. No immediate explanations for these results come to mind. We are therefore forced to a rather general conclusion concerning the effects of the folksinger. The presence of an attractive female at an otherwise all-male party can modify the effects of alcohol observed at similar parties without females. But the nature of this modification is not readily predictable nor understandable.

GENERAL DISCUSSION

In conceptualization underlying the present investigation two major terms were employed—sentience and inhibition—to describe the determinants as well as the effects of alcohol consumption. Before these concepts are given a permanent place in a theory of drinking, it is advisable to assess their appropriateness and adequacy in terms of the present results.

Sentience

The results we have reviewed tend to undermine the use of Murray's (1938) term. Since the experiments in Chapter 1 showed that only physical and bodily references to sex and aggression were affected by alcohol, and since such images are associated with pleasure, it seemed appropriate to apply the concept of sentience. The inclusion of Meaning Contrast was not so obvious. It can be justified if we consider sentience as an Id-need and therefore associated with primary process thinking. Meaning Contrast may be a stylistic manifestation of this process. In the words of Levy (1958), "alcohol diminishes the need of the ego for synthesis, for logical consistency, for unambivalence" (p. 652). But as plausible as this reasoning may appear, we must ask whether new facts are in line with what the concept of sentience suggests. Of the thematic variables, Sensuous Physical Pleasure most clearly fits the definition. We would therefore expect that this variable should be increased by alcohol, if alcohol indeed increases sentience. But despite the fact that special care was taken with this coding category, by choosing appropriate pictures and elaborating on the coding definition, the expected changes did not occur. It seems, therefore, that sentience is not the most appropriate concept under which the effects of alcohol can be subsumed. On the basis of hindsight and knowledge of results to be presented in later chapters we are forced to the conclusion that sentience suggests a state that is more passive and receptive than the state induced by alcohol. It is true that Physical Sex and Physical Aggression suggest a state of bodily physicality, but this state is also associated with an outward impact. In later chapters this impact is conceptualized as power.

Inhibition

The appropriateness of the concept of inhibition in the description of the determinants and effects of alcohol was confirmed by the present results. Expected fantasy changes occurred as a function of the situational arousal of inhibition. The inhibiting setting decreased Physical Sex and increased Time Concern. The situational arousal of inhibition also lowered alcohol consumption. It is also true, however, that other fantasy changes that might have been expected, did not occur. That is, the inhibiting setting had no reliable effects on Sex and Aggression Restraints and Fear. This outcome could have occurred for various reasons. (a) The restraint variables and fear may not be indications of inhibition. (b) There may be different kinds of inhibition, and only Time Concern may reflect the kind involved in the present context. (c) Sex and Aggression Restraints may have failed to be affected for methodological reasons (infrequent occurrence because of inappropriate pictures, or co-occurrence with imagery). Most likely are the second and third reasons. The question of different types of inhibition will be discussed again in later chapters.

Summary and Conclusions

Most of the effects of social drinking on fantasy described in the previous chapter were replicated in the present experiment. Alcohol increased thoughts of physical sex and aggression and decreased thoughts of nonphysical aggression, time concern and fear. The relationships between meaning contrast, and physical aggression, respectively, and amount of alcohol were similar to those obtained earlier. Because of the more adequate control groups, these effects were more unequivocally due to alcohol than in the previous experiments.

The present results strongly support the conclusion that the setting in which drinking takes place can modify the effects of alcohol. An inhibiting setting counteracts some of the major effects of drinking by decreasing variables that are increased and increasing variables that are decreased by alcohol. Specifically, themes of physical sex were fewer and time concern more common in the inhibiting setting. These results support the idea that the absence of positive results in the earlier Experiment I was due to its inhibiting setting. The results also lend considerable weight to the contention made in the previous chapter that certain settings (e.g., an antiseptic laboratory in a hospital full of scientific gadgets) have limited appropriateness for the study of the experiential effects of alcohol.

When sexual cues, in the form of a sexually attractive girl, are part of the setting, the effects of alcohol are also modified, but in less predictable and understandable ways. Subjects who have been drinking in the relaxed setting, in the presence of a girl, express more thematic physical sex than subjects not exposed to the girl. Since the same effect did not occur in the inhibiting setting, we are forced to conclude that sexual arousal after drinking leads to increased expression of physical sex imagery only to the extent that the setting is free from inhibitory cues. No convincing explanations are available as to why the singer decreased nonphysical aggression and time concern.

The attempt to affect alcoholic consumption by varying the drinking context was only partly successful. The presence of the girl increased drinking, but only in the relaxed apartment setting, not in the inhibiting setting. As in the earlier experiments, the predrinking sentience score was positively correlated with subsequent drinking. The present experiment also showed, however, that this relationship does not obtain, or may even be reversed, in settings that are least like party settings.

There are empirical reasons to doubt that the concept of sentience is appropriate to the cluster of thoughts which is stimulated by alcohol, since themes of sensuous physical pleasure—which are clearly implied by sentience—did not increase after drinking. Later chapters will show that the fantasies that are positively affected by alcohol can be more adequately conceptualized as related to power, and that power thoughts can properly be interpreted as a motive which contributes to the desire to drink.

II
MOTIVES FOR DRINKING

The results of the experimental arousal or drinking studies were moderately encouraging in the sense that they supported the notion that some common experiential effects of alcohol could be identified. But this whole approach bothered us because our sample of subjects and of possible codes was obviously so limited. It could reasonably be argued that although we had shown some common effects of social drinking among American male college sophomores, these effects might not be the same among elderly French farmers, Chinese Maoist Red Guards or Navaho sheepherders. It seemed hopeless to try to find out by repeating the arousal experiment in a variety of cultures. So we turned to a technique which had worked in the study of the achievement motive earlier (McClelland, 1961)—i.e., to an examination of folk tales conceived as *collective fantasies*. These materials can be sampled over a wide variety of cultures quite easily.

Although folk-tale data have the advantage of accessibility, they pose some difficult interpretive problems. The thematic differences between pre- and post-drinking TAT productions can be straightforwardly attributed to the effects of drinking in a certain setting. The causes of thematic differences between the folk tales of cultures which use alcohol heavily and those which do not are less easily located. On one hand, it may be that in heavy drinking societies, the use of alcohol exerts an effect on the content of folk tales: tales routinely told at drinking bouts may be shaped by the state of mind of the teller. But it is also possible that these direct effects are very slight: a folk tale may be told on many non-alcoholic occasions, even in societies which drink heavily. Thus if a relationship is found between folk-tale content and use of alcohol, it need not be due to the effects of drinking. In fact, the causal relation may be just the opposite. Folk-tale themes may tap the psychological states which lead to alcohol rather than those which result from it. There is also the possibility that the relationship is spurious; a third variable may lead both to heavy drinking and to folk-tale content of a certain type.

From the outset we knew that correlational studies of folk tales would not allow us to resolve these causal issues firmly. But as the reader will see, we began to think about the associations between folk-tale content and drinking in causal terms. For the most part, although the careful reader will spot exceptions, we adopted the working assumption that folk tales tap the state which leads to drinking, not that which follows from it. This hypothesis allowed us to make some interesting sense out of the data from the folk tales, but it was not the only sense which might have been made. The final work on the causal issue had to wait until we returned to the TAT and the experimental method.

Shifting to a larger corpus of fantasy material in the folk-tale study permitted us to try out a larger number of thematic codes, evidence for any one of which might be too scanty in the four or five 100-word TAT stories we could obtain from a single subject. We had been unsatisfied with our attempt to group our experimental findings under the heading of sentience because we were aware that there were several theories of drinking which, due to our bias or the brevity of the TAT material, our previous studies might not have tested; so we shifted to a machine method of coding to cast as wide a net as possible for even the smallest differences in the fantasies of heavy- and light-drinking societies. It was hoped that the differences that turned up would not only fit our experimental findings, and test alternative theories, but also improve our understanding of the findings we had already obtained.

They did. The folk-tale themes associated with heavy-drinking cultures seemed to suggest that people in these societies were particularly concerned with a certain type of "power" experience. Evidence that the themes should be interpreted in power terms was also found in the network of their correlations with drinking, social structural and ecological variables. Chapters 3 and 4 are crucial to understanding how we arrived at the theory that guided the research and interpretations which comprise the rest of the book.

By a lucky circumstance, another study had been going on in our laboratory at the same time, in which the focus of attention was not alcohol but power motivation measured at the individual level. It seemed a real breakthrough at the time to discover, as reported by David Winter in Chapter 5, that at least certain types of individuals with high power motivation did in fact drink more. The work presented in this section led to the formulation of the hypothesis that power motivation is the key to understanding drinking both at the cross-cultural and the individual level.

Chapter 3

A Cross-Cultural Study
of Folk-Tale Content
and Drinking[1]

by David C. McClelland, William Davis, Eric Wanner,
and Rudolf Kalin

For nearly 25 years scholars have been trying, by correlating amounts of alcohol consumed in particular primitive cultures with other characteristics of those cultures, to find out why people drink. Horton, for example, in his pioneering study (1943), found a correlation between type of economy and insobriety, a finding later confirmed by Field (1962) and by Barry, Buchwald, Child and Bacon (1965). Generally speaking, hunting tribes drink more heavily than settled tribes that depend for a living on agriculture. The difficulties of this type of study are nicely illustrated by the inferences Horton drew from this simple empirical finding.

Since he found that a rating of Subsistence Insecurity was also related to insobriety, it was natural to conclude that hunters were more economically insecure than agriculturalists, i.e., that they had a less adequate food supply. As Barry et al. (1965) write: "Type of Economy is a scale (with Higher Agriculture as 1 and Hunting as 5) intended to represent increasing probability of economic insecurity." In fact, hunting

[1]This chapter is a revised version of an article with the same title which appeared in *Sociometry*, 1966, 29, 308–333.

may have been used as a sign for establishing the other rating (Subsistence Insecurity) which showed a relation to drinking. Then Horton (1943) made a psychological inference—namely, that people with an insecure food supply would be more anxious. From there it was a short logical step to conclude that drinking serves to reduce Subsistence Anxiety.

Later research has called into question both his main assumptions, despite their self-evident quality. Recent students of hunters and gatherers (see Lee & DeVore, 1968) have concluded that far from being in a state of subsistence insecurity, they may have a better food supply than agriculturalists. That is, they often do not have to work as hard and they eat better on the average (more protein in their diet), because in their normal habitats game is plentiful. As part of the present study, a large correlation matrix of cultural variables shows that severity of food shortages is slightly greater in hunting ($r = .16$, $N = 72$) than in agricultural societies ($r = -.31$, $N = 74$, but so is quantity of food available ($r = .18$ vs. $r = -.18$). At the very least, there is serious doubt now that hunters and gatherers have eaten less well on the average than agriculturalists.

Moreover, even if the hunters were less economically secure, it would not automatically follow that an insecure food supply produces more anxiety or that anxiety produces more drinking. Field (1962), who collected various measures of the prevalence of fear in a culture, could find absolutely no relationships to the degree of drunkenness in the society, though it may be argued that he had no direct measure of *subsistence* anxiety.

In fact, this is the key problem in nearly all the studies in this area—the absence of *direct* measures of the intervening psychological variables in terms of which cross-cultural correlations are interpreted. Two further illustrations will make the nature of the problem even clearer.

Field (1962) found that several social structural variables such as patrilocal residence and corporate kin groups correlated positively with sobriety. He suggested that societies with features such as these were highly organized and solidary, creating attitudes of respect along hierarchical lines that tended to control "extremely informal, friendly, and loosely structured behavior at drinking bouts" (1962, p. 72). This may be perfectly true, but note that Field had no direct measures of his dimension of "respect vs. informality" which is the psychological variable he used to explain the observed correlations. So, methodologically Field is not much better off than Horton was.

Bacon, Barry and Child (1965) go even further beyond their data in interpreting them in psychological terms. For instance, they found quite consistently that drinking was heavier in cultures in which children were not indulged and adults were neither emotionally nor instrumentally dependent on others. The picture one gets is of independent individuals who have been rather roughly treated. Yet Bacon *et al.* draw the superficially paradoxical inference that people from these cultures are basically more *dependent* than people from non-drinking societies. They arrive at this conclusion by assuming that all people need to be indulged and that therefore those who are not indulged must have a stronger need for indulgence (or dependency). Alcohol serves to satisfy this need, which explains why independent adults drink more; that is, since the culture does not permit them satisfaction of their dependency needs, they turn to alcohol as a substitute form of satisfaction. Child *et al.* are so convinced, as Horton was, of the virtue of their *interpretation* of their findings that they sometimes refer to one of their operational measures— lack of Instrumental Dependence in adulthood—by its assumed psychological referent ("lack of satisfaction of dependency needs") (1965, p. 26). But surely it is hazardous to jump so quickly from empirical correlations of variables "out there" in the culture to their psychological meaning. It seems doubly so when what is supposed to be going on "inside" is assumed to be the opposite (feelings of dependency) of what is going on outside (independent actions). This is not to argue that any of these inferences is illogical or incorrect. It is to argue strongly for some way of finding out what is going on "in people's heads" so that some of these psychological explanations of cross-cultural correlates of drunkenness can be checked out directly.

Because folk tales provide a method of getting at what people in a culture commonly think about—often at very unreal or fantasy levels— their content should provide a more direct check on some of the psychological explanations of drinking that have been offered. Could one, for example, expect to find among the tribes that drink heavily more tales dealing with subsistence anxiety, with dependency, or with informal rather than formal relationships? Certainly if one did, that fact would lend support to the hypothesis in question. If themes did not occur more often as predicted by a given hypothesis, that hypothesis would become somewhat less credible, though of course folk tales may not get at a deep enough level of personality to test the matter adequately.

In any case, the effort to get a number of folk tales from a sizable sample of cultures seemed eminently worthwhile as a way of providing further information on the vexing problem of what the various cultural correlates of drinking mean psychologically. Other studies have shown that folk-tale themes do correlate with and illuminate the relations among other cultural variables (McClelland, 1961; Wright, 1954; Bacon, Barry & Child, 1965). The study reported in this chapter was consequently undertaken, first to check existing theories of the mental states associated with drunkenness, and second to derive inductively new possibilities overlooked by previous theorists, by analyzing the content of folk tales drawn from cultures in which drinking is heavy or light.

METHOD

The general strategy employed in the present research was to select a representative sample of primitive cultures for which adequate folk-tale collections and information concerning drinking behavior were available. The final sample consisted of 44 cultures.[2]

Selection of Cultures

Since previous studies have been marred by the inclusion of societies that are not independent but are minor variants of the same culture, a special effort was made to make certain that the sample was not only representative but also consisted of cultures differing in language and/or geographical location. Actually as part of a larger study of the relationship of various cultural ratings to drinking, the largest possible sample of such cultures was drawn from Murdock's *Ethnographic Atlas* (1960–1964) ($N = 182$ for some measures). For many of these cultures ratings exist on a variety of variables from kinship type to marriage mode or child-rearing practices. Some 168 such ratings have been assembled from various sources and correlated with various drinking ratings. A few of the most significant of these correlations will be used to help interpret the folk-tale findings; the rest will be reported later.

The number of independent cultures in this sample for which adequate folk-tale collections could be found was only 44. Thirty-six of these came from different sub-cultural areas, or, where this was impossible, from cultures having different linguistic affiliations. For the four pairs of exceptions (Thonga—Basuto; Ganda—Kikuyu; Ifaluk—Ulithi; Palaung—Khasis), where geographical sub-cultural area and linguistic affiliation was the same, it was determined that the members of each pair were separated from each other by a substantial number of other cultures. Because of this geographical distance, and because each member of each pair constituted a distinct culture, it was felt that these collections could be included legitimately in a sample designed to

---

[2]In a previous publication (R. Kalin, W. N. Davis, & D. C. McClelland, 1966) the number was given as 46, but in the final analysis two tribes were dropped: (1) the Jicarilla Apache, because it was considered too similar to the Chiricahua Apache, and (2) the Taulipang, because they are too similar to the Carib, and because their drinking ratings were less adequate. The reliability statistics are based on a sample of 45, because they were run before it was decided the Taulipang were too similar to the Carib to include. This should not matter since independence of cases is not so crucial for determining internal consistency.

maximize independence of cases. That is, easy transfer of folk-tale themes across intervening cultures was considered to be unlikely.

To insure that societies in the sample would be not only independent, but also representative of the major cultural areas of the world, we attempted to select a comparable number of cultures from each major geographical area and to obtain a scattered distribution of the cultures within each major area. To a certain extent, equal representation was realized. Although exact equality was impossible, it was possible to include a substantial number of cultures from most major areas.[3] The distribution was as follows: Africa, nine; Insular-Pacific, seven; Eurasia, nine; North America, 13; and South America, six.

Selection of Folk Tales

A folk-tale collection had to contain at least 4,000 words and about ten separate tales. There were eight cultures for which only nine tales were available, and one collection had only eight tales. However, on the average, each collection consisted of about 8,000 words and 14 tales. Whenever an exceedingly large corpus of tales was discovered, 10 to 14 tales were randomly selected for analysis.

Another rule for selection concerned the reputability of the source. Clearly, it was necessary to select collections that had not been substantially changed during translation. Therefore, the introduction to each collection was checked carefully. If the author made any mention of editing the text, or of changing it in any way, the collection was considered unacceptable. About two-thirds of the collections used in this study were gathered by professional scholars, such as folklorists and anthropologists. The remaining tales were collected by amateurs (e.g., missionaries or government officials) who made no mention of having altered the original versions, and who in most cases, clearly stated that no such alteration had occurred.

Still another criterion for inclusion in the sample concerned the content of the folk tales. We decided to discard any tales that were either originally myths or historical legends from the recent past. Also excluded were tales that consisted primarily of religious ritual or ceremonial instructions. We omitted these because we felt that their content might be particularly remote from the commonplace thoughts and problems of the average members of a given culture.

Drinking Ratings

Folk-tale collections were sought for societies which met the above criteria and for which various drinking ratings were available. Bacon,

---

[3]There were, however, no cultures in the sample from the [Circum-]Mediterranean region.

Barry, Child and Snyder (1965) provide a number of such ratings, which are reduced to four main dimensions by factor analysis. Since we were interested primarily in the quantity of alcohol consumed, we chose two of their ratings which saturated highly on their quantity factor and which had fairly high inter-coder reliability—namely, frequency of drunkenness and general consumption. Though we ran the correlations separately for these two variables, here we report the results only for a combined drinking rating which was simply the sum of these two ratings. The rationale for combining ratings was (1) we were not especially interested here in *how* people drank—whether in sprees or not—though that is a separate and interesting question; (2) the two ratings are highly correlated anyway, $r = +.64$ in the Bacon *et al.* sample and $+.77$ in ours; and (3) a combined rating should give higher reliability than either alone. Other measures of amount consumed, as for example under ceremonial conditions, were not added because of low coder reliability and the low frequency with which most such judgments could be made.

Mode of Analysis of the Folk Tales

The total text to be analyzed consisted of upwards of 400,000 words. Obviously it was necessary to construct a large number of different codes to check all the hypotheses about drinking that have been advanced as well as develop some new ones. Since this presented a nearly impossible task for human judges, we decided to use the General Inquirer, a computer based system of content analysis, developed by Stone and his associates (1966). Generally, the system operates in the following way. First, a dictionary is constructed, containing a number of different concepts or "tags." Tags consist of groups of "entry words" which are thought to be conceptually related. Second, the dictionary is entered into the computer, which stores the tags and their entry words in memory. Third, some text material is read in. The program searches the text for words that match the entry words in its memory. Every match is re-coded as one occurrence of the tag under which the matched entry word is listed. Ultimately, the frequency of each tag in the text is determined and is printed out in raw form and also as a percentage of the length of the text.

The creative (and difficult) part of this procedure is to decide which words are to be grouped under which tags or concepts. Obviously the results obtained depend entirely on how this problem is solved. So the steps taken to develop the final concept list need to be described in some detail.

1. The a priori *Concept List.* First, an attempt was made to define at least a few concepts which might provide operational checks on all the theories that could be found in the literature as to the psychological functions of drinking. For instance, several theories argue that drinking involves anxiety reduction. So we developed several concepts in this area and searched a popular English dictionary to find words that seemed to reflect the concept in question. For example:

Tag (Concept):	*Sample words classified under tag:*
Fear	afraid, dread, fright, flinch, scare(d)-ing, fear
Unable	cannot, incompetent, inept, muddle, ineffective
Fail	fail, flunk, miss, loss or lost
Not	not, no, won't, wouldn't

To get at a more complex concept such as subsistence anxiety, we could use a double classification. That is, the program would first search a sentence for any *food* word (e.g., fruit, snack, bread, meat, supper); and if it found one, it would then search the same sentence again for a word indicating *fear* or deprivation (e.g., not, nothing, etc.). Obviously this provides only an approximation to correct scoring since it would score a sentence such as "He ate so much supper that there was nothing left," even though it probably does not indicate subsistence anxiety. Nevertheless it was possible to estimate from observation that at least 70–90 percent of the coding done by machine was more or less correct in the sense that the words coded appeared in a context congruent with the meaning of the tag.

Concepts of this sort were derived not only from the three theories already mentioned (Horton, 1943; Bacon *et al.*, 1965; and Field, 1962), but also from our own work described in Chapter 1, from a study by Davis (1964) on cultural correlates of drinking, and from general psychoanalytic and psychodynamic interpretations of the significance of drinking (see Knight, 1937). It will be more economical to discuss each of these theories and the tags related to them in connection with the results obtained.

The first *a priori* concept list included 97 single classification tags and 16 double classification or combination tags (that were sums of other tags). It was applied to only half the folk-tale text for each culture at first (1) to provide a measure of internal consistency for each tag from one-half of the text to the other, (2) to cross-validate any correlations with the drinking ratings from one-half of the text to the other, and (3) to provide an opportunity for correcting and improving the concept list based on the results from the first half of the text. For example, in several cases it was found that the words listed under a tag were so infrequent that many of the cultures got no scores on it at all. Such tags were eliminated and the words sometimes distributed under other tags. This resulted in the second *a priori* concept dictionary (consisting of 88 single tags and 29 combination tags) which was applied to the second half of the text in each culture and the scores on each tag correlated with the drinking ratings.

As typical of the results obtained at this stage, here are the correlations for the tags listed above ($N = 45$, $r = .29$ at $p < .05$).

	RELIABILITY (1st half of text vs. 2nd half)	VALIDITY Correlation with drinking ratings	
		1st half of text	2nd half of text
Fear	.20	−.13	−.23
Unable	.17	−.16	.01
Fail	.40	.16	−.11
Not	.65	−.26	−.16

Obviously there is considerable variability from one half of the text to the other, though a fairly large number of the tags show significant reliability (such as "not" above) as Kalin *et al*. have pointed out elsewhere (1966). While a few correlations showed significant validity in the two halves of the text, many more only showed "promise" or borderline validity, and it seemed imperative to improve the *a priori* concept list.

2. *The Empirical Concept List*. Accordingly, the entire concept list was drastically revised, starting this time not with a dictionary of *a priori* tags but with the actual frequency of occurrence of all the entry words in all the tags obtained by the Data Text System (Stone *et al*., 1966). Each half of the folk-tale text for each culture was broken down into the text coming from cultures scoring above and below the median on the drinking rating. Then the frequency with which every entry word appeared was printed out for these four categories of text. Table 3.1 lays out an example of the raw data on which the revision of the *a priori* concept list was based. It will be useful to discuss this illustration in detail to show how and why the concept list was developed in its final form.

Table 3.1—Some word counts for entries under the concept "aggressive implement"

		FIRST HALF OF TEXT		SECOND HALF OF TEXT	
Word	Over-all Frequency	Societies in Which Drinking Prevalence is:			
		Low	High	Low	High
		Percent occurrence			
Arrow	200	.05	.06	.02	.06
Knife	126	.03	.04	.03	.03
Spear	124	.01	.06	.03	.04
		Frequency of occurrence			
Ax(es), hatchet	48	15	10	17	6
Sword(s)	19	0	6	8	5
Club	42	6	16	17	3
Weapon(s)	25	6	2	11	6
Gun, rifle	20	5	1	10	4

In the *a priori* dictionary there were 39 entry words under "Aggressive Implement," one of the tags developed in the area of aggression to provide a cross-cultural check on the results reported in Chapter 1 that thoughts of physical aggression increase during drinking. Seventeen, or 44 percent of the entry words, however, did not occur at all in the approximately 400,000 words of text (e.g., *armament, arsenal, cutlass, pistol, lance*) and certain others occurred very infrequently (e.g., *whip,* five times; and *machete* three times). Leaving such words in has several disadvantages: they take machine time, even though they occur infrequently or not at all; they confuse the *precise* meaning of the concept; and it is impossible to find out whether they are associated with drinking or not. Consequently for the empirical concept list, the following rule was adopted: (1) Delete the entry word if its *total* frequency is less than 20 in the complete text of about 400,000.

The one exception to this rule involves words with frequencies less than 20 that were synonymous with words included in the tag whose frequencies were greater than 20.

Next, consider the ambiguity problem. Many words have several meanings. For example, in Table 3.1 *club* may be an "association" as well as an "aggressive implement." Often we had to resort to the "key word in context" program to find out how frequent alternate meanings were (cf. Stone *et al.*, 1966). This program prints out the 10 words or so on each side of a word such as *club* for a sample of instances, so that a human judge can count the number of times it is used in one sense or the other. That procedure in turn led to the following rule: (2) Delete an entry word with an alternate meaning that occurs more than one-third of the time.

A count of the alternate meaning of *club* as an "association" in a sample of this text showed that it did not occur more than one-third of the time. So it was not eliminated on this ground. As an extreme example, however, we originally classified the word *little* as belonging under the "feminine" tag, but discovered that nearly 90 percent of the uses of *little* occurred in the phrase "after a little while."

Finally there is the key question of validity. Are the words under a given concept used more often in folk tales from high- or low-drinking societies in each half of the text? This point led to the last rule: (3) Include entry words which discriminate well between high- and low-drinking societies, if conceptual sense can be made of groupings of these words.

This process is the hardest to describe because for every new concept it obviously involved judgments which cannot be described in detail here, though they are recorded. Turn to Table 3.1 again for an example. Clearly the top three words in the list tend to be used more in societies which drink heavily, whereas this is not true of the remaining words in the table. What to do? Should all words remain in the tag or not? Our conclusion here and in many similar cases was that our original *a priori* concept was probably imperfect and that it would be worthwhile to attempt to sharpen its meaning wherever such a move was strongly suggested by the data. In this case the three most frequent words, all associated with drinking, seemed to form a concept more nearly described by the term "Entering Implement"—e.g., *arrow, knife, spear*. That is, each is an implement that stabs or enters something. This new concept would seem to exclude *club, weapon*, and *gun* or *rifle*, but it might include *ax* and *sword*. In the end, we included the latter two, even though they did not seem to be associated with heavy drinking. In short, our tag formation was in part empirical and in part conceptual. We did not feel we could exclude a word that belonged with a conceptual cluster just because it did not yield the expected empirical results. So far as possible, a label for the new concept was chosen which denoted the words that appeared most frequently to define it—a procedure adopted to avoid over-interpreting the results in terms of general psychological concepts such as "aggression."

Does this mean that our final concept list can provide definite tests of the various hypotheses in question? In a sense it cannot, because we can never be certain that another group of judges working with the same material would not have grouped the words in some other way that would have supported the hypothesis. All we can say is that we honestly tried to give every hypothesis a chance. And of course there were clearly instances in which it seemed impossible to form any new concept that was meaningful from the results obtained. We had a "left-over" list of 201 words which occurred at least 20 times. We simply could not classify them under any old or new tags in a way that seemed meaningful.

The revised empirical concept list when completed contained 66 single classification tags based on 367 words and seven idioms, and 22 double classification tags. It was applied separately to the two halves of the text and the scores for individual tribes correlated with their drinking ratings as before. One might suppose that this would simply demonstrate whether we had done our job well since we had now defined our tags in part in terms of whether they discriminated between tales from high- and low-drinking societies. But there is more play in the system than that: for instance, it would be quite possible to get the results shown in Table 3.1 for the word *spear* simply by having one tribe above the median in drinking which talked endlessly about spear hunts. If such were the case, a correlation with drinking based on the use of the word in 45 cultures would not be high. As a matter of fact, about 41 of the tags should have had significant relationships to drinking based on the word analyses of the sort shown in Table 3.1. Of these, 11 yielded a correlation significant at the 5 percent level or less. And in several cases a tag whose word entries showed no consistent relation to drinking yielded tribal scores which correlated significantly with drinking. To check still further against the possibility of capitalizing on chance findings, we broke the sample of cultures randomly in half and re-ran the correlations in each half to make sure the correlations were consistent in two independent samples of cultures, as well as in two independent samples of folk tales.

RESULTS

Tables 3.3 and 3.4 organize the correlations obtained between drinking and various folk-tale themes according to several prior hypotheses as to the reasons for drinking. Table 3.2 helps explain the meaning of the various correlations by listing the most frequent words tagged

Table 3.2—Alphabetical list of concepts (with some of the most frequent words tagged under each) and mean relative frequency of occurrence in the total text

Concept (and Words)	Mean	S.D.
Activity inhibition (not, catch, stop)	76.2	22.1
Anal socialization anxiety (dung, excrement+fear or negation) *	.2	.6
Anger (anger, rage, fury)	6.8	5.7
Capability (make, could, can)	62.1	22.1
Change of state (become, feel, change, awake)	32.5	17.0
Child (child[ren], baby, grandchild)	28.3	23.7
Collateral (uncle, nephew, aunt, niece, cousin)	3.9	6.6
Cook (cook, roast, pan)	13.5	10.0
Dependency (ask, carry, help)	37.4	14.1
Drinking (drink, milk, beer, thirst[y])	9.3	9.1
Eating (eat, meat, fat, fruit, hunger)	52.5	25.0
Eating markers (food, feast, meal)	13.9	9.1
Entering implements (arrow, knife, spear)	14.0	10.8
Fear (afraid, fear, fright)	8.1	5.9
First order generation (mother, father, son, daughter)	53.4	31.2
Fish (fish, fisherman)	11.2	17.7
Give (give, let, help)	48.4	20.6
Hunt (hunt, hunter)	6.8	7.5
Kill (kill, slaughter, stab, slay)	13.9	9.9
Negation (not, no, never)	89.1	27.2
Old and dead (old, dead, death)	32.4	19.0
Oral body parts (mouth, stomach, tongue)	9.0	6.7
Scheduling (time, after, before, next)	87.8	27.2
Subsistence anxiety (eating, eating markers, or cook+negation, fear or hunger) *	11.5	7.2
Taking (take, seize, collect)	44.4	16.9
Title (king, priest, queen, prince)	9.5	20.4
Travel and gather (went, go, find, gather)	133.2	45.0
Vertical space (under, above, below)	9.0	6.0
Violent physical manipulation (throw, cut, hit)	34.9	13.3
Want (want, wish, need)	18.6	10.3
War (shoot, fight, war)	11.5	9.6

Note.—The mean shows the average frequency of occurrence in 45 societies per 10,000 words of text.
*Combination tags; same sentence coded for two sets of tags to check for co-occurrence.

under the concepts listed in the several tables. Not all concepts are included here, either because they were of little theoretical relevance and/or because they yielded no significant correlations with drinking.

So far as Horton's subsistence anxiety hypothesis is concerned, the results (Table 3.3, part A) give little support to the notion that tribes which drink a lot worry more about food and being hungry. In fact, they appear to worry less, or at least to refer to fear or being afraid less in

Table 3.3—Correlations with drinking of various folk-tale themes relevant to subsistence anxiety, formal organization and dependency

| | TEXT | | | SAMPLE OF CULTURES | |
| | Over-all | 1st Half | 2nd Half | Odd | Even |
Tags Relevant to :	(N = 44)	(N = 45)	(N = 45)	(N = 23)	(N = 22)
A. *Subsistence anxiety* (Horton)					
Fear	−.44***	−.24*	−.39**	−.48**	−.36*
Subsistence anxiety	.09	.10	.06	.14	.05
Hunt	.38***	.33**	.27*	.57***	.18
Travel and gather	−.18	−.20	−.12	−.03	−.34
B. *Formal organization* (Field)					
Title	−.30*	−.13	−.36**	−.44**	.03
Vertical space	−.12	−.13	−.10	−.08	−.18
Old and dead	−.42***	−.18	−.40***	−.35*	−.49**
Scheduling	−.09	−.17	−.04	.20	−.38*
Activity inhibition	−.35**	−.27*	−.35**	−.53***	−.20
C. *Dependency* (Barry, Bacon, Child)					
Give	−.06	.12	−.15	−.29	.53**
Taking	.21	.18	.17	−.01	.37*
Dependency	−.09	−.06	−.10	−.15	−.06
Want	.16	.19	.07	.08	.21
Capability	−.04	.09	−.20	.01	−.14
Anal socialization anxiety	−.06	−.37**	.07	−.08	−.06

Note.—Significance level is based on the two-tailed test throughout.
*$p < .10$.
**$p < .05$.
***$p < .01$.

their folk tales. This goes even further than Field's data which show no correlations between drinking and ratings by ethnographers as to the presence of certain institutionalized fears such as fear of sorcerers, spirits, ghosts, etc. (1962). If fear or anxiety is a critical factor in drinking, it is so reduced by drinking that it appears *less* often in fantasies from heavy-drinking societies than from light-drinking ones.

The correlations are confusing with respect to another aspect of Horton's argument—namely, the relation of drinking to a hunting and gathering type of economy (vs. a settled agricultural economy). *Hunting* themes do correlate significantly with drinking, but *travelling* and *gathering* themes do not.

Field's hypothesis that formal organizational structure promotes attitudes that lead to sobriety is rather consistently supported by several relevant folk-tale themes (Table 3.3, part B). All of the five correlations are in the predicted direction, and three of them at the 5 percent level of significance. These results strongly suggest that sober societies tend to think more in terms of hierarchy (*title, vertical space,* and *old age*) and social control (*scheduling* and *activity inhibition*).

The Barry, Bacon, and Child dependency hypothesis does not appear to be supported by the folk-tale results, though of course it may be argued that the concepts did not adquately get at the basic psychological processes involved (Table 3.3, part C). Still, if it is really true that people in drinking societies are basically *dependent*, one ought reasonably to expect that their folk tales would show an increased number of themes dealing with *giving, taking, dependency,* or *wanting* (demanding). Or if such ideas are too deeply repressed to appear even in the fantasy of folk tales, then perhaps they should show up *less* often than in the tales told by sober societies. But the data show no regular variations of any kind in these themes as a function of drinking. The *capability* tag was designed to get at the extent to which achievement— "can do"—is emphasized in the folk tales as a means of checking the positive correlation Barry, Buchwald, Child and Bacon report between childhood pressure toward achievement and drinking (1965). But here there is a clear lack of fit between a social pressure and its presumed correlate in the minds of the people practicing it: childhood pressure for achievement is negatively related to the *capability* tag ($r = -.33$, $p < .05$), but it is positively related to the *give* tag ($r = .41$, $p < .05$) and the *want* tag ($r = .37$, $p < .05$). Thus one could argue (as Bacon, Barry and Child do) that pressure for achievement frustrates and accentuates a basic need for nurturance and support, as reflected in the increase of thoughts about *giving* and *wanting* in societies which stress achievement training. *But neither of these states of mind is associated with drinking!* So the explanation for the correlation between achievement training and drinking cannot be sought in these mental effects of achievement training. This is a nice illustration of the way in which direct measures of intervening psychological states of mind can help refine the interpretation of empirical correlations between "external" variables such as socialization practices and various institutional forms.

Bacon, Barry and Child also report a negative correlation between Anal Socialization Anxiety and drinking (1965). Again the presumed mental equivalent—themes of Anal Anxiety—did not show the same result, possibly because their frequency was so low (see Table 3.2), although the correlations in all samples were in the predicted direction.

Table 3.4 checks first on findings reported in Chapter 1 to the effect that social drinking increases the fantasy themes of Sex, Aggression and Meaning Contrast, while it decreases themes of Time Concern and Anxiety. In general, the folk tale results are not dissimilar. Table 3.3 has already shown that in heavy-drinking societies *fear* themes are less common, as is also an inhibitory theme such as Activity Inhibition. Scheduling, which was designed to be the equivalent of Time Concern, unfortunately shows fluctuating results in various sub-samples, though the over-all trend is in the predicted direction.

Table 3.4—Correlations with drinking of folk-tale themes relevant to effects of social drinking and to orality

	TEXT			SAMPLE OF CULTURES	
Themes	Over-all ($N = 44$)	1st Half ($N = 45$)	2nd Half ($N = 45$)	Odd ($N = 23$)	Even ($N = 22$)
D. *Social drinking effects* (Kalin *et al.*, 1965)					
Sex	.27*	Unavailable	—	.38*	.09
Aggression tags					
Kill	.21	.23	.13	−.03	.42**
Entering implements	.35**	.22	.29**	.24	.38*
Violent physical manipulation	.21	.17	.19	.22	.21
Anger	−.30**	−.21	−.28*	−.42**	−.10
War	−.17	.08	−.29**	.00	−.29
Change of state	.35**	.28*	.36**	.19	.49**
E. *Orality themes* (Knight)					
Eating	.35**	.27*	.32**	.47**	.22
Drinking	.24	.14	.24*	.02	.46**
Cook	.09	−.13	.27*	.11	.08
Oral body part	.48***	.34**	.35**	.46**	.53**
Eating markers	−.34**	−.41***	−.05	−.29	−.37*

*$p < .10$.
**$p < .05$.
***$p < .01$.

Themes of Sex and Aggression also show roughly congruent results. Unfortunately the computer could not be programmed to recognize sexual themes, largely because translators or ethnographers use such an extraordinary variety of low-frequency circumlocutions with other meanings in dealing with sexual matters (e.g., *connection* or *intercourse* for coitus). They do not confuse the human reader, but they do confuse the machine; hence scores for sexual content had to be obtained by a human judge. They correlate at the $p < .10$ level with drinking, though the sub-sample variation is disturbingly large. Several sub-types of sexual imagery (affiliative, male-dominated, female-dominated, male rivalry) showed correlations varying from .16 to .21 with drinking, but with the same sub-sample variation, so that further interpretation seems hazardous.

Three out of the five Aggression tags correlated positively and reasonably consistently with drinking; *war* and *anger,* however, correlated negatively, the latter significantly. Apparently the type of aggression most consistently related to drinking is a kind of phallic individualistic acting out, best represented by the use of words such as *arrow, spear,* and *knife.*

Change of state is an interesting tag which relates to drinking consistently, though its connection with the category of meaning contrast used in Chapter 1 is somewhat uncertain. There we scored contrasting statements in the same thought sequence (single sentence or adjoining sentences) about existential matters, as in the phrase: "To be or not to be, that is the question." Although several attempts were made to devise a machine code that would get at the same variable in folk tales, the nearest equivalent that we could find was based on verbs such as *become, turn into,* or *change* which most often indicated a person was going from one state to another (and often contrasting) state. Normally the theme involved a person turning into an animal or vice versa, or it involved a person changing his emotional state, as when he became angry, or hungry, or afraid.

Finally, most psychodynamic theories of alcoholism assume some kind of etiological disturbance at the oral level of psychosexual development. Knight (1937), for instance, argues in fairly standard fashion that the alcoholic has suffered from maternal overprotection (libidinizing the oral mode), thus creating a strong, neurotic need for indulgence which cannot possibly be satisfied in normal ways in adulthood. So the adult regresses to an infantile mode of satisfying his need for indulgence by drinking compulsively. Drinking alcohol also serves to dampen the rage that derives from the frustration of oral dependent needs and the guilt that derives from being so dependent. Hence various tags were designed to get at orality themes.

The results shown at the bottom of Table 3.4 strongly suggest that alcoholic societies may show some preoccupations in the oral mode—at least the *eating* and *oral body part* tags are significantly and positively related to drinking. Incidentally the *drinking* tag was formed precisely to avoid contaminating the *eating* tag with references to whiskey, etc., since it would not appear to be very illuminating to discover that societies that drink more alcohol talk more about it in their folk tales. *Eating markers,* on the other hand, are negatively related to drinking, possibly because they refer to regular, scheduled and organized meal times.

An Inductive Interpretation of the Results

A first run through the findings in terms of prior theorizing has left much to be desired, despite the fact that in nearly every case folk-tale themes have been found that can be used as at least indirect support for some prior psychological theory. Even the dependency hypothesis, which fared badly on direct measures, can be regarded as indirectly supported by the increase in orality themes. For doesn't increased emphasis on eating mean that people who drink a lot are in need of nurturing?

Yet the arguments seem on the whole devious and unconvincing, particularly in the light of some of the negative findings which are also nearly always present. This fact suggested to us that we might start from scratch theoretically and simply attempt to derive whatever theory could be supported by the data of this study. Perhaps the pattern of correlations would be such as to suggest a better interpretation of previous findings than any of the theories so far proposed.

Tables 3.5, 3.6, and 3.7 have been prepared to highlight a re-interpretation of findings in this area suggested by careful examination of the 14 folk-tale tags which correlated significantly with drinking. To make the results more readily understandable, the intercorrelations with certain cultural ratings have also been introduced from the larger study of which this is a part.

For simplicity of exposition, it is useful to start with the relation of drinking to male solidarity, which yields one of the highest correlations obtained ($r = .41$, cf. Table 3.5). Male solidarity is considered to be present or absent depending on whether a culture was rated as showing some ritualization of male activity (Young, 1965) or some separate male housing—for example, for eating or sleeping.[4] Thus the correlation is point-biserial and is, if anything, an underestimate of the size of the relationship. It suggests that perhaps drinking has something to do with gender identity; that is, cultures which do not institutionally stress maleness are the ones that drink. Initially this idea had been reinforced by a finding reported by Davis (1964) to the effect that in a sample of 47 cultures, 10 out of 13 (77 percent) of the tribes practicing couvade were rated high on frequency of drunkenness as contrasted with only 12 out of 34 (35 percent) of those not practicing couvade ($X^2 = 6.48, p < .02$). This fact suggested further that drinking might have something to do with cross-sex identity (lack of strong masculine identity), since couvade males are imitating females in connection with the birth of a child—by sickness during pregnancy, by observing food taboos if the mother does, etc. In fact much of the present study was planned to test this hypothesis. But the data in no way confirmed it.

The most elaborate test involved comparing the frequency with which various tags appeared in the female-role text (sentences containing female pronouns) vs. the remaining text, selecting the few tags that were

[4]Unpublished ratings assembled in J. W. M. Whiting's laboratory, Department of Social Relations, Harvard University, Cambridge, Mass.

more frequently associated with female pronouns (*child*, certain domestic items such as *basket, loom, clothes*, and certain female adjectives such as *beautiful, lovely*, and *pretty*), and then counting the number of male-role sentences for each culture in which female tags appeared minus the other sentences in which the same tags appeared. This created a Man-Feminine combination tag or a measure of the extent to which a culture treated a man in a feminine way in folk tales as cross-culturally defined (always in relation to the general non-male use of feminine tags). The correlation of the Man-Feminine tag with drinking was .05, and many other attempts to relate men behaving in feminine ways to drinking failed to produce relationships of any significance whatsoever.[5] Furthermore in the present sample the relationship of drinking to the practice of the couvade disappears ($r = .09$, $N = 52$).

Thus the lack of male solidarity must be linked to drinking not via cross-sex identity, but in some other way. As the correlations in Table 3.5 suggest, it is more probably one of several interrelated indexes of lack of structural differentiation related to drinking via a connection with folk-tale themes which appear to suggest a kind of magical potency. The argument runs as follows. Low male solidarity, non-lineal descent (i.e., bilateral descent), and lack of a jurisdictional hierarchy at the local level are all related to each other and to drinking. The relationship of local jurisdictional hierarchy to drinking becomes significant ($\chi^2 = 7.2$, $p < .05$) among societies with low extralocal hierarchy.[6] That is, for example, among stateless societies (no extralocal hierarchy) 11 out of 11 of those with no local hierarchy beyond the extended family drink heavily. If there is hierarchy either at the local or extralocal level, drinking is significantly less (only 51 percent of 59 cases above the median in drinking, ($\chi^2 = 7.45$, $p < .01$). In other words, it is the completely non-hierarchical, unstructured societies that drink.

The measures of this lack of structural differentiation are also significantly related to type of economy (Table 3.5, part C), agricultural societies showing more formal organization than hunting societies. Several other indicators not included in Table 3.5 for simplicity's sake also belong in this cluster—e.g., size of local community, sedentary vs. non-sedentary settlement pattern, and class stratification. All these variables, through their linkages to each other and to drinking strongly, suggest that socially less organized societies generally drink more, just as Field argued (1962).

But why? An answer is suggested by a group of four intercorrelated folk-tale themes which are linked both to drinking and to these indexes

---

[5] In our previous paper (see footnote 2) where a relationship is reported between drinking and a Man-Feminine tag, the decisions as to what to code as feminine were made on an *a priori* basis, which now seems to us to be culture-bound and less justifiable than the method used here.

[6] Class O (stateless) societies, from column 33 in Murdock (1960–1964).

Table 3.5—Structural variables and folk-tale themes associated with heavy drinking cross-culturally

VARIABLES	DRINKING		LOW-MALE SOLIDARITY		NON-LINEAL DESCENT		LOW HIERARCHY		HUNT		ENTERING IMPLEMENTS		EATING		CHANGE OF STATE	
	r	n	r	n	r	n	r	n	r	n	r	n	r	n	r	n
A. Indicators of low structural differentiation																
Low male solidarity[1]	.41***	49	—		—		—		—		—		—		—	
Non-lineal descent[2]	.23**	76	.14	55	—		—		—		—		—		—	
Low hierarchy[3]	.20*	71	.26*	52	.28***	173	—		—		—		—		—	
B. "Potency" folk-tale themes																
Hunt	.38**	44	.17	31	.02	44	.31**	41	—		—		—		—	
Entering implements	.35**	44	.44**	31	.31**	44	.21	41	.12	45	—		—		—	
Eating	.36**	44	.29	31	.03	44	.60***	41	.35**	45	.43***	45	—		—	
Change of state	.35**	44	.22	31	.29*	44	.16	41	.00	45	.32**	45	.30**	45	—	
C. Other cultural variables																
Hunting[4]	.30***	76	.26*	107	.31***	182	.30***	173	.22	44	.23	44	.17	44	−.16	44
Agriculture[5]	−.27**	76	−.17*	107	−.30***	182	−.32***	173	−.22*	44	−.11	44	.03	44	.06	44
Non-tropical climate[6]	.49**	54	.23**	88	.26***	137	.12	131	.18	32	.11	32	.01	32	.10	32

[1]Absence or presence of ritualization of male activity (score = 1, 2, 3, or 4 in Young's scale; see footnote 27) or if no rating in Young (1965), presence of men's housing (rating 1 or 2; see footnote 28).

[2]Presence or absence of any unilineal descent groups (Columns 20 and 22 in Murdock; see footnote 11).

[3]Two, three or four levels of jurisdictional hierarchy at the local level (from Column 32 Murdock; see footnote 11).

[4, 5]Percentage dependence on hunting or agriculture (Columns 8 and 11 in Murdock; see footnote 11).

[6]Tropical rainforest and savannah vs. all others, from J. W. M. Whiting (1964).

*p ∨ .10.
**p ∨ ∨ .05.
***p ∨ ∨ .01.

of low structural differentiation (see Table 3.5). *Hunt* is the weakest of these, both in terms of its internal consistency (see Table 3.3) and its relation to the other tags, but it does suggest thoughts of male assertiveness, particularly when taken in conjunction with the *entering implements* tag (*arrow, knife, spear*). What is interesting here is that some of the more directly aggressive tags such as *kill* or *war* are not associated with drinking, a fact which suggests that what is involved is not so much instrumental ego aggression as a kind of primitive assertiveness. What then are we to make of *eating* and *change of state*? If we follow standard psychodynamic thinking, these represent the most primitive types of power imagery—the power to transform something into something else without ego instrumental activity—a kind of magical potency that enhances the actor.[7]

Could drinking represent a means of obtaining magical potency— a kind of primitive "power play"—the desire to find "strength in a bottle"? If so, the further question arises as to why men should be attracted to this kind of magical potency, particularly in relatively unstructured societies. The answer may be in the individualism stressed in such non-solidary societies. For example, hunting societies, which are often unstructured (see Table 3.5), stress achievement in childhood ($r = .26$, $N = 54$, $p < .05$) and self-reliance in adulthood ($r = .44$, $N = 50$, $p < .01$). (See Barry, Bacon and Child, 1957, for definitions of behavior ratings.) In contrast, societies which rank high in male solidarity are rated high in instrumental dependence for adults (Barry, Bacon & Child, 1957) ($r = .41$, $N = 32$, $p < .05$). People help each other, and not so much is left to the individual. Lacking strong organized group support, the individual in an unstructured society may seek magical ways of increasing the strength he needs to face his problems, either by drinking, or actually by using dreams instrumentally to achieve purposes by magical means.

D'Andrade (1961) has coded various societies according to whether dreams are used instrumentally or not. Dreams are considered to be used instrumentally if supernaturals appear therein and give important aid, if religious experts use their dreams in performance of their roles, if magic-helper dreams are required before certain roles may be assumed, or if dreams are induced by fasting or drugs. Unstructured societies (low in local jurisdictional hierarchy) tend to use dreams instrumentally more ($r = .41$, $N = 45$, $p < .01$), and societies that use dreams more tend to drink more ($r = .38$, $N = 28$, $p < .05$).

[7]The *oral body parts* tag could fit in here well enough, since it correlates highly with drinking and fairly highly with the other tags, but it has been omitted from Table 3.5 because it is uncertain whether its significance lies in its oral or in its body part component. For example, it correlates only .12 with the *eating* tag, but .32 with another body part tag (consisting of *hand, foot, leg, arm*, etc.), which also correlates positively with drinking but at a much lower level. Further study will have to elucidate the meaning of the *oral body parts* tag.

Some other correlations give clues as to the more precise nature of the conflicts that are likely to cause trouble in unstructured societies. One set is to be found in the correlations among various behavior ratings, socialization variables and drinking. On the whole in this carefully chosen sample, these relationships are variable for similar measures and non-significant, casting doubt on earlier findings reported by Barry, Bacon, and Child (1957). Frequency of achievement responses in childhood is, however, significantly associated with drinking ($r = .35$, $N = 40$, $p < .05$) but curiously enough so is frequency of obedience responses in childhood ($r = .29$, $N = 52$, $p < .05$) (1957). As might be expected, the two childhood ratings are unrelated ($r = -.08$), so that each contributes independently and significantly to a multiple r of .47 for predicting drinking. In other words, if both types of responses occur together, heavy drinking is more likely than if either occurs alone. But achievement and obedience are response systems which ought often to be in conflict. The individual in such societies would often be in doubt as to whether to assert himself or knuckle under.

And it is precisely in the unstructured societies in which conflicts caused by co-occurrence of the two response systems are most likely to occur. If male solidarity is present, for instance, they tend not to co-occur—frequency of obedience and achievement responses correlate negatively ($r = -.43$, $N = 15$)—whereas if male solidarity is absent, they are positively correlated ($r = .28$, $N = 19$). The difference in correlations is significant ($p < .05$ by Fisher's Z ratio). In unstructured societies a child is likely to have to face the achievement-obedience conflict which later leads to drinking.

The same line of argument may explain the correlation of bride service with drinking ($r = .22$, $N = 76$, $p < .05$).[8] For in such a situation a man must achieve (to earn his bride) but also be obedient, in working for his future wife's family. Furthermore this relationship is limited to non-solidary societies ($\chi^2 = 5.02$, $p < .05$). In societies above the median in male solidarity, there is no relationship between bride service and drinking ($p \sim .50$).

These diverse relationships all point in the same direction: in unstructured societies, a man does not get much organized support or prescription as to what he should do. As a result, he is more likely to face certain conflicts, such as that between achievement and obedience, which create feelings of inability to cope with everything on his own. Hence he turns to alcohol and to dreams for the magical potency he needs to face his individualistic-type problems.

The man in a structured society not only is less often faced with such conflicts, but when they occur, he gets help from others and guidance

[8]Bride service against all other marriage modes, from Column 12 in Murdock (1960–1964).

from his society as to how to behave in a respectful, inhibited way (see below, Table 3.7.).

Before accepting this interpretation too quickly, another simpler one should be examined more carefully. Table 3.5 also shows that cultures living outside the tropics are more likely to drink and show signs of low structural differentiation. They also are likely to be involved in hunting ($r = .35$, $N = 137$, $p < .01$) rather than in agriculture ($r = -.47$, $N = 137$, $p < .01$). Could it be that ecology is the key variable in producing drinking, and that the social structural variables are linked to drinking only because they are associated with climate? Could it simply be that people drink alcohol to keep warm, or that tropical peoples drink less because alcohol makes them uncomfortably warm? This possibility is examined at some length in the next chapter where a more elaborate analysis is attempted relating ecological, social structural, and folk-tale variables to drinking.

Here it is perhaps worth pointing out only how the folk-tale results help to make some interpretations of the data less likely than others. Consider the pattern of correlations in Figure 3.1 drawn from Table 3.5 and elsewhere. In the upper left-hand portion of the figure are a group of variables which are connected in a way that sounds like Horton's hypothesis all over again—that is, climate and type of economy create

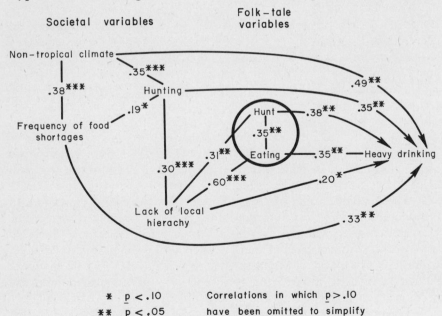

Figure 3.1 Pattern of relationships of societal variables, folk-tale variables, and drinking among pre-literate cultures. *N* varies from 44 to 137.

disturbances in food supply which lead to drinking. But the folk-tale results simply do not bear out such an interpretation; a key theme like *eating* (and other associated tags) is surprisingly not significantly linked to any of the societal variables in this cluster, as it should be if Horton is correct in assuming that the linkage of these variables to drinking is via some concern about eating. Instead *eating* is quite unexpectedly very highly correlated with lack of local hierarchy—which in turn is linked to the cluster of variables Horton talks about via its connection with hunting as a way of life. The only interpretation that occurs to us for such a finding is that the societal variables affect drinking in the way we have proposed—by increasing the concern for magical potency, as reflected in tags such as *eating, hunt, entering implements,* etc. Thus *eating* themes are to be understood as suggesting the power to transform something into something else rather than as suggesting orality-nurturance-dependence. This concern with magical potency is greater in heavy-drinking societies in which a man does not receive much organized institutional support.

Table 3.6 summarizes the findings for three kinship tags which correlate highly with each other and also positively with drinking. They seem to reflect egalitarianism or lack of hierarchical structure in the

Table 3.6—Relationship of egalitarian kin terms in folk tales to drinking and community size

VARIABLE	DRINKING		SMALL COMMUNITIES		COLLATERAL TERMS		FEW FIRST ORDER TERMS	
	r	*n*	*r*	*n*	*r*	*n*	*r*	*n*
Small community size	.27**	58	—	—	—	—	—	—
Egalitarian kin terms								
Collateral terms	.51***	44	.32*	34	—	—	—	—
Few first order generation terms	.27*	44	.20	34	.29**	45	—	—
Few "child" references	.31**	44	.44***	34	.34**	45	.34**	45

Note.—Community size is used, as in column 30 of Murdock; see footnote 11.
  *$p < .10$.
 **$p < .05$.
***$p < .01$.

use of kin terms. That is, drinking societies use more collateral terms such as *aunt, uncle, niece, nephew,* and fewer terms signifying the parent-child hierarchy (*father, mother, son, daughter, child*). Of the several inter-related indicators of structural differentiation, these kin tags are most closely related to community size. So this variable is included in Table 3.6. The suggestion is unmistakable that it is the small, structurally un-differentiated (even in kin terms) bands that drink the most. Field (1962) actually predicted this result when he wrote: "Drunken tribes may have a wide-ranging kinship system emphasizing friendly solidarity among siblings, cousins, and spouses, rather than hierarchical, lineal solidarity between parents and children."

Finally Table 3.7 presents two clusters of folk-tale themes that are negatively associated with drinking and positively with various indicators of social differentiation, particularly local jurisdictional hierarchy and male solidarity. Size of local community also correlates highly with several of these tags ($r = .37$, $p < .05$ with Title and $r = .46$, $p < .01$ with Activity Inhibition), as do other indicators of social structure. The two clusters of tags are presented separately because the correlations within each cluster are higher than between the clusters except for Anger, which belongs in both clusters, and Fish, which is only weakly associated with the Inhibition cluster.

To interpret the results a little, it is not surprising to find that Titles are used more often in folk tales from structurally differentiated societies that do not drink, but it is interesting to note that Fear and Anger fit in this same cluster, both being significantly related to Titles. A likely interpretation is that in a hierarchical social structure Anger is expressed downwards toward subordinates and Fear upwards from subordinates— hence the cluster label of Respect. And Anger also goes with Activity Inhibition; in a very real sense, it is controlled or inhibited aggression. Again it is not surprising to find references to old and dead people in the Inhibition cluster, because both are references to powerful inhibitors on human action. Nor is the presence of Eating Markers difficult to understand, since it includes largely references that suggest control over eating, scheduling of meals, etc. But the Fish tag was a surprise. Why should non-drinking societies tell more stories about fishing? No one's theory would seem to account for it, but its correlation with Activity Inhibition suggested an interpretation. Fishing is psychologically a waiting game (as contrasted particularly with hunting), and therefore stories about it fit in well with the psychological characteristics of sober societies which stress control and scheduling, fear and anger (as controlled aggression).

CONCLUSION

The main results thus fall into place as supporting a somewhat altered interpretation of the significance of alcoholic consumption in cross-cultural perspective. Sober societies, as Field (1962) argued, are better organized, hierarchical, solidary, often agricultural and settled communities which give wide and strong support to a man and which stress inhibition and respect. Societies which do not provide a man with this solid support apparently often put him in a situation of conflict, where he wants or is expected to be assertive and yet must be obedient.

Table 3.7—Folk-tale themes associated with light drinking cross-culturally

Variable	Drinking	Local Hierarchy	Male Solidarity	RESPECT THEMES			INHIBITION THEMES		
				Title	Fear	Anger	Act. Inh.	Old and Dead	Fish
Local hierarchy	−.20*	—	—	—	—	—	—	—	—
Male solidarity	−.41***	.26***	—	—	—	—	—	—	—
A. *Respect themes*	(N=44)	(N=41)	(N=31)		(N=45)				
Title	−.30**	.27*	.32*	—	—	—	—	—	—
Fear	−.44***	.04	.20	.55***	—	—	—	—	—
Anger	−.30**	.12	.42**	.37**	.27*	—	—	—	—
B. *Inhibition themes*								(N=45)	
Activity inhibition	−.35**	.26*	.19	.19	.23	.25*	—	—	—
Old and dead	−.42***	.20	.06	.24	.21	.19	.37**	—	—
Fish	−.36**	.01	.26	−.10	−.12	.36**	.32**	−.03	—
Eating markers	−.34*	−.03	.55***	.11	.10	.28*	.24	.33**	.16

Note.—See Table 3.5 for explanation of "local hierarchy" and "male solidarity."
*p < .10.
**p < .05.
***p < .01.

He solves the conflict by dreams of being powerful in a primitive, non-instrumental, impulsive way, and finds in alcohol a means of promoting these dreams—of buying, at least temporarily, the strength he needs.

It cannot be argued that the findings support this hypothesis in any decisive way as against other interpretations of the data; but at least it seems to fit all the data somewhat better than other theories. Of course fitting a theory to a network of correlations is a notoriously hazardous process. Some of these hazards are considered in the following chapter.

Chapter 4

Power and Inhibition: A Revision of the Magical Potency Theory

by Eric Wanner

MAGICAL POTENCY THEORY AND THE PROBLEM OF INTERPRETATION

In the previous chapter we marshalled a good deal of evidence from the folk tales in support of Field's (1962) hypothesis that corporately organized, solidary societies promote attitudes of respect and inhibition which limit the consumption of alcohol. The correlation of tags such as Activity Inhibition and others (see Table 3.3) with both low drinking and indices of structural solidarity, provide Field with evidence that the social correlates of low drinking act upon psychological attitudes in much the way he had supposed. Even with this psychological addendum, however, Field's hypothesis is hardly an adequate theory of drinking. On the contrary, it is at best a theory of sobriety. Although it delineates a set of social and psychological characteristics which seem to lead a society to avoid the use of alcohol, it does not propose any positive reasons why alcohol should ever be used. As other have noted (see Davis, 1964), it is scarcely feasible to assume a *sui generis* need to drink which emerges wherever attitudes of respect and inhibition are weak or absent. All other theories reviewed in the previous chapter avoid this pitfall by proposing some positive need, state, or motive which is satisfied by drinking. Thus Bacon, Barry and Child (1965) suppose that drinking satisfies covert dependency needs, Horton (1943) that alcohol reduces subsistence anxiety, Knight (1937) that oral gratification is provided, and so on.

Since unfortunately none of these hypotheses received anything but ambiguous support from the folk-tale data, we were led to entertain a new theory of the positive impetus to drink: namely, that alcohol provides a magical means of supplying the drinker with an increased sense of his own potency. To review a bit, our evidence for this proposal centered around a group of tags—Hunt, Entering Implements, Eating, and Change of State—which correlated both with heavy drinking and with indices of low social solidarity (see Table 3.5). We suggested that these tags reflect a heightened concern with a primitive type of non-instrumental assertiveness both ego-enhancing to the actor and peculiarly promoted in those societies that leave the individual on his own in a situation where he is repeatedly forced to prove himself. It was our contention that drinking arouses just those feelings of assertiveness which satisfy such a need for potency.

In effect, then, our proposal adds a positive theory of heavy drinking to Field's theory of sobriety, for we argued that non-solidary societies not only fail to suppress drinking by instilling respect and inhibition, as Field claimed, but also promote a particularly strong need for the type of potent experience which alcohol provides.

To this point our proposal must be considered tentative at best. There remain a number of unanswered, or only partially answered, questions:

1. What evidence is there that drinking arouses feelings of potency?
2. How, in detail, do non-solidary societies foster a special need for potency?
3. And finally, can the folk-tale tags be unambiguously interpreted as indications of such a heightened concern for potent experience?

In large measure, the first of these questions cannot be conclusively answered by the folk-tale study. We have no direct measure of the thoughts and feelings of the various tribal members at drinking bouts. Thus the answer to this question will have to depend largely upon the evidence from subsequent chapters in this volume which show that in our culture at least, drinking does arouse fantasies of potency. Later in this chapter, however, we will investigate the type of behaviors which occur at tribal drinking bouts to see whether they are consistent with the feelings which we claim drinking arouses.

An answer to the second question was outlined in the previous chapter and will be continued here, but notice that both the first two questions are logically subsequent to the third. Unless we can use the folk-tale tags to define the need for potency unambiguously, there is little point in showing how such a need might be either engendered socially or satisfied by drinking. Here the problem is simply one of interpreting tags. We have claimed that the tags—Hunt, Entering Implements, Eating and Change of State—indicate a special type of concern for potency; but tags do not explain themselves and surely other interpretations are possible. A good deal of ink might be expended in justifying our particular interpretation, but unless the issue can be settled empirically there seems little point to such an argument. How can the interpretation of tags be made an empirical matter?

Words are simple to understand in context but notoriously difficult to analyze in isolation. This follows from the well-known but little-understood fact that most words are polysemic and that only the context of surrounding words serves to select the intended meaning. The noun *game* is ambiguous in isolation, but *a game* can only be something to play not something to hunt. Semantic meaning, then, is a matter of the covariation of a number of words in context, not of any single word in isolation. The same point can be made about psychological meaning. Words are not psychologically unique. A word which in one context is the center of pleasant anticipation may in another context be the focal point of some anxiety (the word *money* might be a reasonable example). And notice that there is little way to decide *a priori* upon the appropriate psychological interpretation of a word without looking first at those words with which it covaries in a given context.[1]

All this implies that if we want to support the interpretation that Hunt, Entering Implements, Eating, and Change of State indicate a concern with magical potency, we must show these tags to covary with other sets of tags which indicate a concern for power and a magical mode of implementing such concerns. Unmodified, this strategy would lead to an infinite regression; for how do we decide that these second order sets of tags indicate power and magic? By covariation with still another set of tags? If so, where do we stop?

To avoid such a regression it is necessary to invoke the notion of

---

[1]There are thorny problems involved in defining the notion of "context" adequately. For example, how long is a context? It is clear that if one supposes that semantically equivalent words will "covary in context," then it would not be advisable to choose contextual units as short as a single sentence. *Ham* and *eggs* may covary strongly within single sentence units, but they are not identical in meaning. On the other hand, *swimming pool* and *natatorium* are unlikely to covary in single sentence units, but they are synonomous. The proper length of a contextual unit for a covariance analysis of psychological meaning is simply not known, although one would suspect that it should be rather long. Our contextual unit is the entire folk-tale collection for each society. The average length of these collections is 8000 words.

theme. Although words may be ambiguous, they are not infinitely ambiguous, either semantically or psychologically. Context can only select among the various possible meanings of a given word. Furthermore, contextual selection is not arbitrary; it proceeds by rules which might be called thematic. To illustrate, suppose we know that the two ambiguous nouns *game* and *ball* covary in a given corpus. Knowledge of this covariation provides some purchase on the meaning of each ambiguous word; we can be fairly certain that the sort of "game" involved is a competitive activity, not a quarry, and that the type of "ball" involved in a globular object, not a social event. Similarly, if a group of tags which appear to indicate a concern with magical potency covaries with a group of tags which appear to reflect a concern for power, then we can have increased confidence that both of our interpretations are correct.

Of course, there is room for error in this procedure. To return to our previous example, suppose the correlation between *ball* and *game* was the result of a number of sentences in the corpus such as: "The game was so plentiful that our hunting trip was a ball." Such sentences would clearly invalidate the previous conclusion that "ball games" were being discussed; and the error would be due to a failure to anticipate the possibility that *ball* was being used metaphorically. The point is that covariation can suggest the correct interpretation of either individual words or tags only if the full range of possible meanings of these elements is correctly anticipated. Here the only recourse is to human judges who can assess logical or linguistic covariation rather than mere statistical correlation. That is, even though the covariation of certain tag clusters may support our interpretations of those clusters, we may want to use hand coding, in certain cases, to insure that a set of tags means what we think it does.

Given these ground rules of interpretation, we turn now to an attempt to find out whether there are in fact interpretable clusters of tags which covary with Hunt, Entering Implements, Eating and Change of State in a way which would support the claim that these tags reflect a concern with magical potency.

AN EMPIRICAL REDEFINITION OF MAGICAL POTENCY

The word *potency* has many common associations ranging from reproductive efficacy to the generalized ability to produce results. The core notion seems to be that of strength and power. In Chapter 5 of this volume, Winter shows that fantasy indicating a concern for power consists of images of vigorous expansive activity pronounced enough to arouse direct responses from others, thereby gratifying the ego and (possibly) establishing the basis of reputation. On the face of things, Hunt and Entering Implements appear to be heavily saturated with this sort of vigorous expansive action; but to certify this interpretation we will have to see whether these tags covary with others which also appear to tap this type of concern for power.

But what sorts of covariates would support our claim that drinking is associated only with a particularly magical type of power concern? What, after all does "magic" mean in this context? Originally, we suggested that Eating and Change of State appear to be magical in character, primarily because they represent transformations unsupported by instrumental activity. Instrumental activity, in turn, is traditionally considered an ego function critically dependent on the individual's ability to control impulses and delay gratification long enough to develop planned activity. This interpretation suggests that what we called magical potency refers essentially to an uninhibited way of satisfying power needs. Tags which truly reflect magical potency, therefore, should be negatively correlated with other tags which represent restraint, self-control, and inhibition.

In order to test these interpretive notions, we decided on a factor analysis of a set of tags, including a number which appeared to represent vigorous expansive action and a number which seemed to reflect restraint and inhibition.[2] Factor analysis provides an excellent means of displaying a large number of covariant relations simultaneously. As with most types of cluster analysis, however, factor analysis is sensitive to the domain of variables selected as input. Hence it is necessary to be clear about just how the input variables were chosen. As candidates for inhibition measures we selected just those tags, listed in Table 3.7 of the previous chapter, which had supported Field's hypothesis—that is, that attitudes of inhibition and restraint suppressed heavy drinking. To these we added all those tags which are most strongly associated with male-role text in the folk tales, either by virtue of appearing more frequently in sentences with male-role words than with female-role words or by virtue of being positively correlated with male pronouns and negatively correlated with female pronouns across the folk-tale collections.[3] We chose to limit the domain of the factor analysis in this manner because our measures of heavy drinking refer only to male drinking; thus we felt that those tags which indicate primarily mascu-

---

[2]The factor analytic model adopted was Hotelling's principal components solution as implemented by the *Data-Text* (1967) program for statistical analysis. In this version of principal components analysis the diagonal, elements of the correlation matrix are not replaced by communality estimates.

[3]Specifically, tags were considered masculine only if they were significantly more frequent in male-role text than in female-role text, as indicated by a *t* of at least 2.02, or if they bore a positive correlation with male pronouns of at least .29 and a negative correlation with female pronouns. See Table 4.1 for details.

line concerns in folk tales would be particularly relevant to the state of mind which motivates men to drink.

The masculine tags, together with their most frequent entry words and the measure of association with male text, are listed in Table 4.1. This table provides the first bit of evidence which forces a redefinition of magical potency. For, although Hunt, Eating, and Entering Implements are masculine tags, Change of State is not.[4] For whatever

Table 4.1—Alphabetical list of masculine tags (with most frequent entry words in each) and two measures of association with male text

TAG	Entry Words	t-test[a] (MRT-FRT)	CORRELATIONS[b] Male Pronouns	CORRELATIONS[b] Female Pronouns
Activity change (finish, now, then)		2.37*	.22	−.05
Capability (make, could, can)		3.23**	.20	−.16
Eating (eat, meat, fat, fruit, hunger)		2.99**	.10	.00
Entering implements (arrow, knife, spear)		3.77**	.01	−.04
Having (get, reach, hold, own, have { a, an, any })		−.82	.32*	−.16
Hunt (hunt, hunter)		2.49*	.28	−.05
Oral body parts (mouth, stomach, tongue)		5.87**	.16	−.10
Scheduling (time, after, before, next)		2.87**	.11	−.07
Vigorous activity (run, climb, jump, roll)		1.34	.37*	−.23
Violent physical manipulation (throw, cut, hit)		3.18**	.04	−.07
Want (want, wish, need)		−1.60	.33*	−.18
War (shoot, fight, war)		3.08**	.12	−.06

*$p < .05$ (two-tailed).
**$p < .01$ (two-tailed).
[a]The $t =$ test assesses the differences between the relative frequencies of a given tag in sentences which contain masculine gender words (MRT = male role text) and sentences which contain feminine gender words (FRT = female role text) against the null hypothesis that such differences are zero.
[b]The correlations assess the strength of association between the relative frequencies of each tag and the relative frequencies of pronouns of each gender across the 44 folk-tale collections.

reason Change of State is related to drinking, it is not through any mental state which is peculiarly masculine. Notice also that by no means can all of the masculine tags be interpreted as reflecting power concerns. Thus by putting these tags together in a factor analysis with the inhibition tags, we are trying to find out first whether the magical potency group, or something similar, hangs together as a cluster and second, whether the interpretation of this cluster is supported by positive covariation with a power cluster and negative covariation with an inhibition cluster. Nothing about the way we chose the tags which compose the domain of the factor analysis would necessitate this result.

[4]If anything, Change of State is more a feminine than a masculine tag, although the association is not a strong one: t(MRT-FRT) $= -1.22$; $r = -.06$ with *pronoun male* and .14 with *pronoun female*.

Figure 4.1 displays the first two factors mapped by the principal components of a factor analysis. Together these two factors account for about 44 per cent of the variance common to the input tags. None of the other factors accounts for more than 14 per cent of the communality. Just surveying the clusters for the moment, notice that the tags which we had supposed to indicate magical potency do not constitute a group. Eating and Entering Implements covary, both having high negative loadings on Factor I; but the third member of this cluster

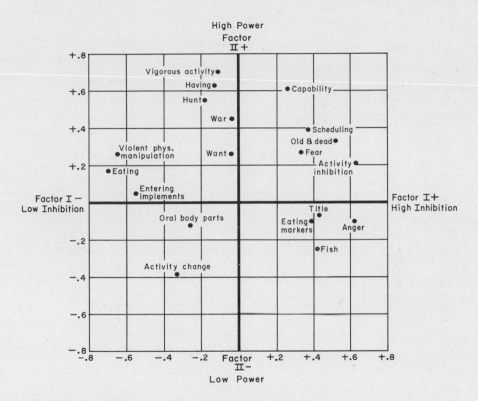

Figure 4.1   Principal components Factors I and II.

is Violent Physical Manipulation, not Hunt. The substantive changes in the magical potency tag group are now three in number: Change of State and Hunt have been lost; Violent Physical Manipulation has been added. Perhaps the theoretical interpretation of this cluster should also be modified. Subjectively, the entry words in Violent Physical Manipulation and Entering Implements (see Table 4.1) suggest aggressive activity which is both vigorous and dramatic and hence related to the kind of self-enhancing power concerns that Winter (Chapter 5) has defined. *Eating* may also be primitive way of enhancing the self, of feeling more substantial. At the same time all these tags have an immediate impulsive character although the loss of Change of State makes their magical quality less evident. On these subjective grounds we will tentatively rename this cluster "impulsive power"; but this name can stick only if this new group of tags covaries positively with a power group and negatively with an inhibition group.

Generally, the inhibition tags load positively on Factor I, but the only high and pure loadings are by Anger and Title. Title may

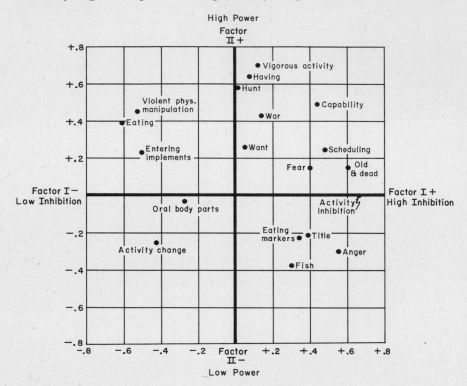

Figure 4.2 Fixed rotation factor analysis: Factor I = Activity Inhibition; Factor II = Power.

reflect the hierarchically arranged social structure which fosters attitudes of respect, and Anger may tap the frustration attendant upon inhibited activity; but neither of these tags appears to provide the clear measure of inhibition we require. To rectify this situation, we decided to rotate the factor axes about 20° counter-clockwise so that Factor I would pass directly through Activity Inhibition. The results of this rotation are displayed in Figure 4.2. Notice first that although the two factors are in a new position with respect to the component variables, the positions of the variables *vis à vis* one another are unchanged.

This fact indicates that rotation is simply a new way of describing the same facts about covariation.

The highest and purest positive loadings on Factor I are now contributed by Activity Inhibition, Old and Dead, and Fear. What sort of inhibition might these tags measure? Taken together, the 17 entry words in these three tags occur some 4700 times in the folk tales. Not surprisingly the single word "not" supplies almost half of this total. To find out how "not" was being used in the folk tales, we hand-coded about 750 sentences in which it occurred.[5] In about 400 of these sentences "not" was used to negate action. Half of the time this inhibition of action was internal ("he would not fight"); in the other half it was external ("he must not fight"). Another 100 sentences displayed cognitive or emotional inhibition ("he did not believe"; "he did not hate her"). A final 200 sentences were irrelevant to inhibition ("it was not there"). Although there is clearly some slippage, the general picture which emerges from the "not" sentences is of controlled activity and guarded beliefs and emotions. These notions are reinforced by the fact that Fear (entry words—afraid, fear, fright) covaries with Activity Inhibition; for fear often involves negative anticipations concerning the consequences of action. And, as noted in the previous chapter, the final covariant in this group, Old and Dead, refers to two powerful inhibitors of human action.

Now notice that the new impulsive power cluster—Violent Physical Manipulation, Eating and Entering Implements—loads negatively on the Inhibition Factor (I). These strong negative loadings (all between −.50 and −.62) provide the first positive empirical support for our assumption that these tags indicate a particular non-instrumental, uninhibited and hence impulsive style. To put it another way, we can now argue that Violent Physical Manipulation, Entering Implements, and Eating reflect an impulsive type of fantasy not only because these tags appear to do so on the face of things but also because they covary negatively with tags which indicate the opposite of impulsivity: namely, inhibition and control.

The same sort of evidence can be provided for our assumption that the impulsive power cluster reflects a concern with the kind of vigorous expansive activity characteristic of power fantasy. Notice, in Figure 4.2 that the impulsive power tags all load on Factor II as well as on Factor I. The highest and purest loadings on Factor II are contributed by the tags Vigorous Activity, Having, Hunt, and War. Consideration of the entry words in these tags suggested to us that this factor might be tapping just the sorts of power imagery that Winter (Chapter 5) describes: "Run," "climb," "jump," "roll," "shoot,"

[5]These sentences were retrieved by the *Key Word in Context* program described in the previous chapter.

"fight," "get," "reach," and "hunt" all suggest vigorous expansive action; "hold," "own," and "have (a, an, any)" may indicate a concern for repuation; and "war" is certainly a way of having impact on others. To check these suspicions, we selected all the folk tales from the five societies which had the highest factor scores on Factor II and from the five societies which had the lowest factor scores on Factor II. This procedure yielded a sample of 60 folk tales. Each of these was then scored by hand for purified Winter *n* Power imagery (i.e., eliminating power images having to do with sex and aggression)[6] and by the "General Inquirer" retrieval program (see Chapter 3 and Stone *et al.*, 1966) for the collective relative frequency of the tags, Vigorous Activity, Having, Hunt, and War. A comparison of these scores shows that these proposed power tags measure much the same thing as purified Winter *n* Power imagery. Twenty (or 69 per cent) of the 29 tales where Winter *n* Power imagery is present are above the median on the relative frequency of the power tags as opposed to only 10 (or 32 per cent) above the median in the 31 tales where Winter *n* Power imagery is absent. The resulting two-way contingency table yields a χ^2 of 8.08, $p < .01$.[7]

This result allows us to have some confidence that Factor II is indeed a power factor. And, to the extent that Violent Physical Manipulation, Eating, and Entering Implements load on Factor II (from .23 to .46), we have empirical justification for claiming that this cluster taps power-related concerns. Thus the label "impulsive power" sticks, and it sticks for empirical reasons.

[6]Winter (Chapter 5) scores power imagery if vigorous expansive action, concern for reputation, or the arousal of emotions in others is evident in the text under consideration. Both sexual and aggressive imagery may fall into any of these three categories. But we have found elsewhere (Chapter 1) that aggressive themes and sexual themes are related to drinking. It is our contention that the type of sex and aggression related to drinking is power-related. To show this, we need a measure of *n* Power which is not confounded with sex or aggression. Such a measure is provided by eliminating sex and aggression from Winter's power imagery categories. Similarly, in the folk tales the "impulsive power" tags are heavily saturated with aggressive words. To show that these tags are power related, we clearly need a measure of power which is not contaminated by aggression. Thus we compared the proposed power tags—Vigorous Activity, Having, Hunt and War—with purified Winter power imagery from which aggressive themes have been eliminated. All hand scoring of purified Winter power imagery was of course blindly, without knowledge of the relative frequencies of the proposed power tags in the 60 tales under consideration.

[7]Thirty per cent error may seem exceedingly large for two variables which purport to measure the same thing. This error must be judged, however, within the context of previous attempts to design *General Inquirer* dictionaries which approximated a hand code. Error of about 20 per cent has been reported for the *n* Achievement dictionary (personal communication, D. Ogilvie) and about 30 per cent for the *n* Affiliation dictionary (personal communication, J. Williamson). The fact that our proposed power tags converge upon a hand code for *n* Power at a level of accuracy comparable to the *n* Ach and *n* Aff dictionaries (described in Stone *et al.*, 1966) is remarkable considering that these dictionaries were built specifically to capture a hand code and our proposed power tags were arrived at inductively.

POWER AND SEX DIFFERENCES

There is further evidence that Factor II is measuring just the sort of self-enhancing power that we have described, although this evidence is of a less formal and more suggestive nature than that provided in the previous section. We noticed in the fixed rotation of Figure 4.2 that very few tags had negative loadings on Factor II; if Factor II was indeed a power factor, we had few if any tags which characterized a lack of concern with power. It occurred to us that this result might be due to our decision to exclude tags associated with female-role text from our factor analysis. That is, if power is defined as vigorous expansive activity which is self-assertive and self-gratifying, then perhaps female orientations which are known to be less self-assertive and more nurturant, (Zelditch, 1955; Osgood, 1964; and Whiting, 1966) would be negatively associated with any factor which is presumed to measure

Table 4.2—Relationship of feminine tags to Power Factor II

Tag (Entry Words)	t-test[a] (PMR-PFR)	CORRELATIONS[b] Male Pronouns	Female Pronouns	FACTOR LOADINGS Factor I	Factor II
Child (children, baby, grandchild[ren])	−5.50**	−.26	.40*	−.223	−.335
Domestic (basket, cloth(es, ing), loom)	−3.64**	−.15	.21	−.009	−.279
Feminine adjective (beautiful, lovely)	−3.63**	−.42**	.12	.287	−.378
First order generation (mother, father, son, daughter)	−4.21**	−.10	.50**	−.064	−.460
Sorrow (cry, weep, sorr[ow, y])	−2.04*	−.26	.38*	−.191	−.390

**p < .01 (two-tailed).
*p < .05 (two-tailed).
[a]See note (a) of Table 4.1.
[b]See note (b) of Table 4.1.

power. To check this hunch we determined, by the same tests we used to define the masculine tags of Table 4.1, which of our folk-tale tags were peculiarly feminine. We then added these tags to the original set that had been factor-analysed, performed a new principal components analysis, and again rotated the first factor through Activity Inhibition. This procedure provided an analysis similar to Figure 4.2, although the plane of the first two factors is slightly altered due to the addition of the new tags. The factor loadings of each of the five feminine tags are presented here along with their measures of association with female text.

Notice first that the content of the feminine tags provides a rough corroboration of previous descriptions of female concerns. The common denominator of the entry words shown above appears to be a concern for others, particularly the young (Child) and the immediate family (First Order Generation, Domestic). Sorrow might indicate a non-assertive emotional response to frustration, although it seems at least as likely that this is an emotion which again proceeds from a concern for the well-being of others. Such a concern for others should be the theoretical opposite of the vigorous, self-assertive activity that we have defined as indicating a need for power; and in fact the negative loadings which the feminine tags have on Factor II demonstrate that this opposition holds empirically as well as theoretically. On the one hand, this result lends weight to our original assumption that Vigorous Activity, Hunt, Having, and War are measuring power concerns; and on the other, it enhances our subjective definition of power by showing that it is an essentially masculine striving.

POWER, INHIBITION, AND HEAVY DRINKING

Recall from the previous chapter that if the folk tales from a given society are high in magical potency themes, that society tends to drink heavily. The correlations of Hunt, Entering Implements, Eating and Change of State with the Combined Drinking score are all between .35 and .38. If the index scores of new impulsive power tags—Violent Physical Manipulation, Eating, and Entering Implements—are standardized and summed, the resulting Impulsive Power Scale correlates .38, $p \leq .05$, with combined drinking. Thus by empirically redefining magical potency as impulsive power, we have clarified interpretive issues without losing any predictive power.

To interpret this new correlation, it would seem that societies which are high on the Impulsive Power Scale tend to drink heavily just because drinking provides an immediate or impulsive way of feeling powerful, of feeling that one is vigorous and can have impact upon others. Table 4.3 provides some corroborating evidence that the members of societies which drink heavily and which are high on the Impulsive Power Scale, do *act* vigorously and do *attempt* to have impact upon others when they are drinking. The measures of drinking-bout behavior are taken from Bacon, Barry, Child and Snyder (1965). Intensity of Exhibitionistic Behavior reaches a maximum at the occurrence of "flagrant boasting and chest thumping, going to absurd lengths to gain attention. . . ." Change in Exhibitionistic Behavior is a measure of the increase in exhibitionism from the dry to the wet state. Extreme Hostility is scored when physical combat occurs; and

Table 4.3—A syndrome of drinking behaviors associated with heavy drinking and impulsive power in folk tales

	Combined Drinking Score		Impulsive Power		Intensity of Exh. Beh.		Change in Exh. Beh.		Occurrence of Hostility	
	r	n	r	n	r	n	r	n	r	n
Impulsive power scale	.38*	44	—							
Syndrome of drinking behaviors:[a]										
Intensity of exhibitionistic behavior	.52*	24	.54	12	—					
Change in exhibitionistic behavior	.57*	20	.47	9	.73**	20	—			
Occurrence of extreme hostility	.42*	41	.44*	28	.36	17	.16	15	—	
Boisterousness	.60**	57	.16	28	.62**	23	.55**	19	.60**	40

*p ≤ .05 (2-tailed).   **p ≤ .01 (2-tailed).

[a]These ratings are explained in the text, but for detailed definitions see Bacon, Barry, Child, and Snyder (1965).

Boisterousness is simply a measure of noise level. Taken together, these intercorrelated behavior ratings portray a loud, self-assertive, often aggressive display. Although the samples supporting several of the correlations in Table 4.3 are small, and although it may be perilous to infer psychological states from overt behavior, this evidence suggests that drinking does provide an immediate means of gratifying the need to feel powerful. At the very least, this drinking-bout behavior looks more like the impulsive satisfaction of power needs than like the reduction of subsistence anxiety (Horton, 1943) or the gratification of dependency needs (Bacon, Barry, and Child, 1965).

Does this mean that any society whose folk tales indicate a high need for power will drink heavily? Apparently not, for when we summed the standardized scores of the tags which provided the highest and purest loadings on the power factor (II)—Vigorous Activity, Having, Hunt, and War—the resulting Power Scale correlated only .06 with Combined Drinking. It seems that only impulsive or uninhibited types of power concerns lead to drinking. Furthermore, when we constructed an Inhibition Scale in the usual way from Activity Inhibition, Old and Dead, and Fear, the result was a negative correlation with Combined Drinking: $r = -.55$, $p \le .01$. These facts led us to suspect that it might be most informative to consider the motives underlying heavy drinking as a joint function of inhibition and the need for power.

To investigate this notion, we divided both scales at the median to provide two dichotomous classificatory variables. The resulting three-way contingency tables are presented in Table 4.4. Notice first that where Power is high, Inhibition is an excellent predictor of light drinking (Table 4.4A). This is not the case where power imagery is infrequent (Table 4.4B): there is a tendency for high Inhibition to predict light drinking, but this tendency does not reach acceptable levels of significance. Due to the small samples involved, and hence to the reduced power of these tests, we must interpret this result carefully. We cannot say that there is a significant interaction between Power and Inhibition, or that Inhibition predicts drinking only when power is frequent. We can say that in our sample at least, the prediction of Inhibition on drinking is enhanced where Power is high.

As summary Table 4.4C indicates, these results imply that while societies which are high in Power but low in Inhibition tend to drink most heavily, societies high in Power and high in Inhibition are most likely to avoid heavy drinking. It is not surprising that 80 per cent of the societies high in Power and low in Inhibition drink heavily, for these are just the societies whose folk tales exhibit the most frequent Impulsive Power (recall that impulsive power tags covary positively with Power and negatively with Inhibition). But why do high-Power,

Table 4.4—Combined drinking as a joint function of Power and Inhibition

A. For those societies above the median on the Power Scale

		Inhibition			
		Lo	Hi		
Combined	Lo	2	10	12	
drinking	Hi	8	2	10	Fisher's except $p = .005$
		10	12	22	

B. For those societies below the median on the Power scale

		Inhibition			
		Lo	Hi		
Combined	Lo	5	7	12	
drinking	Hi	7	3	10	Fisher's exact $p = .185$
		12	10	22	

C. Summary Table: Relative frequency societies with High combined drinking scores under four possible combinations of Power and Inhibition levels.

		Inhibition	
		Lo	Hi
		2	1
	Hi	%hiCD = 80	%hiCD = 16.7
		$n = 10$	$n = 12$
Power			
		3	4
	Lo	%hiCD = 58.3	%hiCD = 30
		$n = 12$	$n = 10$

high-Inhibition societies tend to be such light drinkers (only 16.7 per cent above the median drinking score)? Again the tags which covary with this condition may provide an answer.

Consider Table 4.5, in which, for convenience, the tags are arranged according to the quadrants determined by the fixed rotation factor analysis of Figure 4.2. These quadrants correspond to the cells of Table 4.4C in the obvious way. The tags which fall into quadrant 1, where both Power and Inhibition are high, are Capability and Scheduling. Capability is largely composed of the entry words "make," "could," "can." What is suggested is real ability and effective action. Scheduling (entry words, "time," "after," "before," "next") indicates just how this action is effective: namely, by ordering, arranging, and planning. These words clearly suggest power concerns; certainly effective action is a way of having impact upon others, of actually being strong. But notice that this Effective Power depends crucially on planning and self-control. Conceivably, then, these societies avoid alcohol just because it erodes their controlled abilities to be powerful. This would explain the negligible correlations between the Power Scale and drinking; for while the uninhibited gratify their need to

Table 4.5—Factor loadings from the Fixed Rotation Factor Analysis—arranged by Factor and Quadrant

Cluster	Tag	LOADINGS	
		Factor I (Inhibition)	Factor II (Power)
Defining tags for *Inhibition* factor (I)			
	Activity Inhibition	.659	.000
	Old and Dead	.599	.147
	Fear	.401	.149
Defining tags for *Power* factor (II)			
	Vigorous Activity	.113	.702
	Having	.072	.638
	Hunt	.001	.587
	War	.141	.428
Quadrant 1—*Effective power*			
	Capability	.438	.492
	Scheduling	.478	.255
Quadrant 2—*Impulsive power*			
	Eating	−.612	.396
	Violent physical manip.	−.532	.455
	Entering Implements	−.504	.226
Quadrant 3—*Low inhibition and low power*			
	Activity change	−.433	−.253
Quadrant 4—*Conventional*			
	Anger	.553	−.301
	Fish	.304	−.373
	Title	.387	−.203
	Eating markers	.344	−.221

feel powerful by drinking, the self-controlled avoid what might disturb their ability to *be* powerful.

If this explanation is correct, then both power concerns and inhibitions work together to influence drinking behavior. Certainly Field's (1962) single factor theory of formal restraint still does a good deal of explanatory work; for even where Power is low, inhibited types are less likely to drink heavily (30 per cent above median drinking score) than the uninhibited types (58.3 per cent above). The tags which fall into quadrant 4 characterize the low-Power, high-Inhibition group in a way that might be called Conventional: they respect authority and regulation (*title, eating markers*); they do not act assertively (*fish*) and perhaps show some frustration as a result (*anger*). It may be that these Conventional types drink less than the low-Power, low-Inhibition group (characterized only by Activity change in quadrant 3) because they are both more secure and better socialized.

Apparently, then inhibitions do have a pervasive influence on the use of alcohol, but we have shown that the best predictions of drinking behavior are to be found where a marked concern for power is manifest in folk-tale content. Thus we now turn to an examination of how this concern for self-gratifying impact upon others may mediate the known associations between certain types of social situations and drinking.

POWER, ALCOHOL, AND THE SOCIAL ENVIRONMENT

Recall that at the outset of this chapter we argued with Field about just how the social environment promotes heavy drinking. He claims that heavy drinking in non-solidary societies is the exclusive result of the failure to instill attitudes of respect and inhibition. We added that heavy-drinking societies may also instill a particularly strong need to feel powerful, a need which is satisfied by drinking. To this point we have shown, on evidence which is internal to the folk tales, that the heaviest drinking occurs where fantasy exhibits both impulsivity and a need for power. What sorts of societies promote these states of mind which lead to heavy drinking?

To secure measures of the social characteristics related to drinking, we worked with our sample of 182 societies drawn from Murdock's (1960–64) *Ethnographic Atlas* in a way designed to maximize geographical representativeness, cultural independence, and the number of observations for each of the 168 variables which we thought might have some bearing upon drinking behavior.[8] After examining the correlations between these variables and drinking behavior, we selected 25 variables each of which correlated significantly with the Combined Drinking Score and provided at least 100 observations. Finally, we re-examined the coding schemes of these variables, combining some and altering others in order to provide clear ordinal scales of measurement wherever possible.[9] This procedure left 18 variables which were then factor analyzed by the principal components method. Two factors which accounted for 51 per cent of the common variance were extracted and rotated by the varimax criterion.[10] No other factor accounted for more than 12 per cent of the common variance. The 14 variables

[8]This procedure, partially described in Chapter 3, was worked out by Kalin as follows:
1. A pool of societies which had been rated on variables of interest was selected.
2. To maximize cultural representativeness and independence, no two societies in the same geographical sub-area were chosen unless they were of different cultural types as defined by Murdock (1960–64) or (if no rating of cultural type was available) unless they belonged to different linguistic groups. Exceptions to these procedures were as follows: Ifaluk (If)-Ulithi (If); Carib (Sc3)-Taulipang (Sc15); Balinese (Ib3)-Dusun (Ib5); Aranda (Id1)-Murngin (Id2); Arapesh (Ie3)-Kapanku (Ie1)-Keraki (Ie5)-Kwoma (Ie12): Kurtachi (Ig3)-Lesu (Ig4); Pukapuka (Ii3)-Tikopia (Ii2).
3. To maximize the number of rated cases per variable, those societies within a given cultural type or linguistic group were chosen which has the highest number of rated variables.

[9]Much of this work was accomplished by Mr. Robert Haber.

[10]The varimax criterion provides an orthogonal rotation which approximates simple structure by means of maximizing the variance of the squared factor loadings by column.

which had high and pure loadings on either of the first two factors are presented in Table 4.6. Detailed descriptions of their codes and sources are provided in Appendix VIII.

Our use of factor analysis in this situation is somewhat different from what it was when we were dealing with folk-tale tags. There we were trying to find covarying clusters which would empirically motivate the definition of certain tags; here we are simply trying to locate syndromes of social characteristics which *may* go together to predict drinking. The justification for this procedure runs as follows: any single variable (X) which correlates with drinking may be a valid causal variable, or its relation to drinking may be the spurious result of a third (or fourth, etc.) variable which causes both drinking and X. The only sure way to decide the issue is to re-examine the association of X and drinking with the third (and fourth, etc.) variable partialled

Table 4.6—Social characteristics and practices which predict drinking

	Correlation with Combined Drinking Score		Factor Loadings from Varimax Rotation	
	r	*n*	*I*	*II*
1. Variables loading primarily on Factor I (Socio-economic simplicity scale)				
Degree of Dependence on Hunting	.29**	76	.734	−.208
Open class system	.21*	71	.535	.040
Low degree of Jurisdictional hierarchy	.19	70	.717	.069
Impermanence of settlement pattern	.26**	71	.769	.101
Small size of local community	.26**	58	.740	−.098
Degree of dependence on agriculture	−.26**	76	−.822	.212
2. Variables loading primarily on Factor II (Male institutions scale)				
Presence of male initiation	−.30**	52	.062	.660
Clear initiation impact	−.50***	46	−.030	.687
Strong male solidarity	−.34**	49	−.065	.435
Long post-partum sex taboos	−.36**	50	−.213	.506
Exclusive mother-baby sleeping arrangements	−.24*	48	.135	.510
Large sleeping distance of mother and father (monogamous position)	−.31**	46	−.169	.551
Warm winter temperature	−.43***	54	−.230	.673
Wet climate	−.45***	46	.131	.447

***$p \leq .01$ (two-tailed).
 **$p \leq .05$ (two-tailed).
  *$p \leq .10$ (two-tailed).
   a The following variables were included in the factor analysis but did not load above .390 on either factor: Unilineal descent, Male participation in subsistence, Bride service, Sleeping distance: mother-father (polygynous position).

out or controlled. However, our sample is limited by the 76 societies for which we have drinking ratings. As with most cross-cultural samples, it is simply too small to provide a conclusive test of any association with all other possible confounding variables controlled. It is in this bind that we have used factor analysis as a compromise; for it allows us to locate covarying sets of social characteristics which are associated with drinking. The variables within such syndromes may be causally related to each other, and any one or all of them may be causally related to drinking. Although we cannot always decide these issues, we can speculate about the common effects which such covarying social characteristics may have on individual experience. And note that such speculations are now founded upon the broad base of several variables, rather than upon a single variable whose association with drinking may be spurious.

To see how this works in practice, let us consider the six variables which have high and pure loadings on Factor I. First, it seems quite likely that there are causal relationships holding this cluster together. Thus the development of a fixed, agricultural source of food would seem to be a necessary prerequisite for the emergence of a large, permanent, non-migratory settlement in which the accumulation of a real property can provide a basis for social distinctions of class and a need for fairly complex political jurisdiction. It is not surprising then that we find Degree of dependence on hunting grouped with several indices of social and economic simplicity at the positive pole of Factor I, while Degree of dependence on agriculture has a strong negative loading. Furthermore, the correlations of each of these variables with drinking (reported in Table 4.6) show that it is just the small, migratory, open-class, politically simple, hunting societies which drink heavily.

Facts such as these have been known for some time now, but their interpretation has been a matter of dispute. Horton (1943), as noted in the previous chapter, supposed that the hunters had a less stable source of food than the agriculturalists and that this accounted for all the variance with respect to heavy drinking. Recently, however, Lee (1966) has shown that, on the contrary, so-called hunting societies are not as economically precarious as had been supposed. Their stability is not due to any plentitude of the game sought by men, however, but to the reliable abundance of the vegetable foods gathered by women. Among the Kung Bushman, for example, meat provided by the men is the most highly valued food; but meat accounts for only about 25 per cent of the group's total diet. The reason for this is not hard to find. As Lee has estimated, the probability, on any given day, that a man will return with a kill is about once chance in four. On the other hand a woman's chances of finding vegetable food are close to perfect. Thus hunting societies are buffered against Horton's "subsistence insecurity" by the gathering activities of women. Hunting is still a high risk, low probability venture, but as Lee (p. 6) puts it, "failure in the hunt . . . does not result in deprivation . . . at least not nutritional deprivation." The clear suggestion here is that what the failing hunter is deprived of is status or prestige. Thus Horton's "subsistence insecurity" might well be translated as "status insecurity". The male hunter must take risks to seek the most culturally valued food, meat. Success will certainly provide attention and congratulation, but the odds against him are roughly three to one.

Other aspects of the hunter's situation also have a high-risk, low-probability character. He lives in an open-class system where every individual begins even and must succeed on his own ability. Political hierarchies are simple or nonexistent, so that even if he has ability, it cannot be consolidated into any institutionalized position of wealth or authority. In a sense, a man in such a society must continually reassert himself to maintain a reputation. He is known only by what he can *do*; and he cannot translate his momentary successes into a position of prestige where he might be known simply by who he is.

If these speculations are correct, then societies which are high on Factor I should contain just those individuals who are most deprived of the means of having a lasting impact upon others and who are therefore most concerned with the kind of immediate feelings of self-assertive impact which heavy drinking may provide. To test this proposition we standardized, appropriately weighted (+ or −), and averaged the six variables of Factor I to produce a Socio-Economic Simplicity Scale. As the resulting correlations of Table 4.7 show, the folk-tales from highly simple societies do manifest a strong concern for Power, and particularly the type of Impulsive Power most directly related to heavy drinking. It appears then that individuals who are required by their society to be continually assertive and successful but who are also prevented from gaining permanent prestige, turn to drink as an immediate means of gaining momentary feelings of power.

If this is so, then societies which do not require continual individual assertiveness and which do provide mechanisms through which lasting position can be gained should not be so concerned with finding temporary feelings of impact through alcohol. In this connection, consider the social variables in Table 4.6 which load primarily on Factor II. These eight variables contain indices of male initiation, adult male groups, mother-child families, and a hot, wet climate. Again the covariation among these variables is both well known and a matter of some dispute. Whiting (1964; Burton and Whiting, 1961) has proposed causal links running from hot, wet climates to mother-child sleeping arrangements and polygynously supported, long post-partum sex taboos which are assumed to lead to cross-sex identity in

Table 4.7—Social variables and folk-tale themes related to heavy drinking

	Drinking		Socio-Economic Simplicity Scale		Male Institutions Scale		Power Scale		Inhibition Scale		Impulsive Power		Instrumental Dependence in Adulthood	
	r	n	r	n	r	n	r	n	r	n	r	n	r	n
A. Social syndromes														
Socio-economic simplicity scale	.31***	76	—											
Male institutions scale	−.52***	72	−.30***	175	—									
B. Folk-tale themes														
Power scale	.06	44	.41***	44	−.17	40	—							
Inhibition scale	−.55***	44	−.24	44	.10	40	.18	44	—					
Impulsive power	.38**	44	.32**	44	−.23	40	.22	44	−.32**	44	—			
Conventionality	−.51***	44	−.37**	44	.42***	40	−.33**	44	.47***	44	−.34**	44		
C. Selected behavioral variables														
Instrumental dependence in adulthood[a]	−.41***	39	−.31**	50	.39**	48	−.29	26	.06	26	−.60***	26	—	
Use of dreams[b]	.39*	28	.50***	47	−.25*	47	.44	19	−.51**	19	.54**	19	−.08	19

***p ≤ .01 (two-tailed).   **p ≤ .05 (two-tailed).   *p ≤ .10 (two-tailed).

[a] Rating due to Bacon, Barry, and Child (1965).
[b] Rating due to D'Andrade (1961).

the male child and hence to therapeutic initiation procedures and male solidatiry. Young (1962) has argued that causation runs in the reverse direction: collective action by adult males requires group organization which in turn necessitates both elaborate induction procedures for adolescent males and the supportive work of many polygynous women. Although we have no new evidence which would decide these issues, we are less interested in the causal arguments which divide Whiting and Young than in the descriptive points upon which they agree. Thus, both affirm that adult male groups provide cohesive, self-conscious in-groups to which each of its members owe loyalty. Apparently, then, societies with such institutions do provide members with institutional means of gaining lasting positions in the eyes of others. Such groups also require that the individual limit his own self-assertiveness in the interest of group cohesion. As both Young and Whiting emphasize initiation procedures are a dramatic way of asserting collective authority over the initiate. The initiate has new duties as well as new privileges.

If these assumptions are correct, we should expect societies which have such male institutions to be less concerned with self-assertive impact upon others because such institutions both inhibit self-assertiveness and provide an institutionalized means of gaining prestige. Table 4.7 shows that when the variable loading primarily on Factor II are converted into a Male Institutions Scale in the usual way, societies high on this scale drink little and show small concern with Power or Impulsive Power. Their folk tales are characterized primarily by themes of Conventionality, and we recall that such themes indicate a respect for authority and regulation which covaries positively with Inhibition and negatively with Power.

It would appear then that adult male groups plus their attendant initiation procedures reduce heavy drinking by fostering self-control and by providing institutional means of consolidating prestige. The Male Institutions Scale must be interpreted cautiously, however, because, as previously noted, it contains indices of mother-child families and a hot, wet climate as well as indices of solidary male groups. Either of these factors might influence drinking behavior independently of male solidarity. Thus, for example, in mother-child families the father tends to be relatively remote from the young child; and there is some evidence that the need for impact on others is a predominantly masculine striving (see Winter, 1967 and the section on power and sex differences in this chapter). If so, then the child whose father is relatively distant may simply lack the opportunity to incorporate such a concern with power at an early age. It is difficult to make a comparable case for climate, for its is unclear how climate could have any direct influence upon either power concerns or inhibition. Nevertheless such effects might operate through totally independent channels: body temperature, storage and spoilage factors are all possibilities.

To disentangle these issues, we divided the Male Institution Scale into three subscales: one which included only indices of Male Groups (presence of male initiation plus clear initiation impact plus strong male solidarity); one which indicated Wet Hot Climate (warm winter temperature plus wet climate); and one which provided an indication of Father Distance (long post-partum sex taboo, exclusive mother-baby sleeping arrangements, and large mother-father sleeping distance). Each scale was divided at the median, and the relationship of each scale to drinking was examined with each of the other scales controlled. The six resulting three-way contingency tables are summarized in Table 4.8.

Notice first that at every level of Male Groups and Father Distance, societies in wet, hot climates are less frequently above the median drinking score than societies in dry, cold climates. Climate does indeed have an independent effect upon alcohol consumption, a fact which raises the possibility that the scale we have named Male Institutions is actually related to drinking only through the effect of climate. This does not appear to be the case, however; for within each of the levels of climate, those societies with strong male groups tend to use alcohol less heavily than those societies without such institutions. Father Distance, on the other hand, appears to have little if any independent effect upon drinking within the levels of either Climate or Male Groups. Thus the notion that drinking behavior depends upon some subtle transfer of power concerns between a father and his young son receives no support. In fact these data suggest that the crucial experiences with respect to drinking occur later in life when the adolescent learns to take his place in a regulated adult male community.

To summarize, the composite picture of the social situation which leads to Impulsive Power and heavy drinking is that of a society with two contradictory demands; it both requires its individuals to be assertive, and frustrates that assertiveness by failing to provide mechanisms for consolidating assertive behavior into permanent prestige. Sober societies, on the other hand, require more self-control of the individual and provide means by which personal position can be consolidated. The apparent result is a less power-oriented, more inhibited, Conventional state of mind, and consequently less use of alcohol. This picture is reinforced somewhat by the correlations between the "selected behavioral variables" of Table 4.6 and the two major social scales. For notice that highly simple societies tend to be low in Instrumental Dependence and high in the Use of Dreams. Thus individuals in such societies must not only assert themselves but also make such assertions without support from others. The odds against

Table 4.8—Relationship between three components of the Male Institution Scale and the Combined Drinking Score

Controlled Variable	Level (number) of societies at indicated level)	Independent Variable	Level (number of societies at indicated level)	Percentage of Societies Above Median Combined Drinking Score	P = level[a]
Male groups	Strong (21)				
		Climate	Wet hot (12)	8.3	
			Dry cold (9)	44.4	
Male groups	Weak (31)				
		Climate	Wet hot (14)	28.6	
			Dry cold (13)	76.5	$p < .02$
Father distance	Distant (27)				
		Climate	Wet hot (15)	6.7	
			Dry cold (12)	66.7	
Father distance	Close (27)				
		Climate	Wet hot (11)	36.4	
			Dry cold (16)	68.7	$p < .01$
Climate	Wet hot (26)				
		Male groups	Strong (12)	8.3	
			Weak (14)	28.6	
Climate	Dry cold (26)				
		Male groups	Strong (9)	44.4	
			Weak (17)	76.5	$p < .14$
Father distance	Distant (29)				
		Male groups	Strong (17)	23.5	
			Weak (12)	41.7	
Father distance	Close (27)				
		Male groups	Strong (6)	16.7	
			Weak (21)	61.9	$p < .10$
Male groups	Strong (23)				
		Father distance	Distant (17)	23.5	
			Close (6)	16.7	
Male groups	Weak (33)				
		Father distance	Distant (12)	41.7	
			Close (21)	61.9	$p < .50$
Climate	Wet hot (26)				
		Father distance	Distant (15)	6.7	
			Close (11)	36.4	
Climate	Dry cold (28)				
		Father distance	Distant (12)	66.7	
			Close (16)	68.7	$p < .20$

[a]The probability levels reported here each refer to a pair of tables which exhibit the relationship between drinking and some independent variable across both levels of the controlled variable. These probabilities were computed by determining the p-level for each table individually (most often by Fisher's method), finding the corresponding chi-square values and summing. The probability of the resulting χ^2 was evaluated with two degrees of freedom.

success in such ventures may well lead to the use of dreams as a means of gaining prominence and the use of alcohol to gain feelings of prominence. Low-drinking societies, on the other hand, have social means of promoting loyalty and cooperation. Societies high on the Male Institutions Scale do tend to aid one another instrumentally. The results of such loyalty and cooperation seem to be a reduced concern with self-assertive, impulsive power and, consequently, little use of alcohol.

In our sample, these two types of social situations tend to be negatively correlated (Socio-Economic Simplicity correlates $-.30$, $p \leq .01$ with Male Institutions). Thus the more complex a society, the more likely it is to have male institutions. This association may well be due to the fact that our sample is skewed toward simple, homogeneous cultures. Certainly technologically advanced, heterogeneous cultures such as our own vary tremendously in the degree to which they provide cohesive, loyalty-promoting groups; but it is doubtful that advanced societies do this job as well as those agricultural societies with strong initiation procedures and solidary male groups. On the whole it seems that societies such as our own are more like hunters in this respect; for our large, heterogeneous cultural systems both require and thwart individual assertiveness. Again, of course, there is a great deal of local variation which may give rise to the possibly erroneous notion that the genesis of heavy drinking is an individually unique and largely idiosyncratic matter. We have suggested that, in simple societies at least, this is not the case; and it remains to be seen whether or not heavy drinkers in our society have situational predicaments and attitudes of mind in common with each other and with the heavy drinkers in elementary societies.

CONCLUSIONS

To summarize, we have now provided some answers to the three questions which initiated this re-examination of the theory of magical potency. A procedure for empirically validating our interpretation of the magical potency tags was undertaken, and in the process magical potency was re-defined, both substantively and theoretically, as impulsive power. We then showed that the heaviest drinkers among our societies are just those whose folk tales manifest the most impulsive types of power concern and that their behavior at drinking bouts strongly suggests their use of alcohol to satisfy the need for impact upon others. Finally we delineated two social syndromes: one which promotes both impulsive power concerns and heavy drinking by simultaneously requiring and thwarting individual assertiveness; and another which inhibits both drinking and its associated state of mind by promoting loyalty and cooperation.

Having provided these answers to our original questions, the theory of impulsive power now rests on less tentative grounds than did the earlier version of this theory presented in the previous chapter. No other known theory of cross-cultural drinking provides an equally adequate account of the facts we have presented. It remains to be seen, of course, whether we have located a state of mind which universally motivates the use of alcohol. In particular, there may be limits on the extent to which the collective fantasy of folk tales is uniquely associated with the private fantasy of the individual who drinks heavily. Thus the chapters which follow explore these more molecular relations between individual motives and heavy drinking.

Chapter 5

The Need for Power in College Men: Action Correlates and Relationship to Drinking[1]

by David G. Winter

This chapter presents the first evidence from our research that power concerns are related to drinking at the level of individual behavior. It traces the development of a new scoring system for power motivation (n Power), and then reports data which suggests that under certain circumstances drinking is a behavior characteristic of young men high in n Power.

Actually, this research was not originally designed to study drinking, although it was carried out at the same time as the work on folk tales and the social-structural correlates of drinking discussed in earlier chapters. Rather, our concern was to develop an improved measure of n Power (Winter, 1967 and 1968a), using the technique by which motives are experimentally aroused and then measured in

[1]This chapter is based on the author's Ph.D. thesis, Harvard University, 1967. The author is indebted to David C. McClelland for suggestions, encouragement, and guidance; to George H. Litwin, Douglas Bunker, and David Kolb for assistance with the arousal experiment; to Stanley H. King and the staff of the Harvard Student Study for the use of data collected by the study; and to Arthur S. Couch for theoretical and practical assistance in the analysis of data. This research was in part supported by a Public Health Service Fellowship (MH-21,404) from the National Institute of Mental Health.

fantasy (cf. Atkinson, 1958). Two previous attempts to measure power motivation in this way (Veroff, 1957; Uleman, 1965) had yielded unclear patterns of results (cf. Skolnick, 1966; McClelland, 1966). Sometimes the Veroff system related to aggressive leadership, and sometimes it related to a defensive fear of being manipulated by other people. In any case, no relationship between either the Veroff or the Uleman systems and drinking had been reported. The new measure was designed to clear up some of these uncertainties about power motivation, and only in the process of validating the new measure did the relationships to drinking emerge. Therefore, before going further, it will be useful to give a brief description of the development of the new measure of *n* Power.[2]

AROUSAL PROCEDURES AND DEVELOPMENT OF THE *n* POWER SCORING SYSTEM

Ninety-one Harvard Business School males who had volunteered for an experiment announced as a study of "the human response to communication content in mass media" were randomly assigned to two adjacent rooms, as they appeared at the set time. The aroused group ($N = 47$) was shown a film of President John F. Kennedy's inauguration, while the control group ($N = 44$) was shown a relatively neutral film, in which a businessman described scientific demonstration equipment. Immediately after the films, both groups wrote stories to the following six pictures of the TAT type:

1. Soldiers in field dress, one pointing to a map or chart.
2. Boy lying on a bed reading a newspaper.
3. "Ship's captain" talking to a man in a suit.
4. A couple in a restaurant drinking beer, guitarist in the background.
5. "Homeland": man and youth chatting outdoors.
6. A couple sitting on a marble bench with heads bowed.

The assumption was that the Kennedy film would arouse a concern for power, broadly defined in its rational-legal, traditional and charismatic aspects (c . Weber, 1947). A scoring system was devised through an extended process of comparing some TAT protocols chosen randomly from each group and also integrating some *a priori* ideas about power. This system was modified after comparing more protocols from

[2]The term *n* Power will hereafter refer to the new system. References to the other systems will be labelled as "Veroff system" or "Uleman system," in order to keep the three systems straight.

each group, scored blindly. (See Winter, 1967, for details.) A brief summary of the system is given below; this is the version with which the research reported in this chapter was conducted. A further revision, incorporating some of the experience gained in this book is reproduced in Appendix I.

A brief summary of the n Power system

POWER IMAGERY—to be scored first

Power Imagery is scored if someone in the story (called "the actor") is concerned about his impact; that is, about establishing, maintaining, or restoring his prestige or power in the eyes of the world. A person or a group of persons, or an abstract unit such as a country can be an actor. This generic definition can be divided into three criteria which can be used for scoring Power Imagery.

1. The actor demonstrates or increases his impact or his prestige through taking direct, vigorous, expansive action, Actions can be planned, fantasied, remembered, or they can actually take place. They do not have to be successful. Examples include attacks, exploitative sex, vigorous arguments, vigorous work or exercise, and wild or drunken parties. Other more subtle examples include giving help or advice, creative writing that is intended to create public attention, and a concern about getting a job or position that reflects or improves prestige. Some illustrations are:

> "They plan to attack an enemy base."
> "He is trying to seduce his secretary."
> "Her husband went with her to help her."
> "The guy is trying to impress his date."
> "The boy has just had finals—they were rough; there is a feeling of peaceful exhaustion."
> "They are tired after returning from the beer blast."

Not scored: Routine action, such as teaching, military activity, or arguments. Imagery is not scored if the story goes on to deny the impact of the actor, or if he remains weak, indecisive, fearful, or passive. Sex is not scored if it involves love and romance. Challenges that are avoided, evaded, or where the person challenged gives in and is polite or cooperative are not scored, because in such cases the actor does not demonstrate his impact.

2. The actor takes some specific action which is sufficient to arouse and focus the feelings (positive or negative) of someone else ("the respondent"). Such feelings include idealization, fascination, ecstasy, happiness, great interest or enthusiasm, worry, shame, crying, fear. Some illustrations are:

> "The man has taken the woman to a small romantic cafe. She is enchanted and shows her delight."
> "As he told the tale, Mary began to weep."
> "The pro gives a demonstration, and the boy is thrilled."

Such feelings must be in response to a specific action by an actor; strong feeling in response to a natural disaster or a depression is not scored.

3. The actor is concerned about his reputation. This concern is often manifested in a desire to control or find out information which could be evaluative. Some illustrations are:

"He will lose the captaincy of the ship and will be bitter."

"The young man knows the right spots in town to be seen in, and how to be seen in these spots."

SUBCATEGORIES—to be scored only if the story has been scored for Power Imagery.

Prestige of the actor (positive or negative)—PA+, PA—

Scored if the story mentions aspects of the actor which reflect high or low prestige: titles such as general, commander, professor, adjectives such as famous, prominent, very skilled, well-educated. Negative prestige, phrases such as "cheap punk," "has bad breath," or "is a cheapskate" can also be scored.

Feelings of the respondent (positive or negative)—FR+, FR—

Scored if someone other than the actor has strong emotional feelings. FR+ is scored if the respondent is trusting, devoted, feels respect, is happy, etc. FR— is scored if he feels fear, worry, hesitation, doubt, etc.

Self-perception of the actor (positive or negative)—SPA+, SPA—

Scored if the actor has some feeling or perception about himself, related to his efforts to increase his prestige, or if he anticipates such feelings. Illustrations are:

"Seeing her smile reassures him that his efforts have paid off."

"Nothing will be accomplished, and the father realizes that he has failed to help his son."

Act

Scored if there is overt activity by the actor, in the story, which is designed to establish, maintain, or restore his impact. There must be an actual statement of action within the story, apart from the original statement of the situation or the outcome of the story. Planning or retrospection are not scored for act.

Set

Scored if the actor acts in an extraordinary situation: if the setting of the story is dramatic or important; if adjectives of prestige are applied to the situation; if a prestigeful institution is mentioned; or if the actor acts against someone of high prestige. Illustrations include:

"They are on the forefront of the Allied push in the Pacific."

"He takes her to a fancy restaurant/nightclub."

"The newspaperman is trying to get the lowdown for a real scoop."

Thema

Scored if the power sequence is elaborated to become the major plot of the story. Not scored if there is any counterplot, such as achievement, affiliation, success, or relaxation.

Imagery and each of the nine subcategories can be scored only once per story, and are given a score of +1 when they occur. Thus the score for a single story can range from 0 to +10.

ACTION CORRELATES OF THE *n* POWER SYSTEM

The first investigation of the action correlates of *n* Power was made using data from the Harvard Student Study of the college careers of 83 men from the Harvard Class of 1964. The Study had administered six-picture TATs to these students during the first week of their freshman year, under relatively neutral testing conditions. The following pictures were used:

1. "Ship's captain" talking to a man in a suit.
2. Boy lying on a bed reading a newspaper.
3. Young man greeting older couple.
4. Teacher talking to student.
5. Man and woman standing on roof.
6. Young man on a street reading a book.

These TATs were scored for n Power, and were also scored for the Veroff and Uleman systems. The Study had collected a wealth of information about the college life, activities and performance of these students, their family background, and their attitudes and opinions. A few students had been interviewed intensively over a period of four years. The research program was designed to explore the characteristics of n Power by relating TAT scores to the data collected by the study. Actually, such a plan proved rather quixotic, inasmuch as the data were stored on IBM cards as thousands of separate variables. Since the data were obtained for purposes quite different from studying n Power, questions had been asked and activities recorded in ways which sometimes made it difficult to pull apart the power-related significance on a student's response. For these reasons, it was necessary to select, rearrange, and combined variables from the available data. (See Winter, 1967, for the complete account of the data analysis.)

The first stage of data analysis, then, involved exploring the relationships between n Power and numerous highly specific variables. Obviously if a large number of variables is investigated, some relationships will emerge as significant purely by chance. In an initial exploratory study, one can frame hypotheses in advance as a protection, but there is no final way to proceed other than by investigating a wide range of variables. Often it is the unexpected relationship, if it proves to be stable and appears in other investigations, that turns out to be the most interesting and fruitful. Hence these findings need to be confirmed with thorough additional research. Such research is currently under way in order to replicate the present findings (Winter, 1968a and 1968b).

One obvious *a priori* hypothesis is that students with high n Power would tend to be officers in student organizations, even though many recent writers might argue that, on the contrary, the contemporary college student finds few power satisfactions in such student organizations (Kenniston, 1968; Peterson, 1968). One would also predict that competitive sports is another obvious outlet for n Power. Table 5.1

shows the initial relationships between n Power and office-holding and participation in sports. n Power tends to be related to these two activities, although the relationships are not at usual levels of significance. In part this is due to the rather small proportion of students who were either officers or atheletes.[3] The relationship between n Power and *either* holding office *or* participating in competitive sports was more nearly significant.

Table 5.1—Office-holding, competitive sports, and n Power[a]

| | | Persons holding office in a student organization: | | |
		At least one	None	Total
	High	7	20	27
n Power	Medium	6	18	24
	Low	3	25	28

$$\chi^2 = 2.42, \ df = 2, \ p = .30$$

| | | Persons participating in competitive sports:[b] | | |
		At least one	None	Total
	High	8	21	29
n Power	Medium	6	19	25
	Low	3	25	28

$$\chi^2 = 2.70, \ df = 2, \ p \sim .25$$

| | | Persons holding office or participating in competitive sports: | | |
		At least one	None	Total
	High	11	16	27
n Power	Medium	12	12	24
	Low	6	21	27

$$\chi^2 = 4.30, \ df = 2, \ .20 > p > .10$$

[a]The totals vary slightly due to absence of information on two subjects.
[b]Competitive sports are defined as participation at the varsity level in any sport for which Harvard maintained a team: e.g., football, soccer, squash, wrestling.

This raises a fundamental point about the concept of motive or need, a point to which we shall return several times in this chapter. As Murray (1938) and Frenkel-Brunswik (1942) used the term, a motive refers to a basic or abstract personality disposition which can express itself in a variety of specific behaviors apparently unrelated. Each of the behaviors is an alternative way of satisfying the basic motive or need. In many cases it is impossible or very unlikely that a person would engage in a great number of the behaviors. For example, as Wittenborn (1955) points out, a hungry man might eat chicken or he might eat steak; but it is unlikely that he would eat both at the same time. In the case of the college student, it is probably unlikely that he will have enough time to be a varsity athlete and an officer in a student organization. Moreover, he may not have the experience, skill, or physique for either activity. Thus on theoretical and practical grounds,

[3]Winter (1968a) found highly significant correlations between office-holding, sports, and n Power in a sample of middle-class adult males.

we were led to look for other things that were related to *n* Power, and we were also led to combined variables and clusters of variables in order to define a wide range of power-related activities.

Table 5.2 presents some of the other early results concerning *n* Power and the spending patterns of students, the possessions that they own or have direct access to, and their dating behavior. Note, first, that *n* Power is not related to the total amount of money that students report they have to spend. It is significantly related, however, to the amount that they spend on alcohol and on supplies for their rooms. Here was the first direct relationship between *n* Power and alcohol at the individual level. To be sure, buying liquor does not mean consuming it; it could be that these students simply had more parties. But this relationship led us to explore the area further.

n Power was also related to the amount spent on room supplies. Further examination of the possessions that they owned or had access to as freshmen revealed that these room supplies and other possessions

Table 5.2—Spending money, possessions, dating, and n Power

I. Correlations of amount of money spent for various things with *n* Power

Item	Correlation with n Power	Item	Correlation with n Power
Total spending money per month	−.02	Transportation	−.17
Dues	.04	Supplies	.27 *
Dating	−.01	Miscellaneous personal	
Books for courses	−.08	expenses	.15
Phonograph records, etc.	−.02	Gambling	−.09
Clothes	−.06	Cigarettes	.13
Laundry	.02	Alcohol	.24 *
Recreation	.09		

$N = 83$, * $= p < .05$

II. Possessions owned or having direct access to, and *n* Power

Item	Percent having n Power High	Med	Low	$\chi^2 (df = 2)$	p
1. Car	61	58	50	.73	n.s.
2. Motorcycle	7	4	4	.44[1]	n.s.
3. Motorscooter	18	21	7	2.19	∼.35
4. Fully-equipped bar	29	29	7	5.04	<.10
5. Television set	54	38	18	7.73	<.05
6. Refrigerator	86	75	64	3.42	<.20
7. Cleaning equipment	64	58	43	2.76	∼.25
8. Harvard beer mug	50	46	36	1.24	n.s.
9. Wine glasses	54	50	32	2.94	∼.25
10. Hat (not a cap)	29	25	7	4.59	=.10
11. Musical instrument	25	33	46	2.49[2]	∼.30
12. Body-building equipment	36	46	36	.75	n.s.

Correlation of *n* Power with prestige possessions scale (1 point for each of items 1-10 above) = +.28 $p < .05$.

Table 5.2—continued

III. Dating behavior and *n* Power

Correlations of various questions about dating with *n* Power

Item	r	p
Number of hours dating per week	−.04	n.s.
Rated importance/frequency of the following activities on dates:		
"Playing around" in the room	.21	<.10
Studying together	.23	=.05
Watching TV	.26	<.05
Movies	.23	=.05
Classical music concerts	−.02	n.s.
Dances	−.14	n.s.
Taking walks	−.07	n.s.
Making love	.24	<.05

Percent reporting that they have petted with a girl (freshman year)

	High	82%	
n Power	Medium	91%	$\chi^2 = 5.66$, *d.f.* = 2, *p* < .07
	Low	64%	

1. The expected frequencies are too small to yield meaningful chi-squares.
2. Reverse direction; i.e., those low in *n* Power tend to have more often.

seemed to fit together into a group that we have called "prestige possessions." Thus it seems very likely that a college sophomore who has a car, a motorcycle or motorbike, a fully-equipped bar, a television set, a refrigerator, and a hat will be considered by his peers as having a good deal of prestige or impact. At least this is the message that advertisers in young men's magazines try to convey. Therefore we constructed a scale of prestige possessions, in which each of the items showing a tendency to relate to *n* Power counted one point if it was owned. The correlation between *n* Power and the scale score was significant ($r = +.28$, $p < .05$).

Finally, in the area of dating, *n* Power shows a slight relationship to petting behavior on dates, and to the rated importance or frequency of "making love" as a date activity. While it is hazardous to rely on self-reports as a reliable measure of sexual behavior, it seems plausible that *n* Power would relate to more aggressive sexual behavior.

Table 5.3 shows that *n* Power is related at a high level of significance to power behavior; that is, to holding office or being an athelete or having many prestige possessions. Neither the Veroff nor the Uleman system is significantly related to this combination of power behaviors. Moreover, if we consider the six persons high in *n* Power who nevertheless do not show any power behavior, we find that they tend to have scores on the M-F scale of the MMPI that are significantly higher (i.e., more feminine) than those with high *n* Power who do show power behavior. In other words, those high in *n* Power who do not show any of the three power behaviors so far discussed may be less attracted to the American stereotype of "masculine" interests and style (c. Kagan and Moss, 1962). Hence they would tend not to pursue such interests, and we would have to examine their behavior in greater detail in order to discover how they might express their *n* Power.

So far we have discovered two unexpected kinds of behavior that may be related to *n* Power, at least among college students: the possession of prestigeful objects, and aggressive sexual behavior. The interesting point is that neither of these actions seems to involve skill or experience in the same way as does holding office or sports. If you want to play football, you need physical ability, and probably experience in secondary school. But if you want to express your *n* Power through having a lot of things that your peers admire, then all you have to do is scrimp on other purchases and buy them, or pick roommates who have them already. Sexual activity might require more skill or experience, but this doubtless varies tremendously with the particular partner. Surely there is no obstacle to *reported* sexual activity.

Table 5.3—Power behaviors, masculine interests, and n Power

		Persons showing power behavior: holding office in competitive sports, or having above the median prestige possessions		
		Power behavior	No power behavior	Total
n Power	High	22	6	28
	Medium	20	4	24
	Low	12	16	28

$\chi^2 = 12.50$, $df = 2$, $p < .005$

Multiple correlation of *n* Power with office-holding, competitive sports, and prestige possessions = $+.33$, $p < .05$.

		MMPI M-F Scale Score		
		above median	below median[a]	Total
Subjects high in *n* Power, and	show power behavior	9	13	22
	do not show power behavior	5	1	6

$p = .074$ (Fisher exact test)

[a]Median calculated for the group of subjects high in *n* Power.

Thus the early results suggest three conclusions: (1) There is a tendency for *n* Power to predict such social behaviors as office-holding and sports, but (2) *n* Power has other forms of expression such as prestige possessions, alcohol, and possibly sex. Finally, (3) although all of these behaviors are more or less unrelated to each other (see Table 5.4 below), they do go together as alternate expressions of a common power motive. These preliminary conclusions encouraged us to continue the analysis of data using more complicated and sophisticated multivariate techniques.

The first step was to read through the extensive interviews that the staff of the Harvard Student Study had conducted with a selected group of students, looking for additional differences in the activities and life-style of those scoring high as compared to those scoring low in *n* Power. This procedure suggested one important domain of behaviors, namely vicarious power-related experience. Such experience would include watching sports, watching television, and reading *Playboy* and other magazines that in their articles and their advertisements attempt to present experiences of power, potency, and prestige to their readers. Note in Table 5.2, part III, that *n* Power relates to watching television and movies on dates. Careful reading of some interviews also suggested that some students high in *n* Power might be more vigorous and persistent about approaching and arguing with faculty members. Unfortunately, there were not very many systematic measures of such behavior available for all students, and so we had to use reported frequency and intensity of interaction with the student's housemaster.[4]

The second step was to search through the available data for several different variables that could be a part of each of the clusters of power-related behavior that had been isolated through the early analysis and through studying the interviews. These variables were then combined into scale scores, as noted below. The scales were an attempt to give more precise empirical specification to the various hypothesized aspects of power motivation.

THE POWER-RELATED BEHAVIOR SCALES

Office-holding: One point for each organization in which the student holds an office; president or other major office rated as two points.

Competitive sports: One point for each varsity participation in a sport for which Harvard maintains a team.

Prestige possessions: One point for owning or having direct access to each of the possessions listed as numbers 1–10 in Table 5.2, Part II. Note that some items are included that show only trend differences between high and low *n* Power subjects.

Vicarious experience: Made up of three subscales, each standard-scored before being combined: (1) The number of hours per week

[4]Most upperclassmen at Harvard College live in Houses, each of which has a senior professor as a resident housemaster. Often the housemaster is the faculty member whom a student knows best, or at least sees most often during his three years in the House.

reported as spent at spectator sports; (2) A subscale with one point for each of the following: attending Harvard sports, Boston sports, Harvard football game, Harvard-Yale football game, and Harvard "away" football game; (3) A subscale with one point for each "vicarious" magazine (such as *Playboy, Rogue, Gent, Dude,* etc.) that was regularly read. In addition, one point was added to the whole scale if the student regularly read *Sports Illustrated.*

Interaction with housemaster: Points given for both intellectual and social conversations with the student's housemaster, on a 0–3 scale of frequency for each.

Sex: First, only students who were not engaged or going steady were considered, because we wished to distinguish sexual behavior that may actually involve love or dependence from a more exploitative kind of sex. There were three subscales, each standard-scored before being combined: (1) A subscale with one point each for reported kissing, petting with a girl above and below the waist, and intercourse; with additional points for having done each over an extended period of years before college. (2) A subscale with points for ranking either "sex" or "the enhancement of my reputation" as motives for dating; and (3) a subscale with points for dating pick-ups, going to girls' dormitories to try to date "availables," and for "bird-dogging" at parties, when reported as dating practices.

Drinking: Two subscales, each standard-scored before being combined: (1) the total amount spent per month on alcoholic beverages; and (2) the reported frequency of drinking, on a 0–2 scale of frequency.

Table 5.4 gives the correlation of all of these scales with each other and with *n* Power. It is immediately apparent that while several of the scales are interrelated, only one (Prestige possessions) has any significant first-order relationship to *n* Power. Indeed, the drinking scale, which is of principal interest here, is almost completely unrelated to *n* Power. Of course such low first-order correlations are not unexpected, and need not destroy our principal hypothesis about drinking. Just as it is unlikely that a hungry man would eat both chicken and steak at the same time, so is it rather unlikely that a college student would be simultaneously an officer, an athlete, a heavy drinker, a vigorous talker with his housemaster, and a sexual hero. Such a person might be one version of the American Dream, but it seems implausible that he would be a very common figure at Harvard College. Therefore, to test the principal hypothesis about the scales as alternative expressions of power concerns, a principal components factor analysis was performed on the domain of *n* Power and the behavior scales. The resulting loadings and scores were then rotated, according to Kaiser's Varimax criterion for simple structure by variables (see Couch, 1967).

Table 5.4—Intercorrelation of the behavior scales and n Power

	Sports	Prestige Possessions	Vicarious Experience	Interaction With Master	Sex	Drinking	n Power
Office-holding	.04	−.02	−.16	.03	−.32*	−.03	.13
Competitive sports		.04	.33**	.29*	.13	−.01	.13
Prestige possessions			.33**	.04	.38**	.30*	.28*
Vicarious experience				.11	.51**	.18	.05
Interaction with housemaster					.00	.01	.12
Sex						.40*	.08
Drinking							−.01

The *N* varies slightly for each correlation.

* = significant at the .05 level, given the *N*.
** = significant at the .01 level, given the *N*.

Table 5.5 shows the rotated factor loadings, while Figure 5.1 illustrates the plot of rotated Factors I and II. Most of the behavior scales form themselves into a bi-polar Factor I, with office-holding slightly (but not very strongly) toward one pole, and drinking, sex, and vicarious experiences—which we shall term the "stud" cluster of behaviors—at the other. Sports and interaction with housemaster do not appear to load on either factor. Factor I seems to measure some dimension of impulsive expression vs. impulse restraint. It seems reasonable to take it as a close parallel to the Inhibition dimension referred to in the previous chapter. Certainly a person has to inhibit impulses towards drinking and sex, and he cannot spend much time in vicarious experience, if he wants to run an organization. Moreover, it seems reasonable that drinking, sex, and reading *Playboy* tend to cluster together.

n Power, however, loads virtually completely on Factor II, whereas none of the behavior scales, except prestige possessions, has any important loading on this factor. So it would appear that the factor analysis confirms the results of Table 5.4, in that *n* Power now appears completely orthogonal to most of the interesting behaviors

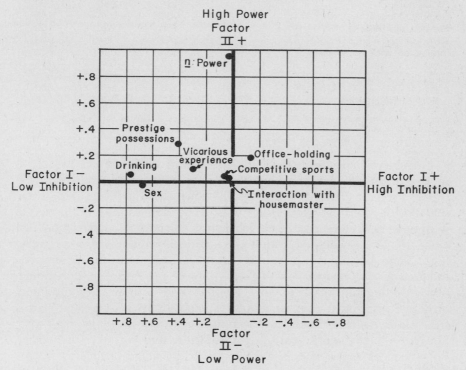

Figure 5.1 Plot of rotated factor analysis showing loadings of *n* Power and behavior scales.

that we had hypothesized as power-related. Yet *n* Power and Inhibition (the bi-polar Factor I) are independent; that is, it is possible for a person with high *n* Power to be either high or low on Inhibition. If the two poles of Factor I (office-holding and the stud cluster) are in fact alternate and perhaps mutually exclusive manifestations of *n* Power, then we would predict that, as *n* Power increases, subjects will tend to be farther toward *either* the right pole (Factor I− or office-holding) *or* the left pole (Factor I+ or the stud cluster). A look at a plot of the individual subjects by their scores on Factors I and II, as shown in Figure 5.2 shows this to be roughly the case. To assess the strength of such a tendency, we computed the correlation between *n* Power and the *absolute score* (plus or minus) on Factor I. The resulting correlation was +.22 ($p < .05$), indicating that as a person's *n* Power increases, he manifests more office-holding *or* more stud behaviors.

Table 5.5—Rotated factor loadings of behavior scales and n Power

| | Loadings on Factor | | |
Variables	*I*	*II*	*III*
Office-holding	−.134	1.80	.087
Competitive sports	.056	.034	.241
Prestige possessions	*.409*	*.285*	.162
Vicarious experience	*.299*	.084	.048
Interaction with housemaster	.026	.030	*.833*
Sex	*.671*	−.031	−.145
Drinking	*.772*	.044	−.021
*n·*Power	.028	*.952*	.063
Sum of squared loadings	6.249	6.856	5.231

Note: This table has been extracted from a larger table containing other variables. All loadings above .300 are italicized.

Thus we have confirmed, at least tentatively, that *n* Power is a motive in the original sense that Murray (1938) and Frenkel-Brunswik (1942) used the concept, and we have shown that drinking, along with sex and vicarious experience, are important manifestations of concern with power. To be sure, the correlation coefficient of *n* Power and the absolute score of Factor I, although statistically significant, is not very high. There may be two principal reasons for this, apart from measurement error: (1) Persons very high in *n* Power may be able to combine office-holding and stud behavior, although such activities are unrelated or negatively related for most people. The possibility is supported by the fact that five out of the seven officers who are high in *n* Power are also above the median on at least one of the three stud variables (drinking, sex, vicarious experience). Such persons will tend to be located in the middle of Factor I and high on Factor II, although actually they are high on *both* poles of Factor I. (2) Some persons high in *n* Power but in the middle of Factor I may be expressing their power through some behaviors that we have not thought to measure. Included here would be those with a high MMPI M-F scale score (Table 5.3). Indeed, there is a whole range of behaviors among adults, from politics to the army to violence, that may not be readily available to college students with a high *n* Power. Perhaps this fact might account for the current discontent with campus activities and college life that is expressed by many students (cf. Keniston, 1968; Peterson, 1968; and also foot-note 3).

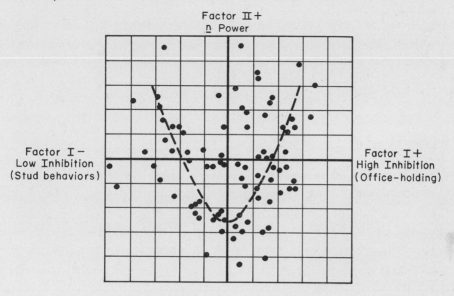

Factor II+
n Power

Factor I −
Low Inhibition
(Stud behaviors)

Factor I +
High Inhibition
(Office-holding)

— — — — Central tendency of subject distribution,
showing increasing absolute score on Factor I
as score on Factor II increases.

Figure 5.2 Distribution of subjects, plotted by scores on Factors I (Inhibition) and II (*n* Power).

In any case, we have achieved a preliminary confirmation of the relationship between *n* Power and drinking, at least an an alternate form of the relationship between *n* Power and office-holding. Yet, predictions that a person will do either *A* or *B* are confusing and of limited use. Is there any way in which we can find out which mani-festation a person's *n* Power will take? In other words, under what circumstances will *n* Power relate directly to drinking?

PATTERNS OF POWER MOTIVES
AND POWER BEHAVIORS

The most obvious place to look for factors which will lead to the expression of *n* Power through drinking rather than through office-holding is in the characteristics of the power-related fantasies themselves. Research on *n* Achievement has come to distinguish two aspects of the achievement motive: the "hope of success" and the "fear of failure," each of which involves certain categories of fantasy (Clark, Teevan & Ricciuti, 1956; Heckhausen, 1968). In the case of the power motive, might there not be a similar distinction between the "hope of impact" and the "fear of impotence"? Perhaps these two aspects of *n* Power, if they can be shown to exist, will directly relate to the different kinds of power behavior.

Our first step in drawing out distinctive aspects of power fantasies was to perform a factor analysis of the scores for power imagery and the subcategories of the *n* Power system. Since we were working with a preliminary version of the new scoring system, we also had the TATs scored for the Veroff and Uleman systems of measuring *n* Power, and included all of these additional subcategories in the matrix. Table 5.6 gives the resulting factors of the three combined scoring systems, rotated according to the Varimax criterion. For the sake of clarity, only the four factors with the highest sums of squares after rotation are reproduced here, although the factors are labelled with their original numbers (I, II, III and VI).

Factor I involves most of the Veroff scoring system, particularly statements of concern about controlling the means of influence (imagery), need, instrumental activity, and blocks in the world. It is negatively related to consulting others to gain power and to positive perceptions of the self. In terms of the fantasy characteristics, this factor seems to represent an individualistic concern with overcoming blocks to gain influence, but without any particular positive inner affect.

Factor II contains criterion 2 of the new system for power imagery—arousing strong emotions in others (especially positive emotions), without dread or self-deprecation. It seems to represent a more confident, socially-oriented, power fantasy pattern.

Factor III involves forceful, vivid action (new system criterion 1 for power imagery) by prestigeful people in a dramatic setting, which often creates negative emotions in the minds of others. This pattern seems to represent a kind of threatening, tyrannical power, at least in fantasy. Nevertheless, all of the first three factors seem to suggest a relatively confident actor who is able to take effective action, sometimes while overcoming blocks.

Table 5.6—Rotated factor loadings of the three
n Power scoring systems

Variable	Loadings on Factor			
	I	II	III	VI
Veroff System:[a]				
Imagery	.658*	.296*	.284*	.476*
Stated need	.567*	.019	−.194	.041
Goal anticipation—positive	.243*	−.004	.066	−.115
Goal anticipation—negative	−.017	−.169	.050	.352*
Instrumental activity	.624*	.308*	.300*	.485*
Block—personal	−.071	.071	−.087	.134
Block—world	.649*	.064	−.097	−.036
Goal state—positive	.060	.092	.048	.102
Goal state—negative	.010	.048	−.167	.675*
Thema	.409*	.226	.237	.442*
Uleman System:[a]				
(Imagery—not given points)	.048	.913*	.106	.219
Prestige	.233	.031	.333*	−.123
Organization	.008	.086	.063	.505*
No self-deprecation	.032	.872*	.149	−.023
No reminiscense	.026	.931*	.120	.157
No dread	−.017	.798*	.066	.035
Counter-reaction	.397*	.085	.203	−.075
Consultation	−.511*	.177	−.020	−.005
Threat	.071	.209	.124	.447*
Separation	.009	.133	.025	−.014
Winter System:[b]				
Imagery—Criterion 1	.116	.132	.776*	.110
Imagery—Criterion 2	.098	.246*	−.119	−.216
Imagery—Criterion 3	.018	.104	.133	.242*
Prestige of actor—positive	.028	.059	.647*	−.147
Prestige of actor—negative	−.126	.192	.288*	.284*
Feelings of respondent—pos.	.000	.470*	−.201	−.419*
Feelings of respondent—neg.	−.166	.019	.313*	.076
Actor's self-perception—pos.	−.339*	.112	.274*	−.094
Actor's self-perception—neg.	.169	−.088	.049	.507*
Act	−.031	.054	.712*	.150
Set	.126	.035	.739*	−.062
Thema	−.225	.154	.702*	.153
Sum of squares	2.560	3.886	3.439	2.548

$N = 83$

Note: This table has been extracted from a larger table containing other factors. These four factors have the highest sums of squares. All loadings above .250 are starred.

[a]See Veroff (1957) and Uleman (1965) for details and scoring definitions.
[b]These categories are described and illustrated at the beginning of this chapter.

Factor VI, however, is quite different. Here the fantasy pattern involves most of the negative categories. Characters in the stories are concerned about their reputation, and while they may take some action, they have negative anticipations of the result. They are of low prestige, and look on themselves that way. They usually fail to gain power and are unhappy about it. The Uleman categories of "Organization" and "Threat" also appear in the factor. It seems plausible that the actors are in fact threatened by powerful organizations, and that thereby they generally lose their power and are bitter about it. At the very least, they are concerned about their reputation—perhaps their reputation *vis-à-vis* the organization. This factor, then, strongly suggests the negative aspect of *n* Power, or fear of loss of power.

This rather speculative interpretation of the four principal factors derived from the *n* Power scoring systems has laid the groundwork for the correlations of each fantasy factor score with the behavior scales, as reported in Table 5.7. What is immediately apparent is that

Table 5.7—Correlations of the scoring system factors and the behavior scales

Behavior scale variables	Scoring System Factors[a]			
	I	*II*	*III*	*VI*
Office-holding	.14	.16	.07	−.07
Competitive sports	−.07	.06	.07	.00
Prestige possessions	−.08	.03	.27 *	.22 *
Vicarious experience	−.11	.13	.08	.28 *
Drinking	−.03	.05	−.02	.34 **
Sex	.01	−.06	−.06	.42 **

$N = 83$ $* = p < .05$ $** = p < .01$
[a]Sub-categories which define by high loadings are given in Table 5.6.

Factor VI, which we have tentatively suggested as representing fear of losing power or fear of failure in an attempt to gain power, does in fact significantly relate with all three of the behavior scales that constitute the stud cluster: drinking, sex and vicarious experience. It appears, then, that when high *n* Power is constituted principally of fearful, negative images of failure and threat, then the power motive will express itself in actions which at first do not appear to be inherently powerful, such as drinking or reading *Playboy*. Yet, all of these actions can create a relatively immediate, certain, and riskless *subjective feeling of power*. Such feelings are not the substance of social power of course; but they may be a second-best alternative for the man who is both highly concerned about power and highly threatened or made fearful by it.

What factors predict office-holding, which is our rather inadequate measure of "real" social power among Harvard College men? Factors I and II both have the highest positive relationship, although neither correlation is significant at usual levels. If both factors are combined, then the multiple correlation is higher and just significant ($R = .21$, $p \sim .05$). Hence it seems that office-holding is best predicted by individualistic concerns about overcoming blocks to gain influence, or by a confident concern with arousing strong effects in others. Factors I and II together, then, may represent the "hope of impact" in the power motive. Factor III relates to having prestige possessions, as does

Factor VI. The men who gather such things around them, it appears, have fantasies of vivid and dramatic action which strongly affects others. Perhaps they feel that prestige possessions will help them to create such actions and effects. Probably the possessions do help. Whether these people ever carry out vivid actions themselves is beyond the scope of the present data to answer. Factor III, then, cannot easily be assigned either to the hope or to the fear aspect of power.

This attempt to establish different patterns within the general domain of power fantasies has been only a preliminary step, but it was an important and encouraging step. Actually, the situation may be more complex. Some recent research on *n* Power (Winter, 1968b) suggests that the model of Atkinson (1957), in which motives interact with expectations and incentives to produce action, may also clarify the conditions under which *n* Power leads to drinking, vicarious behavior, and sex rather than to office-holding and organized social power. Under conditions of low expectancy of achieving real social power, the person with high *n* Power may turn to the vicarious substitute, or subjective "short cut," mentioned above. On the other hand, a high fear of failing to gain power, or a fear of losing power, may cause one to have very low expectancies of succeeding in the world. Whether different patterns of fantasy or different cognitive expectations can best account for the different forms of power behavior —and indeed, whether the fantasy patterns and the expectations are themselves intimately related—will require a lot more research to answer.

SUMMARY

This research on *n* Power has, first of all, increased our understanding of power, through delineating a domain of behaviors that are all related to an underlying power motive, although the relationships are sometimes complicated and not fully understood at present. Indeed, we would hesitate to label the scoring system as "*n* Power" if it did not relate to obvious social power actions such as holding office. *n* Power is not, however, simply a redundant term for powerful actions. For one thing, it is measured quite independently from the measurement of action. More fundamentally, *n* Power is a motive. That is, it is an underlying genotype or personality disposition that draws together and relates a wide variety of actions, many of which do not appear at first to be power-related. Under some conditions, the power motive leads to drinking, sex, vicarious powerful experiences, and having prestigious possessions. Why is this so? Apparently all of these rather subjective actions are at least capable of giving the same sort of psychic satisfaction that objective social power can give. In such cases the satisfaction may be less intense and less "real"; but it is also less threatening and more completely under the control of the person who performs the action. External social reality impinges on our social behavior, but our vicarious, subjective experiences appear to be more under our own control. Figure 5.3 illustrates the overall organization of the two aspects of *n* Power and power-related behaviors.

Figure 5.3 Two aspects of n Power

Generic definition	Concern with creating impact through vigorous, strong action, through concern with reputation, or through arousing and focusing the strong emotions of others.	
	Leads to a domain of power-related actions: organized social power and expressive subjective power.	
	Related to a strong father-identification. Possible pathologies of aggression and paranoia.	
Differential description	Positive.	Negative.
	Hope of getting power and creating impact.	Fear of losing power.
Fantasy pattern	Concern with creating effects in others through strong acts; also concern with means of influence.	Explicit concern with own reputation; also mention of superior/subordinate relationships.
	Prestige, dramatic settings; positive expectations; positive feelings aroused in others; instrumental actions.	Negative anticipations, emotions about outcomes; low prestige and view of self; threats, organizations.
Action characteristics	Organized power within a social structure.	Expressive, subjective, "potency" behaviors.
	Holding office, competitive sports, (prestige possessions).	Drinking, exploitative sex, vicarious experience, prestige possessions.

These conclusions may help to resolve the controversy about whether fantasy is directly related to action, or whether it is a substitute for action (see Lazarus, 1961, 1966; McClelland, 1966). Do we rehearse in fantasy the things that we actually perform in action? Or is our fantasy a substitute for the actions that we would like to perform but do not? Consideration of these results with the power motives suggests that very often there is a direct relationship between fantasy and action. Sometimes, however—especially when the fantasy is tinged with threat, fear and failure—the related actions involve power of a subjective, expressive sort. It is as though they were quick short-cuts to the goal. They may achieve that goal subjectively, although to the external observer they may often appear to lead to the very opposite of the goal.

In such cases we must distinguish the outer public "actuality" from the inner "reality" (see Erikson, 1964).

What can we conclude about the relationship between an individual's power concerns and his drinking, at least among our sample of Harvard College men? Although there is no direct, first-order correlation between the two, drinking is one important part of a cluster of actions which is a principal manifestation of the need for power. We have termed this cluster the stud cluster, since it includes drinking, sex, and vicarious power experience. It appears to represent low inhibition or *impulsive* forms of potent actions. As expressions of power concern, all of these actions appear to be an alternative to obtaining social power through ways that involve inhibition and conscious control, such as by holding office.[5] Furthermore, from these data we also suggest that drinking is a direct and first-order correlate of power concerns when these concerns are negative, threatening, or fearful. Along with the other low-inhibition stud behaviors, drinking may be directly related to fantasies of losing power, or fantasies of the power of another over the self.

---

[5]It is possible to check directly whether inhibition at the level of fantasy leads to less drinking, as the results of the folk-tale research discussed earlier in this book would suggest (see Chapter 3). Moreover, Winter *et al.* (1963) suggest that the "classic personal style" is a personality disposition organized around the concept of inhibition, particularly inhibition in fantasy.

III
DRINKING AND THE NEED FOR POWER

Having at last formulated a theory of drinking from our exploratory studies, we wanted to subject it to tests in order to see if it would hold up on closer scrutiny. As a first step, we had to go back and re-examine the results of our experimental arousal studies to see if the fantasy effects of drinking could be recoded in power terms without causing them to disappear. At the same time we repeated the drinking study on a sample of older men, from a different social class background in still a different setting, with pictures more suggestive of power themes, to make sure that our earlier arousal findings had fairly wide generality at least within our culture (Chapter 6).

With these results confirming the theory that drinking increases power concerns, we returned to the question left hanging at the end of Chapter 1. Will people who show the experiential characteristics produced by drinking, even when they are *not* in a drinking situation, be the very ones who tend to drink more? In other words, will the type of power concern aroused by drinking also provide a clue as to why some men drink more than others? The answer to this question, provided in Chapters 7 and 8, once again convinced us we were on the right track in thinking the power motive crucial to understanding drinking. More than that, we began to understand that drinking was only one way of expressing the power motive and that a full understanding of drinking required a knowledge of alternative manifestations of the power drive, as traced out in some detail in Chapter 8.

Finally we wanted to perform an experiment to see whether the power theory or the widely held nurturance theory of drinking would predict who would drink more in an experimentally controlled situation. Interpreting networks of intercorrelations, however significant, as in Chapter 8, is always a difficult enterprise because there are so many alternative ways to make sense of them. If we really understood the motive underlying drinking, as we thought we did by this time, we ought to be able to produce a power-oriented situation which would make men drink more. Alternatively, a situation rigged to heighten nurturance concerns, we felt, should not increase drinking if our general line of reasoning was correct. The results of this experiment, reported in Chapter 9, clearly support the theory that drinking is related to the vicissitudes of the power motive rather than to concerns about nurturance.

Chapter 6

The Effects of Drinking on Thoughts About Power and Restraint

by David C. McClelland and Sharon Carlson Wilsnack[1]

The findings presented in the last three chapters point to a connection between high-power/low-inhibition fantasies and heavy drinking. In Chapter 3 it was shown that the folk-tale tags associated with heavy drinking could be interpreted as signifying an interest in magical, non-instrumental potency, while the tags associated with sobriety indicated a kind of inhibited respect for social order. In Chapter 4, further analyses of the folk-tale data suggested a distinction between impulsive power fantasies, on the one hand, associated with low inhibition and drinking, and effective power fantasies on the other, associated with high inhibition and sobriety. The data presented in Chapter 5 confirmed the importance of this distinction at the individual level; heavy drinking belonged to a cluster of activities which could be characterized as impulsive expressions of power (e.g., the stud cluster) as contrasted with more organized expressions of power like office holding.

[1]We are grateful to the following assistants who did the recoding on which this chapter is based: Nicholas and Duncan McClelland, Robert Frye, Mary Thomas, Ross Goldstein, and Dan Goleman.

None of these findings deals primarily with the *effects* of drinking on fantasy. In the folk-tale study, for example, it is not clear whether heavy drinking produces power-related fantasies or whether people who tell tales on power themes tend to drink more. Either might be true, or both.

To investigate the matter, we must return to our arousal studies reported in Chapters 1 and 2. They may not clearly separate cause and effect if heavy drinkers drink more on a given occasion, yet they eventually will permit a comparison of the effects of drinking on those with histories of heavy and light drinking. They demonstrated that alcohol consumption decreased restraining thoughts like Time Concern and increased themes of Physical Aggression, Physical Sex, and Meaning Contrast. The decrease in restraining thoughts seems to parallel closely the folk-tale finding that heavy drinking is associated with low frequencies of such folk-tale tags as Fear, Scheduling, and Activity Inhibition. That is, if the folk tales are told while drinking, they may contain fewer such thoughts, because as we have found in the case of individuals, drinking reduces the frequency of restraining thoughts. Yet we still need to check within the confines of one study to see whether to such different measures of restraint as Activity Inhibition and Time Concern are similarly affected by drinking. It will also be important to discover whether a low level of such thoughts not only follows heavy drinking but also precedes and helps predict it.

Interpreting the themes which increase with drinking presents more difficult problems. Our first hypothesis was that the "physical" nature of the increases in the imagery of Sex and Aggression meant that drinking heightened sentience. But as Chapter 2 concluded, a more direct measure of sentience—Sensuous Physical Pleasure—did not increase with drinking. Can the increases alternatively be interpreted in power terms?

Physical Aggression presents no problems because by definition it is designed to "have a strong vigorous impact." So all instances of Physical Aggression would also be scored as power-related in the Winter coding system for *n* Power. Winter also codes as power-related *exploitative* sex in which a man is trying to seduce or sleep with a girl when no element of love or romance is mentioned. That is, the man appears to be using the girl to satisfy is own desires in a power-oriented way. It occurred to us that most such exploitative sex stories would also be scored for Physical Sex, so that instances of the latter as obtained in Chapters 1 and 2 might turn out to be generally power-related. At least it seemed worth checking to see whether the shifts obtained with the coding definition of Physical Sex would also be obtained if the exploitative or power-related definition of Sex Imagery were used.

The Meaning Contrast code at first glance did not seem obviously power-related. To examine the problem further, some 100 randomly selected stories that had been scored for Meaning Contrast in the studies reported in Chapter 1 were read for power content. The results were encouraging. In a high percentage of the cases the affective contrast occurred at a point in the story where a character experienced a sudden or drastic, real or perceived difference in his position of power or prestige. In one type of story a strong man suddenly lost all or a weak person became dramatically powerful or famous, often without doing anything, by a twist of fate. In a slightly different type of story a character held beliefs, fantasies, or aspirations of strength and greatness which were in sharp contrast to his actual position of weakness or inadequacy. Or in still another type of story, the contrast was between a weak party, usually a helpless individual, and a strong party, usually a demanding, threatening, omnipotent authority or institution. Thus in a large percentage of the cases, stories of Meaning Contrast appeared to involve a *power* contrast which would have led them to be scored anyway in a coding system for *n* Power.

It was decided, therefore, that an attempt should be made to see if drinking would have the same effects on such categories if they were re-defined in power terms. Furthermore, if drinking does increase power fantasies, it should do so even when the fantasies are *not* related to the previously discovered shifts in Sex, Aggression, or Meaning Contrast. So we designed a new coding system which not only redefined these categories in power terms, but included other power categories not related to Sex or Aggression or Meaning Contrast.

A second objective of our re-analysis of earlier findings was to pursue the question of whether the types of power fantasies increased by drinking, if any, were those which also predict who will drink the most. Thus, for instance, thoughts of Sex and Aggression Power might not only be increased by drinking; they might also, if they appear in a "dry" TAT, predict heavy drinking, as a finding in Chapter 1 suggests.

Studying this issue has involved a complex series of interrelated coding decisions in which various *n* Power sub-scores have been derived and tested successively to see (1) whether they predicted customarily heavy drinking and (2) whether they increased with drinking. The studies of prediction are summarized below in Chapters 7 and 8, the studies of drinking effects in this chapter.

Essentially there were three major attempts to partition the *n* Power categories in ways to reflect states of mind that could be both the cause and the effect of heavy drinking. (1) The Sex and Aggression vs. Other Power distinction was made initially to see whether the effects of drinking were power-related; (2) a distinction between weak and strong power categories was derived from the data in

Chapter 5. There it was shown that the power-related thoughts associated with drinking or the stud cluster of activities included primarily negative sub-categories, suggesting fear of losing power. On the other hand, certain "strong" sub-categories like instrumental activity seemed associated with acts of effective power like becoming an officer in an organization. (3) A distinction between personalized and socialized power was suggested by the discovery that the first two methods of partitioning the *n* Power score did not successfully predict heavy drinking. This distinction is explained in full below in Chapter 8.

The task in the present chapter is to investigate the effects of drinking on these various ways of partitioning power-coding categories, on the assumption that the effects of drinking on power fantasies may be similar to the types of power fantasies which predict heavy drinking. Obviously there is no reason why the two phenomena have to be the same or even positively related. It is conceivable that the state of mind which leads people to drink would be precisely the opposite of the state of mind they are in after drinking. But our correlational studies encouraged us to think that cause and effect might be related, and the work in this chapter on effects was guided throughout by the data we were gathering on the categories which predicted drinking.

PROCEDURE

Derivation of the expanded set of coding categories for various types of power-related thoughts involved essentially three steps which will be only generally summarized here. Complete details are given in Appendix I; many of the coding distinctions had no lasting significance, as they were superseded by later ones.

(1) Whenever a coder decided a story contained Power Imagery according to Winter's criteria (see Appendix IV), he next decided whether the theme of the story involved primarily Exploitative Sex, Physical Aggression, or some other theme. Sub-categories in the Winter *n* Power coding system were then recorded as they occurred, under whichever type of power theme had been checked for the story as a whole. This separated the types of power imagery by primary intent rather than by specific image. For example, if a story centered on a seduction plot, all the power categories related to this theme were classified under Sex Power; and even though incidentally the hero might have hit someone in pursuit of the girl, the imagery was not counted under Physical Aggression. The purpose of keeping the three power-coding systems separate was to see if each of them, particularly the new Other Power themes, would increase after drinking.

Themes of Exploitative Sex were those in which sexual desires and activities were described, love and affection were not specifically mentioned, and the physical aspects of sex were at least suggested. Usually seduction, rape, going to bed with someone or some physical aspects of sex was mentioned (see Chapters 1 and 2). *General* sexual references (e.g., "they are having an affair") were not scored unless sexual activity was further elaborated.

Themes of Physical Aggression were scored in practically the same way as described in Chapters 1 and 2, with minor modifications described in Appendix I.

All other power themes were classified under Other Power.

(2) Sub-categories in various n Power coding systems (see Table 5.6) were classified as Strong or Weak (or neither) depending on their factor loadings reported in Chapter 5. That is, since Factor II scale scores correlated ($r = .16$) with the one measure of organized power available—namely, oflce-holding—sub-categories loading high on Factor II were classified as signifying a Strong or organized way of thinking about power. Analogously, Factor VI scores correlated ($r = .34$) most closely with drinking and other impulsive activities in the stud cluster. So types of power fantasies loading high on Factor VI were classified as indicating an impulsive power orientation and summed to get a Weak Power score. The exact way in which categories were classified, combined or omitted to get these two scores is described in Appendix I.

(3) As demonstrated in Chapter 7, classifying individuals simultaneously by their n Power and Activity Inhibition scores proved a good way of predicting average liquor consumption. Individuals with high n Power drank a lot if they were low in inhibition and much less if they were high in inhibition. It proved possible to derive empirically a code reflecting the differences in the *types* of power imagery used in writing stories by these two kinds of people. A full explanation of this new coding system and how it was constructed and cross-validated is given in Chapter 8. For the present, a general description of the two types of power orientations must suffice. The inhibited subjects produce power themes which are more often altruistic, that is, oriented toward exercising power *on behalf of others*—as in teaching, helping, etc. Furthermore they seem more cautious in thinking about power: ways of attaining power goals are more often specified (instrumental acts); actors doubt their ability to win; and so-called victories are often seen to be flawed, as in the Meaning Contrast stories reinterpreted above as involving Power Contrasts. These categories were summed and called socialized power or s Power; taken together they imply a type of power that is oriented toward social ends in a socially acceptable manner.

The uninhibited subjects, on the other hand, appear to think of power in more personalized or selfish terms. They describe power as a struggle between two opponents in which one must pursue his own interests in order to win out over the other. These categories were summed up and called personalized power or p Power; they imply a type of power that is used to promote personal goals.

Finally, to discover the usefulness of the category for predicting individual behavior, an Activity Inhibition score was obtained simply by counting the number of instances of the word *not* in the stories, in a fashion exactly parallel to the machine code used to get such a measure from the folk tales (Chapters 3 and 4). Contractions as in *wasn't* or *did'nt he* were not counted, as they less often signified inhibition of activity. Also a "purified" score was obtained in which *nots* were eliminated if they did not inhibit an activity—as in "he was not there." However, the purified score was not used in the final analysis because it was of lower frequency (and hence reliability), because it was not the same score as the one used in the folk-tale research and because it behaved more or less as the "impure" Activity Inhibition score did anyway.

All of the scoring systems described were learned by several coders and their agreement in scoring the same stories checked. Agreement coefficients on major categories such as presence of power imagery ranged around .90 to .93. On sub-categories which were scored at least 10 times, agreement coefficients ranged from .67 to .90 with medians ranging from .77 to .85, depending on the judges compared. In general, if judges could not be trained to agree on presence of a category at a level of .65 or higher, the category was abandoned or redefined.

All of the protocols from the drinking parties described in Chapters 1 and 2 were available. Samples of them were re-coded according to the various schemes just described to check out various specific hypotheses. Stories were also available from drinking parties for older men conducted in a working-class bar, as described in Chapter 7.

RESULTS

The first task is to determine whether fantasies of Sex and Aggression, when limited to those which were power-related, increased with drinking in the same way as they did when they were defined as Physical Sex and Physical Aggression. For comparative purposes, mean scores for the two ways of coding Sex and Aggression are presented together in Table 6.1 for the wet and dry fraternity parties described in Chapter 2. The mean scores for Physical Sex and Physical Aggression have been taken from Tables 2.3 and 2.4 to contrast with similar scores when the Sex and Aggression imagery is in a power-related context. Results for TAT II and TAT III have been summed; as noted in Chapter 2, the nature of these parties was such that not much more drinking occurred between TAT II and TAT III, so that these two sets of three stories each might as well be regarded as a more stable measure of whatever states of mind the subjects were in after the parties had been going on for an hour or so.

The results are encouraging. The new power-related Sex measure yields the same significant increase after drinking as the earlier Physical Sex measure. The Aggression Power score also increases after drinking, although the difference is not at a high level of significance—as in fact it was not when the stories were coded according to the earlier definition for Physical Aggression. The differences in mean levels is due to

Table 6.1—Effect of drinking on mean frequencies of Sex and Aggression imagery coded in two ways
(TAT$_{II}$ + TAT$_{III}$, 6 pictures)

Party condition, No Singer present	N	Average alcohol consumed	SEX		AGGRESSION	
			Physical[a] mean	Power-related[b] mean	Physical[a] mean	Power-related[b] mean
1. Apartment, dry	17	0.0	1.18	1.35	.47	2.30
2. Apartment, wet	27	4.8[c]	2.48	2.55	1.22	3.14
Drinking effect 2–1			+1.30	+1.20	+.75	+.84
p value, pd[d]			<.01	<.05	<.05	<.15

[a]Coding definitions as used in Chapter 2. Every reference to Physical Sex or Physical Aggression is counted in each story.

[b]Sum of all categories in Sex-related Power stories or Aggression-related Power stories (sub-totals 3 and 4 in Appendix Table 1.2).

[c]Ounces of 86-proof alcoholic beverage consumed during the period between TAT I and TAT II. Between TAT II and TAT III an average of 2.2 oz. was consumed.

[d]Predicted direction.

the fact that the Aggression Power code includes many sub-categories (see Appendix Table 1.2) such as High and Low Prestige, Actor failure, etc., whereas the Physical Aggression code counts only as many instances of actual Physical Aggression as occur in the stories.

These results were not unexpected, since the coding definitions were so similar. It is of more importance to determine whether the Meaning Contrast category can be shown to be power-related and whether alcohol increases types of Power Imagery beyond those reflected in the Sex and Aggression categories. To check whether Meaning Contrast stories were power-related, a tally was made for each story from three conditions according to whether it contained both types of imagery, one or the other, or neither. The three conditions were: apartment, dry, no singer ($N = 17$, three administrations of three stories each or 153 stories); apartment, wet, no singer ($N = 27$, 243 stories) and apartment, wet, singer ($N = 26$, 234 stories). Ninety-one out of these 630 stories were scored for Meaning Contrast. Of these 91 stories, 64 or 70 per cent were also scored for Power Imagery, indicating that over two-thirds of the Meaning Contrast stories involved Power themes of some kind. And in only three of these stories was the Power Imagery scored for a different section of the story from the one used to score Meaning Contrast. Of further interest is the way in which Meaning Contrast stories which were not scored as Power-related were affected by drinking. That is, it would be unfortunate not to score these stories by insisting on a power theme if they were the very ones that tended to increase most with drinking. To check this possibility, only the 477 stories from the two wet conditions were analyzed, as shown in Table 6.2. Sixty-five instances of Meaning

Table 6.2—Percentage of Meaning Contrast scores related and unrelated to Power occurring before and after drinking

	N	DISTRIBUTION OF INSTANCES OF THE SCORING CATEGORY	
		Before drinking TATII	After drinking TATII + TATIII
Meaning Contrast, no Power	18	44%	56%
Meaning Contrast, Power	47	21%	79%

$$\chi^2 = 3.4, \; p < .10$$

Contrast occurred in all these stories. But if we consider only those 18 that did not occur in power-related stories, they appeared to be almost as likely to occur before drinking as after, whereas a much higher proportion of the 47 power-related Meaning Contrast stories occurred after drinking. In other words, the Meaning Contrast stories appear to have greater validity as indicators of prior drinking if they are power-related. The result suggests that little will be lost by insisting that Meaning Contrast images be power-related and in fact that something might even be gained.

Three of the main fantasy effects of drinking previously identified —Sex, Aggression and Meaning Contrast—can apparently be re-defined in power-related terms without much loss of validity. That is, the redefined categories show much the same trends after drinking as the earlier categories.

However, a new and more significant question raised by the notion that drinking increases power concerns is this: *Do Other Power themes also increase after drinking?* In our earlier arousal studies, did we overlook the fact that not only thoughts of Physical Sex and Aggression (now seen as power-related) were increasing, but also other types of power-related thoughts, not involving sex and aggression at all? The increase in power-related Meaning Contrast images after drinking shown in Table 6.2 suggests that such might be the case, but a more direct test of the hypothesis is needed.

Unfortunately the studies of fraternity men reported in Chapters 1 and 2 are not ideal for checking the hypothesis, because the pictures used to elicit stories were not chosen with Other Power themes in mind. They were selected to get at themes of Sex, Aggression, and Meaning Contrast. Furthermore, in the Chapter 2 studies, the sets of pictures were not rotated before and after drinking; quite by chance, the set of pictures for TAT II contained cues that elicited more Other Power stories than the set for TAT I. Thus, any effects of drinking on Other Power themes was obscured by the fact that more Other Power themes were written by all subjects—even those in the dry conditions— to these pictures.

So the stories written by students participating in the large parties described in Chapter 1 were coded for Other Power themes. In this case the pictures were rotated across TAT administrations so that any variations in picture cues were equalized for stories written before and after drinking. Only the stories from TATs I and II were coded, because it was suspected that Other Power themes might increase maximally after smaller amounts of drinking and give way to Sex and Aggression Power themes after more drinking (as at TAT III). The mean Other Power Scores for TAT I and TAT II are summarized in Table 6.3 for random halves of the samples of students attending the

Table 6.3—Mean Other Power scores in fraternity parties (Chapter 1)

	N	TAT*I*	Mean oz. 86-proof beverage consumed	TAT*II*	Percent gaining 2 or more points	
Dry	19	1.21	0.0	.95	11%	$\chi^2 = 2.95$**, $p < .05$, pd.
Wet	18	1.78	7.2*	2.22	39%	
diff.		+.57		1.27		
t		—		1.92		
p		n.s.		<.05, pd.***		

*Estimated from average for total sample (see Table 1.1).
**Corrected for continuity.
***Predicted direction.

large dry and wet parties respectively. While the students in the two samples wrote stories at the outset with comparable amounts of Other Power in them, those students who subsequently drank alcohol filled their stories with significantly more Other Power themes at the second TAT administration than the students attending the dry party. Since the difference at the outset was in the same direction, it is perhaps more conservative to note that whereas only 11 per cent of the students at the dry party wrote TAT II stories two or more points higher in Other Power scores than their TAT I stories, 39 per cent of the students at the wet party gained two or more points in the Other Power scores. In short, this analysis supports the hypothesis that Other Power thoughts increase with drinking just as those of Sex and Aggression Power do. Or to put it another way, the increase in thoughts about power which occurs after drinking is not restricted to concern with Sex and Aggression Power. This is a genuinely new finding over what was reported in Chapters 1 and 2.

The power-scoring categories as explained above, were also partitioned into Strong and Weak Power sub-totals in an attempt to find scores which would predict heavy drinking. The question then arises whether these sub-totals are also increased by drinking. Table 6.4

Table 6.4—Effect of drinking on Strong and Weak Power sub-totals for TAT*II* + TAT*III*

	N	Average alcohol consumed	Weak Power	Strong Power
1. Apartment, dry	17	0.0	3.59	2.00
2. Apartment, wet	27	4.8[a]	5.41	1.44
Drinking effect 2–1			+1.82	−.56
p value			<.05	n.s.

[a]Between TATII and TATIII an average of 2.2 ounces of 86-proof alcoholic beverage was consumed.

provides a partial answer. The Weak Power sub-total is significantly higher in TATs written after drinking in the apartment setting described in Chapter 2. The Strong Power sub-total is insignificantly lower. Although one is tempted to conclude that drinking elevates negative or weak aspects of power fantasies more than strong or positive aspects, the interpretation is not that straightforward. As Appendix Table 1.2 suggests, more of the Weak categories are scored for Sex and Aggression Power and more of the Strong categories for Other Power. For example, in the bar study to be reported in the next chapter, when the theme of the stories was Sex or Aggression Power, an average of .96 Weak and .34 Strong categories were scored. When the stories dealt with an Other Power theme, an average of .84 Weak and 1.82 Strong categories were scored. Thus the results in Table 6.4 in a sense replicate and are not independent of those in Table 6.1, which showed Sex and Aggression Power to have increased after drinking in the apartment setting. As for the failure of the Strong Power sub-total to be larger after drinking in this study, one must remember that since the picture cues were not rotated and TAT II elicited a large number of Other Power themes, even in the dry condition, the measure may have been insensitive to possible changes in Strong or Other Power themes induced by drinking.

 As to determining which sub-score should be best for predicting drinking, the arousal studies are indeterminate. It can be argued that either a Sex and Aggression Power sub-total or a Weak Power sub-total might predict drinking, since both can be shown to increase after drinking.

 Findings reported in Chapter 8, however, show that neither sub-total in fact predicted drinking very well. Instead, a new way of partitioning the *n* Power score was more successful in differentiating the type of power imagery which was positively associated with heavy drinking from the type which was not. Particular care was devoted, therefore, to discovering how these two new types of power concerns were affected by increased amounts of drinking. Table 6.5 assembles data from two sources—the large fraternity cocktail party described in Chapter 1, in which picture cues were rotated, and the working-class bar study described in Chapter 7. In the former instance, two sets of stories were obtained after drinking (TAT II and TAT III) and in the latter only one set. As in Figure 1.1, a given subject might

Table 6.5—Frequencies of personalized and socialized power themes after consumption of increasing amounts of alcohol

ALCOHOL CONSUMED

	Light .1–3.9 oz. N = 8	diff.	Moderate 4–6 oz. N = 16	diff.	Heavy 6.1–12 oz. N = 24
mean p Power	.63	*	1.88		1.50
% 2 or more	13%		44%		50%
mean s Power	.38	*	1.94	*	.71
% 2 or more	0%	*	56%	*	17%
mean Power contrast	.00		.44		.13
% p > s Power	25%		31%		50%

B. Bar, older men

LIQUOR CONSUMED

	.05–.07 oz. N = 14		.08–13.9 oz. N = 13		over 14 oz. N = 12	Correlations with liquor consumed
mean n Power	5.14		5.08		8.50	.35 *
mean p Power	1.21		1.54		2.50 **	.30
% 2 or more	29%		38%		75% **	
mean s Power	1.64		1.69		1.42	−.15
% 2 or more	29%	+	54%	+	25%	
mean relative s Power	+.26		+.39		−.66	
% high[1]	36%	*	77%	*	33%	
% p > s Power	21%		23%		58%	
mean p-s Power	−.43		−.38		+1.08	.36 **

+$p < .10$ pd; *$p < .05$; **$p < .01$ for heavy minus light consumption
[1]Obtained s Power score (y) minus s Power score predicted on the basis of *n* Power score (x), where $y = .211x + .286$. Subjects relatively high include 17 who had a higher s Power score than predicted plus the next two smallest negative deviations from prediction.

appear in two means in Table 6.5 if he had had different amounts to drink before TAT II and TAT III. Some of the protocols from subjects who drank more than 12 oz. of 86-proof alcohol were missing and could not be recoded, but since they were shorter and the points they established more variable anyway (see Chapter 1), it seemed better to omit what scrappy information the remaining protocols could provide.

Personalized or p Power includes power stories in which the actor is after personal power and must contend with an opponent to get it. In the fraternity cocktail party, it first increased significantly as students drank more, and then levelled off. Although the mean shows a slight decrease with still higher drinking, it is belied by a slightly higher proportion of the subjects telling stories with two or more instances of p Power in them. In the bar study, where older men were involved, it was necessary to define light, moderate, and heavy drinking at higher levels, since these men were used to drinking more heavily and more often than the students were. In any case the p Power score increases steadily and significantly for the older men as they drank more, up to a median of around 17 oz. of 86-proof liquor consumed in the course of an hour and a half or so in a bar. The same trend appears for the total n Power scored, which correlates .35, $p < .05$ with amount of liquor previously consumed, although in the mean analysis, the effect is most marked in those who drank 14 or more oz.

By way of contrast the socialized or s Power score, reflecting more socialized power concerns, increases significantly with moderate drinking, in both samples, and then decreases significantly with still further drinking, again in both samples. In the bar study the effect reaches only marginal levels of significance for the raw s Power scores. The raw scores are partly determined, however, by their correlation with the total n Power score ($r = .45$, $p < .01$), which tends to rise significantly and linearly with amount of liquor consumed ($r = .35$, $p < .05$). What we are interested in is whether s Power rises or falls *relative* to the total n Power score. Two instances of s Power in a record scoring three on over-all n Power obviously has a very different meaning from two instances in a record scoring 13 on over-all n Power. So s Power scores were predicted from the n Power total on the basis of the regression equation relating the two variables and a corrected s Power score obtained which indicates whether it was high (positive deviation from regression line) or low *relative* to the amount of power concern expressed in the protocol. These relative scores increase significantly with moderate drinking and fall significantly with further drinking. The same correction could not be applied to the cocktail party scores because the total n Power measure was unavailable. In any case, the effect appeared clearly with the uncorrected scores.

What is particularly interesting about this finding is that it closely parallels the results for the Meaning Contrast category reported in Chapters 1 and 2, which also increased and then decreased with drinking. The s Power sub-total contains a Power Contrast category, redefinining Meaning Contrast in Power terms; and, as Table 6.5 shows, it behaves just like Meaning Contrast in the fraternity party— increasing with moderate drinking and then decreasing with heavy drinking.

What is particularly helpful about this finding is that it integrates the Meaning Contrast result into a more general theory. Previously it stood alone and was difficult to interpret as part of a Sentience or Inhibition syndrome. Now it appears to be part of a more general effect of moderate drinking, which is an increase in socialized or controlled power thoughts. To elaborate a little, the s Power categories suggest a power concern which is controlled by altruism (exercising power in behalf of others), by the realistic employment of instrumental activities, by realistic doubts about one's adequacy, and, last but not least, by irony or humor. Many of the stories scored for Meaning or Power Contrast after drinking involved absurd statements about exaggerated prowess, totally in contrast with reality, like the story of the young man who fell into a wheat thresher, got mangled, became a movie star and married Elke Sommer. These "typically alcoholic" fantasies are seen here as a form of power concern which is in fact checked or controlled by irony or obvious absurdity. With heavier drinking these s Power thoughts give way to more typically p Power concerns, and the world is seen as a jungle in which a man must fight to win over threatening opponents.

As Table 6.5 shows, s Power thoughts dominate at low levels of drinking, but at high levels of drinking the number of subjects for whom the p Power score is greater than the s Power score is notably higher. Thus if we combine the samples in Table 6.5, p Power is more frequent than s Power for 23 per cent of the light drinkers and 53 per cent of the heavy drinkers, a difference which is statistically significant ($\chi^2 = 5.1, p < .05$).

One other finding of interest turned up when we investigated the effects of drinking beer on fantasies. We were led to make this separate analysis by the discovery reported in Chapters 7 and 8 that heavy beer-drinkers do not have the same personality dispositions as heavy liquor-drinkers. So presumably drinking beer might have somewhat different effects on fantasy.

It does, as Table 6.6 shows. Even though only 11 men chose to drink beer, its effects can be shown to be significantly different from the effects of liquor drinking. The more beer consumed, the greater the *n* Power score, a finding which parallels the increase in *n* Power after drinking liquor. The orientation of the power concern, however, is quite different. Beer drinking increases s Power thoughts, while liquor drinking increases p Power thoughts. Thus the p-s standard score is very differently affected by drinking beer vs. drinking liquor. Heavier beer consumption decreases it (shifts it in an s Power direction), whereas heavier liquor consumption increases it (shifts it in a p Power direction). The difference between the two correlations with the *p-s* score ($r = -.40$ for beer and $+.36$ for liquor) is significant ($t = 2.05$, $p < .05$). Thus the hypothesis that beer and liquor drinking are differently related to motivational variables is confirmed, at least in this culture.

Table 6.6—Correlations of amount of beer and liquor consumed with subsequent power concerns

	Amount of beer consumed N = 11	Amount of liquor consumed N = 39
n Power	.78 **	.35 *
p Power	.05	.30
s Power	.58	−.15
p-s Power[1]	−.40	.36 *

*$p < .05$;   ** $p < .01$
[1] Difference between standard scores for p Power and s Power.

To return to the query with which these studies began, we now have a clearer idea of why so many people drink in moderation, in view of the fact that inhibitory thoughts do not seem to decrease much until drinking is heavier. Generally speaking, a few drinks seem to increase socialized power thoughts. More drinks shift these thoughts to a greater concern with personal dominance. Why? To begin with, one should recall that in these experiments the amount consumed is not varied independently of drinking history. So the shifts in power imagery just discussed may be due to personality differences between those who regularly drink a lot as contrasted with those who tend to drink little. Habitually heavy drinkers obviously drink more; in those studies the reported frequency of having four or more drinks correlated .45, $p < .01$ with amount consumed on this occasion. So any interpretation of the results must take into account not only the possible effects of alcohol *per se*, but also the personality characteristics of those who tend to drink more of it. These two possible determinants of the effects of drinking on power fantasies are studied separately in the next chapter. On the basis of findings reported there and general common sense, it seems reasonable to conceive of the fantasy effects of drinking as a joint product of stable personality dispositions interacting with expectations aroused by the situation and by the action of alcohol on the body, roughly following Atkinson's model (1957).

Physiologically, alcohol has short-term immediate effects on the body which produce sensations of increased strength: it is absorbed through the stomach wall directly so that it rapidly increases blood sugar and hence energy available; it stimulates in some degree the production of adrenalin which mobilizes the body for action; it produces vaso-dilation which increases sensations of bodily warmth; it blocks off debilitating sensations from aches and pains. (See Chapter 12.) All of these effects make the person feel temporarily stronger or more powerful. Such feelings may arouse or make more salient whatever power concerns a man has developed over his lifetime. His power concerns in turn interact with his characteristic level of inhibition or control and also with the cue value of the setting for power and for inhibition. If we leave aside for the moment individual differences in levels of power concern and inhibition (to take them up later in Chapter 7), we can outline how the situation influences the fantasies induced by alcohol as follows.

In normal settings, the physiological effects of drinking stimulate socialized power thoughts, which are here assumed to be pleasurable in the sense that men who are expected to be strong and assertive like to feel strong and assertive. This explains why people like to drink. The more inhibited the settings, the more power thoughts induced by drinking proceed along socialized lines. The evidence for this conclusion is somewhat indirect but fairly convincing. It consists in the first instance of the sole increase in the Meaning Contrast category reported in Chapter 1 for the most controlled discussion group; and, as we have noted, Meaning Contrast is essentially an s Power category. Further it consists of the evidence reported in Chapter 2 that Physical Sex increases less after drinking in an inhibiting classroom than in a relaxed apartment setting. Physical Sex is, as we have shown, nearly always Exploitative Sex, which by definition would be coded as part of p Power. Thus, we can infer that drinking in inhibiting settings tends to decrease p Power thoughts as it increases s Power thoughts.

If drinking continues to higher levels, it begins to reduce inhibitory thoughts like Time Concern and Fear-Anxiety. This in turn shifts power thoughts away from their initial socialized orientation (s Power) towards a less inhibited type of thinking about personal dominance (p Power). It will be recalled that the distinctions between s and p Power were originally derived by comparing the power orientations of more and less inhibited people. So it seems logical to interpret the shift from s to p Power after heavier drinking as being due to alcohol's known decrease in inhibitory thoughts at fairly high levels of consumption.

The exact nature of these shifts will obviously depend on the personality characteristics of the sample of men investigated, their usual level of alcohol consumption, and the nature of the setting in which they are drinking. But it seems clearly established that drinking increases primarily power thoughts of various types at the same time that at somewhat higher levels of consumption it is decreasing inhibitory thoughts.

RELATION OF TWO MEASURES OF INHIBITORY TENDENCIES TO DRINKING

Time Concern and Activity Inhibition, as noted in the introduction, appear to be tapping a similar inhibitory tendency since both have been shown to be associated with lower drinking. They have not, however, been used in the same study. Activity Inhibition is a code developed for the folk-tale study which correlates with a low drinking rating for a society, whereas Time Concern is a code developed for individual TATs; it decreases after drinking and tends to predict drinking at a low level of confidence. Although it proved difficult to find an exact analogue of the Time Concern code for the General Inquirer analysis of folk-tale content, it was easy to code individual TATs for Activity Inhibition, since the score consists essentially of the number of "nots" in the text. The question to be resolved then is: do the two measures of inhibition when applied to the same individual stories intercorrelate positively and predict low drinking equally well? A second related question is whether Activity Inhibition, like Time Concern, is decreased by drinking; that is, does drinking decrease both measures of inhibitory tendency in a like manner?

To answer these questions a sample of protocols from the studies reported in Chapter 2 was coded for Activity Inhibition and for Time Concern. The sample consisted of all subjects in the apartment, wet, no singer condition ($N = 25$) and subjects selected from the three other drinking conditions to represent those with heavy or light drinking histories (nine from the classroom, wet, no singer condition, nine from the classroom, wet, singer condition, and 15 from the apartment, wet, singer condition). That is, since we were not concerned to see how well each measure of inhibitory tendency would predict drinking history, it was considered desirable to include primarily those subjects with the largest differences in reported drinking habits as measured by the problem drinking score (see Kalin, 1964).

The first findings from this analysis came as something of a surprise. The presence of the folk singer while the first TAT stories were being written lowered the amount of Activity Inhibition in them.

Sixty-seven per cent of the students wrote stories with no instances, or only one instance of Activity Inhibition when the singer was present, as contrasted with 47 per cent of the students writing such stories when she was absent ($\chi^2 = 4.5$, $p < .05$). The effect of the singer on Time Concern was similar—50 per cent expressed none when she was present, 41 per cent when she was absent—but it was not significant. Consequently it seemed desirable not to include the subjects from the conditions with singer present because the Activity Inhibition expressed would not have the same diagnostic significance for individual differences in inhibition levels as it would when the singer was absent.

In Table 6.7 the two Inhibition scores are related to each other and to two measures of tendency to drink heavily when the singer was not present. It will be recalled that in a prior analysis of *all* the subjects in these studies (Chapter 2), the amount of Time Concern in stories written at the outset of a session is significantly related to low subsequent drinking on that occasion. In Table 6.6 this same trend appears, though at a lower level of significance than usual. In contrast, the Activity Inhibition score for these same protocols does *not* predict low subsequent drinking in the bar.

**Table 6.7—Relation of two Inhibition scores on TAT[i]
to each other and to drinking history and consumption
at bar (Parties with no singer present)**

	N	Drinking history % heavy drinkers[1]	Bar consumption % heavy drinkers[2]	Activity Inhibition % high (2 or more)
Time Concern				
High score (1 or more)	20	65%	40%	45%
Low score (0)	14	36%	57%	64%
χ^2		2.8*	1.0	1.3
Activity Inhibition				
High score (2 or more)	18	39%	50%	
Low score (1 or 0)	16	69%	44%	
χ^2		3.0*	.1	
Interaction χ^2		5.6**	.9	

$* = p < .10$ $** = p < .05$

[1]Anyone reporting that he drank at least 7 oz. of hard liquor on an average occasion or that he drank 6 oz. of hard liquor at least 4 days a week or that he drank at least 4 cans of beer on an average occasion. $N = 18$.

[2]Anyone who drank 6 oz. or more of 86-proof alcohol during the entire party on this occasion. $N = 16$.

Activity Inhibition, however, is associated ($p < .10$) with lower reported habitual drinking, a fact which seems to jibe with its association with low societal levels of drinking in the cross-cultural study. The association gains added credibility from a similar finding for a different group of subjects reported in Chapter 7, where it is demonstrated that men with more instances of Activity Inhibition in their protocols reported significantly less often that they were heavy drinkers. (See

Table 7.3.) In contrast, Time Concern is associated in the *opposite* way with drinking history in Table 6.7 so that the two measures appear not to tap the same inhibitory factor. The interaction chi-square is highly significant, indicating little chance that Activity Inhibition and Time Concern would ever relate to reported drinking history in the same way. As one would expect from these relationships, the two measures of inhibition tend to be inversely related to each other. While the levels of significance of some of these relationships are low, one conclusion seems inescapable: the two scores are *not* measuring the same inhibitory tendency. Time Concern appears to reflect the constraint a person feels on a particular occasion which controls his subsequent drinking on that occasion. In commonsense terms, if he is worried about time or under time pressure, he does not drink as much; he presumably wants to get on to something else. Time Concern is a measure of a situation-bound restraining tendency.

Table 6.8—Effects of drinking on Time Concern and Activity Inhibition (N = 58)

	TAT I		TAT II		p diff. TAT II-I	
	Time Concern	Activity Inhibition	Time Concern	Activity Inhibition	Time Concern	Activity Inhibition
Percent present	55%	67%	36%	59%	< .05	n.s.
Percent 2 or more		41%		29%		n.s.

	TAT III					
Percent present	34%	59%				
Percent 2 or more		22%				
p. diff.* TAT III-I						
presence	< .05	n.s.				
2 or more		< .05				

*Based on chi-square tests.

Activity Inhibition, in contrast, appears to be a measure of more stable individual differences in self-restraint under normal testing conditions; that is, it is a general measure of the tendency of the individual to restrain himself on a variety of occasions in a variety of situations. Thus it tends to go with lower reported average drinking. Apparently the general tendency to restrain oneself and the restraint felt in the experimental situation are simply uncorrelated so far as this sample is concerned.

Further evidence for this conclusion is provided in Table 6.8 which contrasts the effect of drinking in a party atmosphere on the two measures of inhibition. As expected from all previous analyses, Time Concern decreases significantly in TAT II or TAT III, after drinking, as compared with TAT I. Since the sets of TAT pictures were not rotated, it is possible that this decrease is due to the greater drawing power of TAT I for Time Concern rather than to the effect of drinking on TAT II and TAT III. Yet, the fact that both TAT II and TAT III produce less Time Concern than TAT I makes it less likely that the decrease could be due just to picture differences, especially in view of all the prior research showing a similar decrease when pictures are rotated. Though Activity Inhibition also tends to decrease somewhat, only one of the four tests of significance reaches the .05 level. Thus it is a good deal less certain that thoughts of Activity Inhibition tend to be diminished by alcohol. Further data reported below (see Table 7.5) support the inference that while drinking tends to decrease Time Concern, it does not significantly affect Activity Inhibition. Once again the simplest interpretation appears to be that getting caught up in a drinking party tends to diminish situation-bound time concerns (the person forgets what he was going to do), but does not affect basic personality differences in inhibition or restraint reflected in the Activity Inhibition measure.

Chapter 7

The Influence of Unrestrained Power Concerns on Drinking in Working-Class Men

by David C. McClelland and William N. Davis[1]

In Chapter 4 we reported that societies which drank a lot tended to fill their folk tales with themes of physical assertiveness and to mention inhibition of activity less often than other societies. In Chapter 5 the need for power in individual fantasies was found to be related to heavy drinking in college students; it was inferred that folk-tale themes of assertiveness might better be conceptualized as part of a syndrome of thoughts and actions expressing a concern with power. This lead was followed up in Chapter 6, where it was demonstrated that in fact drinking increases power thoughts, and at higher levels of consumption decreases retraining thoughts. So it is possible that the results obtained in the cross-cultural study may merely reflect the fact that heavy-drinking societies are more likely to tell their folk tales while drinking; hence their collective fantasies (folk tales) may show the same effects of alcohol consumption that individual fantasies do.

There is, however, another possibility that also needs to be

[1]We are grateful to Mal Slavin, John Muller, Robert Stolorow, Steve Tulkin, and Robert Aylmer for helping carry out this study, and to Krayna Tulkin for secretarial assistance.

investigated. Individuals who have a heightened need for power and a low level of inhibition may for some reason consume more alcohol. Unrestrained assertiveness may be a cause as well as an effect of drinking. If it is, the question naturally arises as to how the cause and the effect interact. Why would people with high levels of unrestrained power thoughts tend to drink more in order to increase their unrestrained power thoughts? Do such individuals react in some special way to alcohol—a reaction which leads them to drink more often? And more heavily?

These are the questions which the present chapter attempts to answer. The investigation will parallel closely at the individual level the study of cultures reported in Chapter 4. Here, as there, we will be concerned with finding out whether individuals who drink heavily, like societies that drink heavily, are found predominantly among those whose fantasies show a high concern for power and a low incidence of inhibition. The critical difference is that at the individual level, cause and effect can be separated and their interaction studied. One can collect the fantasies of men when they are not under the influence of alcohol, and relate them to the individual's characteristic level of alcohol consumption. Then those same individuals can be tested after some social drinking to see how their fantasies have been affected. In this way we can not only study the effects of alcohol on the fantasies of persons who differ in their characteristic levels of the expression of power and restraint, but we can also see if the fantasies are in some way different for individuals who report that they characteristically drink heavily. One of the obvious points of interest here is the possibility that the findings may give us insight into why some people become alcoholic. Is there a peculiar combination of predisposition and effect that leads some individuals to drink more often and heavily?

To get a sample of heavy or problem drinkers, we chose to work with older men and to measure the effects of drinking in a "working-class" bar. There are, to be sure, problem drinkers among college students, and these problem drinkers are likely to grow up to be alcoholics (see Chapter 10). But it seemed desirable to work with a sample of older men whose drinking habits had become stabilized and whose reported consumption would be less influenced by youthful exuberance or experimentation. Older men of an upper-middle-class background, however, like the college students, do not frequently go to all-male drinking parties; characteristically they go to cocktail parties at which both sexes are present. Thus it was necessary to conduct our research in a working-class bar where men still habitually drink socially in the evenings with other men. The reason for leaving women out of the picture is apparent from the findings reported in Chapter 2: their presence simply complicates the results, which are already difficult enough to understand. Working with men from a lower-class background was not only a practical necessity; it also had an advantage. It gave us the opportunity to see whether the results obtained with college students would also characterize males differing in habits, values and attitudes, and drinking under conditions quite different from the weekend fraternity cocktail parties studied previously. Some theorists argue that people get out of drinking whatever they expect they ought to get out of it. It could be argued, therefore, that the unrestrained assertiveness we have found to characterize the thinking of college students is precisely what one would expect to find in fraternity cocktail parties, which indeed may be organized to promote such an atmosphere. Would the effects be the same in a working-class bar? And would the same type of person drink heavily under the two conditions?

PROCEDURE

Recruitment of Subjects

In order to obtain adult male subjects it was decided to post a notice in an employment agency. The notice explained, essentially, that the authors of the present study were interested in studying the effects of a barroom atmosphere on average people; that people who participated would be paid $15 for spending a few hours in a bar drinking at a normal rate, and telling a few imaginative stories.

Unfortunately the initial attempt to obtain subjects was completely unsuccessful. Within a week's time only a few men had expressed any interest in the notice. As a result it was decided to place an advertisement in a newspaper. The ad ran for two days and read: "Work in the evening and make $15.00. About three hours of interesting work participating in a psychological study. Must be between 25 and 55. Call _____."

In contrast to the original attempt, placing an ad in the paper resulted in a deluge of phone calls and interested parties. A receptionist received most of the calls and explained in detail the nature of the study. It was specifically mentioned that the study involved the use of alcohol and that it would take place in a barroom. If the caller was a man between 25 and 55 and he expressed an interest in participating after the study was described, he was asked a number of biographical questions. These included: name; age; occupation; education; marital status. Had he ever been hospitalized for any physical or mental illness? In general, did he think he was in good health? Was he currently being treated, or had he ever been treated for alcoholism?

Potential subjects were excluded for any previous hospitalization for an illness which could be exacerbated by drinking (e.g., diabetes), for psychiatric reasons, or for being currently in treatment for alcoholism or a member of Alcoholics Anonymous. However, if someone had received some treatment in the past but was *not* now, and *not* now a member of Alcoholics Anonymous, and *was* now drinking, he was accepted. The goal was to include as many problem drinkers as we could without running risks of harming the subjects in any way through an evening spent in normal drinking in the type of bar most of them were accustomed to frequenting.

When a potential subject was screened and found acceptable, he was told to report to a local employment agency (the same one where the initial notice had been posted) between 7:00 and 8:30 on an evening determined in advance. As enough subjects became available for one experimental session, other acceptable subjects were told to report to the employment agency at a later date in preparation for the next experimental session, and so on until a sufficient number of applicants had been selected.

There were several exceptions to this general method of obtaining subjects. They occurred when someone heard about the study and came directly to the employment agency to inquire. If a place was available and if the brief biographical screen did not present any difficulties, he was accepted.

Explaining and Carrying Out the Drinking Sessions

When subjects arrived at the employment agency, they were met by one of the authors (W.D.) and by the agency proprietor. They were then asked to fill out an "Activities Questionnaire" which contained items referring to behavior found to be related to drinking and to power concerns (cf. Chapters 5 and 8, Appendix II) and items referring to drinking behavior (see below).

When subjects had completed the "Activities Questionnaire," the nature of the study was fully explained to them again, and they were given an opportunity to ask questions. At the time, particular emphasis was placed on the imaginative stories they were to tell. Every subject was shown a TAT picture (one not used in the present study). It was explained carefully what kinds of stories he was expected to tell: imaginative, dramatic ones that included something about who the characters are, what led up to the situation, what the characters were thinking, what they wanted, and what would happen. Subjects were also told that they would have only to tell their stories, not write them, because assistants of the experimenter would be there to write down what they said.

Methods for payment and for transportation to and from the bar were then discussed. Subjects had to agree to accept in payment a check dated the day after they came to the bar, and they had to agree to accept a cab ride to their home at the conclusion of the session. The latter rule meant they could not drive their own cars to the bar. Both these conditions were emphasized in an attempt to prevent any complications arising from subjects becoming intoxicated at the bar. By dating their checks the next day, we made it difficult for them to leave the bar, cash their checks and continue drinking that night. By requiring that they accept a cab ride home, we made certain that they would not be driving while intoxicated or otherwise running risks of getting into trouble after the drinking session.

Subjects had to pay for their own transportation to the bar. However, the drinks they had and the cab fare home were paid by the experimenters. In addition, they received a check for $15 for participating in the study.

At the conclusion of the preparatory session in the employment agency, subjects were told where the bar was and when they were to come to it, and were asked to sign a voluntary participation sheet. Without exception, the experimental session in the bar was held the night after subjects came to the employment agency. They were asked to arrive at 8:00 and were told that the study would run until about 10:00. The voluntary participation sheet restated what each subject was expected to do while participating in the study. It declared that a subject had no reservations about what he was expected to do, and that he was not currently in treatment for alcoholism or trying to refrain from drinking.

The bar in which all the experimental sessions were held was located five or six blocks from the employment agency on a busy street. It might be characterized as an average working-class bar. It was not a cocktail lounge, nor was it a "seedy" establishment. The bar contained two rooms, one with a long bartop, bar stools, a television set, and a pin ball machine, and one with a large number of tables and booths. All the experimental sessions began in the latter room although subjects were free to pass from one room to another, watch TV or mingle with the other customers if they chose to do so.

The experimenter paid between three and five assistants, depending on the number of subjects expected, to help him during the experimental sessions. Generally speaking, there was one assistant for every two subjects. All of the assistants were graduate students in clinical psychology well versed in the administration of the Thematic Apperception Test (TAT).

As subjects arrived at the bar for an experimental session they were introduced one by one to an assistant who was free at the time. Each assistant then took the subject to whom he had been introduced to a relatively isolated part of the room. After a few minutes of small talk, he asked the subject to tell stories to a special set of four pictures (TAT I), using the standard TAT instructions to tell an imaginative story with a beginning, a middle, and an end. The assistant wrote the stories down as they were told. As soon as he had completed administering a TAT, he went back to the experimenter to see if any more testing was necessary. Usually each assistant tested two subjects. The room in which the TATs were administered was typically deserted at this point in the evening.

Just before the subject told his last story, a waitress took orders for drinks. The waitress was paid to record how many and what kind of drinks the subjects ordered. The drinks were made at the bar and served exactly as they were for any other customer.

When the pre-drinking TAT was completed, the subjects were allowed to drink whatever they wanted and as much as they wanted and to do whatever they pleased. That is, they were free to talk among themselves, watch television, play pin ball, or talk to other customers. The understanding was that they were to behave as they normally would on such an occasion. The drinking period lasted approximately an hour and a half. During this time the bar typically became somewhat crowded with perhaps 20 or 25 people by the bar itself and another five or 10 in the adjoining room.

At about 9:45 they told more stories to a second set of four pictures (TAT II), again under standard instructions. For the most part, experimental assistants tested the same subjects they had previously. A last call for drinks was made just after the story-telling began, and after that no more drinks were served.

Shortly after TAT II was completed for all the subjects, two, or if necessary three, cabs were called and all the subjects were placed in them on a pre-determined basis, according to the geographical location of their homes. One assistant rode with each cab and was responsible for paying the driver at the end of the trip.

A day or so after each experimental session the subjects who participated in that session were mailed a "Situation Questionnaire," along with a letter of thanks for their help with the project. The Situation Questionnaires contained questions referring to the subjects' experience while in the bar. They were asked, in an open-ended way, whether the bar they were in for the study was similar to the kind of bar in which they typically drank; whether they drank the same kind and amount of liquor that they usually drank; whether they talked to others as much as they normally did; whether they acted as they normally would; whether they felt about the same as they normally do when drinking in a bar. All these questions were intended to get some

themes related to power motivation, since by this time it was hypothe-sized that many of the earlier findings concerning the effects of alcohol on fantasy could be subsumed under a general concern for power. Two of the pictures in each set suggested stories about sex and aggres-sion respectively; two others dealt with more general power-related themes. The pictures and related themes are described in Table 7.2, and reproduced in Appendix VII.

Table 7.2—Power-related themes sampled by relevant pictures in TAT*I* and TAT*II*

A. BAR *I* (*N* = 50)

Power-related Themes		Relevant pictures	
	TAT*I*		TAT*II*
Authority impact	Prominent man talking to re-porters on board a ship		Army officer apparently in-structing subordinates
Exploitative sex	A businessman eyeing his sec-retary's legs as he dictates		Couple in a night club
Aggression	"Mad scientist" peering at test tube in a strange light		Boxer, shadow boxing
Prestige supplies	Nicely dressed businessman walking past a poorly dressed man who is looking at him		Working-class man eyeing a Cadillac parked on the street
n Power mean		4.72	6.14
SD		4.61	4.02
p Power mean		1.08	1.62
SD		1.24	1.47
s Power mean		1.30	1.40
SD		1.74	1.55

Note: The order of presentation of pictures was scrambled within but not across sets.

B. BAR *II* (*N* = 108)
Same pictures as TAT*I* for Bar *I*

n Power mean		3.80
SD		3.29
p Power mean		1.23
SD		1.41
s Power mean		.93
SD		1.38

See Appendix VII for picture reproductions.

Pictures were randomly presented within sets to eliminate any peculiar serial position effects which might overshadow the influence of the alcohol variable. The sets of pictures (TAT I and TAT II) were given to all subjects in the same order in Bar I and were not counter-balanced because it was feared that they would be seriously uneven in pulling power for various themes. In that case set variance might outweigh the variance attributable to individual differences in drinking history. Primary interest, in short, was not in the effects of alcohol on fantasy, but in the way individuals with different drinking histories responded to the same pictures after drinking. The first TAT was designed to give a measure of individual differences on the power/inhibition dimensions under dry conditions rather than a "before" measure with which an "after" measure could be directly compared.

The stories were typed on separate sheets which were coded on the back for TAT set, picture, sequence within set, tester and date. All sheets were then scrambled and coded "blind" by several scorers who did not know the conditions under which the TAT was obtained. Percentage agreement among the coders for the same stories ran between 86–95 percent for the more frequent categories and between 40–100 percent for the infrequent categories. The scoring systems of major concern for this chapter are the personal and social power systems mentioned in Chapter 6 and derived in Chapter 8; the Activity Inhibition score, which is simply the number of "nots" in the protocol, as in the folk-tale study; and the n Power score. The latter was a revised version of the n Power score used by Winter in Chapter 5. It was based on a re-analysis and integration of the results from all the power arousal studies and is fully described elsewhere (Winter, 1968). Correlation between n Power scores obtained by two different coders from the same individual records was .90.

RESULTS

Table 7.3 presents the correlations between the drinking variables and the power and inhibition codes, considered singly. They are not strongly encouraging. In the first bar study the n Power score correlates significantly only with the quantity/frequency index for drinking liquor. n Power is certainly not associated with amount of beer consumed on an average occasion, and the correlation with the amount of wine consumed on an average occasion is even slightly negative. Nor does it predict consumption of liquor at the bar in the experimental social drinking party. In the second bar study all of the n Power correlations with the drinking variables are small and insignificant, though some slight reassurance might be extracted from the fact that its relationship to the quantity/frequency liquor index is in the right direction. The Activity Inhibition code fares somewhat better. Rather consistently, it is negatively associated with the frequency and quantity of drinking measures in the two studies, although only for liquor and not for beer. Finally Time Concern is of little or no predictive value. It even relates to quantity of liquor and wine consumed on an average occasion positively. Once again its status as a variable indicating an immediate situational concern is confirmed by the negative though insignificant correlation with amount of liquor consumed at the bar.

$-.08$

3 .23
.16+ .07

.02
.06 .05

.22

$-.13$

: or more often vs. all others.

.t the start of a party
ʒ.
er and wine drinking
that fantasy related to
to do with drinking these
is actually related *positively*
atively* to the *n* Power score.
edicted by any combination of

ing, however, is at least in the
ies, particularly for the quantity-
ng. Thus it becomes of particular
ble classification of individuals by
/ that the heavy drinkers are dis-
those whose protocols are high in
Inhibition frequency, as was the

parallel the presentation for the
lts are surprisingly similar. For
dian in *n* Power, the Activity
es in determining who will be a
low the median in *n* Power, like
Activity Inhibition score makes
e shows, the individuals in the
re higher on the frequency and

/

**High
(4 or**

Low

*Quan
a week (s
[1]Frequer
year; 3 =
scale app'
[2]Quant
4 = 6–8 d

quantity
other thre
whom we
index. In th
in the high
drinkers on q
three quadrant
or 17 percent. 1
fact, the proporti

quadrant is significantly larger than the next highest proportion of heavy drinkers—in the low-power/low-inhibition quadrant, which also contained the next largest proportion of heavy-drinking cultures in the folk-tale study.

In the study of individuals in Bar I there is an inhibition effect which is significant regardless of the power score; individuals with a high activity inhibition score are much less likely to be classified as heavy drinkers regardless of their power score. This is confirmed by the significant negative correlation in Table 7.3 between Activity Inhibition and the QF index. In the second bar study the inhibition effect is somewhat less marked, but is significant in the predicted direction (see Table 7.3). In general the proportion of heavy drinkers in Bar II, as we have already indicated, was significantly less than in Bar I; thus the relationships, while the same as those in Bar I, are somewhat attenuated. The major finding is the same—namely that the percentage of heavy drinkers in the high-power/low-inhibition quadrant is significantly greater than in the other three quadrants (30 percent vs. 10 percent, $\chi^2 = 6.83$, $p < .01$). This strongly confirms the hypothesis, derived from the folk tale study, that unrestrained assertiveness characterizes individuals, like cultures, that tend to drink a lot. And the finding cannot here be interpreted as being due to the effects of drinking on fantasy. It should be recalled that, especially in the second bar study, the fantasy protocols were collected in an employment agency, on an entirely different occasion from the one in which some of the subjects drank in the bar. Thus we would appear to be justified in concluding that people who characteristically think a lot about power and little about restraint are likely to drink liquor heavily. But not beer: using the same QF index, the proportions of heavy beer-drinkers in the high-power/low-inhibition quadrant vs. all others are 36 percent vs. 33 percent in Bar I, 37 percent vs. 35 percent in Bar II.

But why should high-power/low-inhibition people drink a lot of liquor if drinking produces the very state of mind which seems to characterize them generally even when they are not drinking? This in turn raises the further question of whether drinking does something special to the fantasies of heavy liquor-drinkers as compared with the fantasies of more normal drinkers. In an attempt to answer, we classified the individuals in the first bar study on the basis of their reported drinking history into three groups—the heavy drinkers referred to in Table 7.4; moderately heavy drinkers who drank fairly heavily but rarely, or frequently but lightly; and light drinkers who drank very little and not very often. Included in the analysis were only those 39 men who drank liquor during the social evening in the bar, since we were specifically interested in what liquor did for people with heavy drinking histories. All of our data to date have suggested that wine and beer drinking appear to have a somewhat different psychological significance.

Table 7.5 presents the means for various types of power and inhibition imagery for men with different drinking histories both before and after drinking in the bar. Unfortunately direct comparison of mean scores of TAT I and TAT II is not meaningful, because different picture cues were used on the two occasions and the sets of pictures were not rotated. It is possible, however, to get some idea of the effects of drinking on the thoughts of men with different drinking histories by comparing the differences in the percentage of men with different histories who shift up or down after drinking. For instance, while the

Table 7.5—Mean frequencies of Power and Inhibition themes before and after drinking[1] for men varying in drinking history

| | | DRINKING HISTORY: QF INDEX | | | |
		Light[2] (N=11)	Moderate[3] (N=14)	High[4] (N=14)	r with H vs. ML[5]
average bar consumption		8.1 oz.	11.7 oz.	12 oz.	
n Power	TAT$_I$	4.45	4.07	6.07	.30*
	TAT$_{II}$	5.45	5.93	7.00	.18
	% gaining	55%	57%	57%	
p Power	TAT$_I$	.72	.71	1.71	.44**
	TAT$_{II}$	1.00	1.50	2.57	.36*
	% gaining	27%	64%	64%+	
s Power	TAT$_I$	1.18	1.07	1.07	.10
	TAT$_{II}$	1.73	1.35	1.71	.16
	% gaining	36%	36%	36%	
Activity Inhibition	TAT$_I$	4.73	2.43	1.43	−.34*
	TAT$_{II}$	2.82	3.14	2.50	−.11
	% losing	63%	21%	21%++	
Time Concern	TAT$_I$	2.09	2.36	2.00	.23
	TAT$_{II}$	1.73	.86	1.43	
	% losing	45%	79%	50%	

*$p < .05$ **$p < .01$
+χ^2 H vs. L = 3.4 $p < .10$ ++χ^2 H vs. L = 4.8 $p < .05$
[1]Only those drinking liquor on this occasion.
[2]Men reporting they usually had up to 2 drinks, 2–4 times a month or 3–5 drinks less than once a month.
[3]Men reporting they usually had 3–5 or more drinks up to 2–4 times a month or up to 2 drinks 2–3 times a week or more often.
[4]Men reporting they usually had 3–5 or more drinks 2–3 times a week or more often.
[5]Dichotomous correlation of fantasy scores produced by men with a heavy [H] drinking history vs. all others (those with moderate or light [ML] drinking histories).

men with heavy drinking histories are considerably higher in *n* Power before drinking, no greater proportion of them gained in *n* Power after drinking than of those with a light-drinking history. Some kind of ceiling effect may of course be operating here. It may be easier for those with a light-drinking history to gain in an *n* Power score because they start so much lower in *n* Power.

of their own free will to drink varying amounts on this occasion, despite differences in drinking history. Thus, the effects of drinking history could be studied with drinking controlled, and vice versa, as shown in Table 7.6. This table gives the mean *n* Power scores after drinking for the four categories of men formed by the double classification. The number of cases is small in each cell, and it was not possible to include any really light drinkers, because too few of them drank enough on this

Table 7.6—Effect of drinking history and alcohol consumed on total n Power scores in TATII

| Drinking history | LIQUOR CONSUMED PRIOR TO TATII | | mean n Power |
	Moderate 08–13.9 oz.	Heavy 14–20 oz.	
Moderate[1]	$N = 4$ mean $= 4.8$	$N = 6$ mean $= 7.0$	6.1
Heavy[2]	$N = 7$ mean $= 4.7$	$N = 5$ mean $= 9.6$	6.8
Mean *n* Power	4.7	8.2	
% scoring 6 or more	27%	82%	

$$\chi^2 = 6.8, \, p < .01$$

[1]Men reporting they usually had 3–5 or more drinks up to 2–4 times a month or up to 2 drinks 2–3 times a week or more often.
[2]Men reporting they usually had 3–5 or more drinks 2–3 times a week or more often.

occasion to provide a group matched in this respect to heavier drinkers. Yet the results seem fairly clear and informative. From an inspection of the row means in Table 7.6, it appears that *drinking history*, independent of amount consumed, has no effect on *n* Power score after drinking. On the other hand, the amount of liquor consumed markedly increases the *n* Power score, as already noted in Table 6.5, but now we can observe that this effect is independent of drinking history.

So far as the p Power score is concerned, both determinants appear to have an independent effect. Table 7.7 reports an analysis of variance for the p Power scores corrected for disproportionate subclass numbers. As the column and row means show, drinking history has an effect regardless of consumption level, and amount of liquor consumed has an effect regardless of drinking history, although it is significant only at the 10 percent level. These findings support the conclusion drawn from Table 7.5 that heavy drinkers not only have higher power scores to start with, but that after drinking they show an even greater tendency to see power relationships in egoistic terms—one man must win out over another in order to survive or extend his influence. This is true not only because they tend to drink more, but also independently of the amount they consume. Thus we are now in a position to say that the significantly greater increase in p Power score after heavy drinking reported in Table 6.5 is determined (1) by the greater amount of liquor consumed and (2) by the fact that those who drink more have a personality disposition in which drinking accentuates the p Power score, independently of the amount consumed.

Certainly the interaction effect of drinking history and consumption level is fairly strong, although it does not reach an accepted level of significance. The five customarily heavy drinkers who also drank a great deal on the present occasion had the very high mean p Power score of 3.40. Since heavy drinkers by definition normally do drink more, it is obvious that they will continually get themselves into states of mind in which their p Power thoughts are elevated in frequency. On the other hand, drinking history has no notable effect on *n* Power scores independent of amount consumed (see row means, Table 7.7).

Table 7.7—Effect of drinking history and alcohol consumed on mean p Power scores in TAT_{II}

Drinking history	LIQUOR CONSUMED PRIOR TO TAT_{II}		
	Moderate 08–13.9 oz.	Heavy 14–20 oz.	Mean p Power
Moderate[1]	N = 4 mean = .75	N = 6 mean = 1.83	1.40
Heavy[2]	N = 7 mean = 2.00	N = 5 mean = 3.40	2.58
mean p Power	1.55	2.55	

F value for drinking history = 4.63 $p < .05$
F value for consumption level = 3.69 $p < .10$
F value for interaction = 1.83 $p < .20$

[1]Men reporting they usually had 3–5 or more drinks up to 2–4 times a month or up to 2 drinks 2–3 times a week or more often.
[2]Men reporting they usually had 3–5 or more drinks 2–3 times a week or more often.

Since total *n* Power goes up with heavier drinking, and since s Power correlates significantly ($r = .45$, $p < .01$) with total *n* Power score, it would be difficult to find a hypothesized decrease in s Power themes, as already noted. That is, since there are more power themes of all sorts after heavier drinking, the *opportunity* to tell an s Power story increases. But the question to be answered is whether a person takes advantage of the opportunities to tell an s Power story less often after heavy drinking than after light drinking. To find out if this is so, it is necessary to use the regression equation to predict the expected s Power score based on a given total *n* Power score, then to calculate whether the obtained s Power score is above or below what is expected for a given level of *n* Power. Table 7.8 presents the results of this analysis for the same sample of men.

Clearly the men who drink more have s Power scores which are significantly more often below what they would be predicted to be on the basis of their total *n* Power scores, whereas those who drink more

Drinking in the Wider Context of Restrained and Unrestrained Assertive Thoughts and Acts

by David C. McClelland, Eric Wanner, and Reeve Vanneman[1]

Ever since the factor analysis of folk-tale themes reported in Chapter 4, evidence has repeatedly cropped up suggesting that there are two types of power thoughts which ought to be distinguished. One generally is associated with low inhibition or impulsivity. In the folk-tale study it was represented by such categories as Entering Implements (spear, arrow), Eating, and Violent Physical Manipulation (cut, chop). The other type of power imagery, associated with high levels of Activity Inhibition, was represented by a set of categories suggesting organization or planning, such as Capability, War, and Scheduling. These two types of power imagery we relabelled Impulsive and Effective Power Concerns, respectively.

Since heavy drinking was clearly associated with Impulsive Power, we have made several attempts to get measures of these two types of power concerns at the individual level. The first attempt was based on

[1]This chapter in particular has been the product of nearly everyone associated with the project. The names listed as authors include those responsible for most of the analyses and interpretations of data. We are particularly grateful to Nicholas McClelland, Mary Thomas, Ross Goldstein, and Dan Goleman for recoding the TATs according to the various schemes described.

picking out those power themes which were associated with impulsive assertive activities, like drinking, in contrast to the more socialized ones like office holding, in the study of college students reported in Chapter 5. Since the categories associated with the Impulsive Power or "stud" cluster of assertive activities seemed to be more negative (low prestige, actor failure, etc.), we labelled their sum the Weak Power sub-score. The sum of the remaining categories like High Prestige and Instrumental Activity was labelled the Strong Power sub-total. See Appendix I for exactly how these two scores were obtained.

The second method of partitioning the n Power categories was described in Chapter 6. It arose out of our effort to discover whether drinking affected not only concerns with sex and aggression but other power concerns as well. It seemed logical to partition n Power scores not by sub-category but by the total thematic content of a story. If the story had to do with sex or aggression primarily, all sub-categories coded in it were thrown into what might be referred to as an Id Power score, and if not, they were summed to get an Other Power score. The distinction seemed to fit the folk-tale factor analysis fairly well; certain aggressive folk-tale themes like *cut* and *chop* belonged in the Impulsive Power quadrant, whereas Other Power themes (with the exception of war) seemed to predominate in the Effective Power quadrant (e.g., scheduling, capability). It also made theoretical sense if one could think of Sex and Aggression Power concerns as a more primitive type of assertiveness, developmentally speaking, which gradually became more socialized with age into what we were calling Other Power concerns.

Neither of these methods of partitioning the power-scoring system, as we shall see in a moment, turned out to be very useful for predicting which type of people would drink a lot or engage in more socialized types of power activity. Thus it became necessary to develop still a third method of distinguishing two types of power concerns. The clue as to how to proceed was provided by the findings reported in Chapter 7 showing that among individuals, as among societies, those high in power concerns drank heavily if they scored low in Activity Inhibition, but not if they scored high in Activity Inhibition. Why not try to discover directly how the power concerns of these two types of individuals differed? It might be possible to identify which types of power themes led to heavy drinking and which types did not. Then one could check further to see if the two types of power concerns so determined would have any more general utility in predicting a broader range of activities which people engage in.

The procedure we followed was simple. Two sets of stories told by men to the first group of pictures in Bar I were selected for comparison. The first set of stories were written by individuals who scored above the

sign that the individual writing such a story had an impulsive power orientation.

The same is not true of another category—Zero sum conflict—which appeared promising in Sample 1. It does not appear appreciably more often in the records of those low in Activity Inhibition in the two cross-validation samples. So Zero sum conflict was discarded from the set of categories originally diagnostic of impulsive power concerns.

The only other category that appeared more commonly in the records of those low in Activity Inhibition was what is labelled Opponent block in Table 8.1. To receive a score for this category, stories had to picture someone in a power struggle with identified specific other persons (or forces) who were trying to defeat him. In a sense this is only a slight modification of the Zero sum conflict story in which it is made clear that if one person wins, the other must lose. The Opponent block category is more general in the sense that there is still a power struggle between two people described, but it may not be made clear that the outcome is zero-sum. While the mean difference is in the wrong direction for Sample 1, the correlation with Activity Inhibition is negative, as it should be, and the cross-validations in Samples 2 and 3 are strongly in the predicted direction. Thus the p Power score consists of the sum of instances in which the power goal is personalized and in which assertive attempts are carried out against the active opposition of an adversary.

Cross-validation for the four categories which make up the socialized power code was more consistent, as shown in Table 8.1. In all three samples, those with scores high in Activity Inhibition described power more often in socialized terms, mentioned more often that the proponent may have some weaknesses in himself, specifically described instrumental acts relevant to attaining power, and mentioned that power is flawed or deceptive, or treated it ironically (power contrast). The full descriptions of these scoring categories are given in Appendix IV.

The over-all picture that the s Power scoring system suggests is of a type of power concern which is more socialized, in the sense that it is expressed in terms of plans, self-doubts, mixed outcomes and concern for others. As the figures at the bottom of Table 8.1 show, the total s Power score is significantly associated with the Activity Inhibition score in both Bar Study I and Bar Study II, as indeed it should be, considering how it was derived. The total p Power score is significantly less associated with Activity Inhibition, though the correlation is significantly *negative* only in Bar Study II. The total *n* Power score, which is coded independently of the p and s Power scores, seems to have a slight positive correlation with Activity Inhibition in both studies, although this may be due to the fact that both scores have a positive correlation with length of the story. (See Table 8.2.)

The two new "faces" of power as represented by the p and s Power scoring systems seem to have some promise, at least to the extent that they distinguish between power themes written by inhibited and uninhibited people. What is perhaps surprising about the nature of these coding systems is that the primary distinction is not between impulsive vs. controlled power but between a "personalized" vs. a "socialized" power concern. That the distinction between these two types of records would take this form was not predicted, but it is theoretically interesting, and we looked forward with some interest to seeing whether it would in fact enable us to predict what types of assertive activities people would engage in.

First, however, it is worth examining the pattern of intercorrelations among the different ways of partitioning *n* Power scores. Four interesting points emerge from the intercorrelation matrix provided in Table 8.2.

1. Correlations with protocol length are generally positive but so low that it seemed unnecessary to make any corrections in the power sub-scores for those who produced longer or shorter stories.

2. The Sex Power sub-total is *negatively* related with the Aggression Power sub-total and the Other Power sub-total. Even the Aggression Power sub-total is not significantly positively correlated with the Other Power sub-total. How can we contend that these are all measures of the same power drive system? Shouldn't we think instead of three independent power drives?

While this method of partitioning the power coding system was ultimately abandoned, the question raised by the lack of relationships among these three sub-scores proved to be an interesting theoretical one. For it occurred to us that one possible explanation for the lack of relationships might be that if a person started telling one type of power story—centering, let us say, on violence and robbery—he was by definition in this scoring scheme unable to get credit for power categories under either of the other two sub-totals. (See Appendix Table 1.2.) But there was still the problem of demonstrating that the different sub-scores might legitimately be considered to tap the same power drive. The only way to find out if this is so is to see whether each of the sub-scores correlates in the same way with a common set of independent activities; that is, the Sex Power score and the Aggression Power score might be alternative manifestations of the same power drive, as shown by the fact that each would correlate with a set of outside variables in the same way. Both might, for instance, be positively correlated with office-holding and speeding, and negatively correlated with watching

$$\begin{array}{ll}\text{p Power} & .38,\ p < .01 \\ \text{s Power} & .60,\ p < .01 \\ \text{p-s Power} & .48,\ p < .01 \\ n\ \text{Power} & .51,\ p < .01 \end{array}$$

What is surprising about these test-retest correlations is that generally such reliabilities for thought codes of this type run lower (see McClelland, 1958); that the range of scores is rather narrow, which should attenuate such correlations, at least for the p and s Power values; and that drinking occurred between the first and second TATs, a fact which might well be expected to reduce test-retest reliability, especially in view of certain specialized effects of drinking (see Chapter 6). That the reliabilities are high in spite of these factors suggests that these codes may be stable measures of individual differences.

4. Finally, the correlations in the Activity Inhibition column in Table 8.2 suggest that the earlier methods of partitioning the power codes may not be particularly successful in predicting who will drink heavily. Sex Power, Other Power, Weak Power, and Strong Power all correlate to a moderate degree positively with Activity Inhibition, which we know from Chapter 7 is a negative predictor of heavy drinking. Thus it is only when we get to the distinction between personalized and socialized power sub-scores that we find a significant difference in the correlation with Activity Inhibition which has some promise of differentially predicting drinking. As already noted in Table 8.1, the difference in these correlations with Activity Inhibition is even greater for Bar Study II.

RELATIONS OF TYPES OF POWER CONCERNS TO VARIETIES OF ASSERTIVE ACTIVITIES

The men who participated in the bar studies, as has been said earlier, filled out extensive questionnaires concerned with their participation in all sorts of assertive activities, including drinking, sports, office-holding, and the vicarious power satisfactions of watching violent TV shows or reading "sporty" magazines. The questionnaire, which was adapted from one given to the sample of college students described in Chapter 5, was modified for Bar Study I and modified further for Bar Study II. It is described in Appendix II. The interpretive problem was to find some method of classifying the various assertive activities according to whether they theoretically represented an impulsive vs. restrained or a personalized vs. socialized type of power action. The solution seemed to call for a factor analysis of the activity variables to see which ones belonged together, in the hope that clusters of activities identified in this way could be clearly seen to represent one face of power or the other. And indeed the factor analysis of the activity variables for the first bar study yielded the readily interpretable results we had hoped for. The principal component factors were rotated according to the varimax criterion to yield a three-factor solution in which the factors were more or less clearly defined by loadings on different variables as shown in Table 8.4. To make the table easier to read, only factor loadings of ±.40 or greater are for the most part recorded. Exceptions are made for variables of particular theoretical interest.

Factor I appears clearly to be a "power" dimension inclusive of a wide variety of assertive activities such as current participation in sports, fast driving, running successfully for office, reading "sporty"

Table 8.4—Factor saturations of activities variables and their correlations with n Power and Activity Inhibition Bar Study I, N = 50

	Factor I (Assertiveness)	r with n Power	Factor II (Restraint)	r with Act. Inh.	Factor III (Gregariousness)
Sports participation[1]	.77	.24 +			
Fastest speed driven	.75	.33 *			
Office holding	.68		.10		.26
Time with women	.61		.25	.22	
"Sporty" magazines	.51	.29 *	.28		
Cost of desired car	.43				−.35
Ave. *liquor* consumed	.43	.24 +	−.59	−.27 +	
Violent TV shows	.42		−.14		.25
Ave. *wine* consumed	.41		.22		−.50
Time hanging around			−.76		
Freq. 4 or more drinks			−.45	−.35 *	.45
Ave. *beer* consumed			−.34	−.21	.37
Age	−.44	−.24 +	−.52		
Time TV viewing	−.40		−.27	−.27 +	.39
Time working			.45		
Years of sports participation[1]					.48
Attend. college sports					.47
Attend. pro sports					.69
Watching TV sports					.60
Time dancing					.41

saturations below ±.40 and r's below ±.20 omitted, except where theoretically important

Correlations with factor scales[2]

	Assertiveness scale	Restraint scale	Gregariousness scale
n Power	.35 *		
Activity Inhibition		−.19	−.27 +

+*p* < .10   *p* < .05

[1]Non-contact sports only.

[2]Sum of variables (standard scored) loading ±.40 or more on the factor.

[3]Rotations were stopped at three factors because of the clear break between the amount of variance accounted for by the third and fourth principal components. Latent roots for the first four principal components were 6.45, 4.83, 4.03, 2.70. The first three factors together accounted for 34 percent of the total variance of the 45 activities.

magazines (such as *Playboy*, *Sports Illustrated*), interest in ow.
costly car, and the consumption of large amounts of liquor and v
Loaded negatively on this factor are spending a lot of time watchi.
TV and being old, both of which suggest being less assertive or powerful
in action. The *n* Power score is not only substantially correlated with a
number of these activities, as Table 8.4 shows, but is also correlated
significantly with an Assertiveness Scale built from Factor I. This
scale was obtained by computing the signed sum of an individual's
standardized scores on the activities items loading $\pm.40$ on Factor I.

Factor II, although it is not as well defined on the positive as on
the negative side, appears to represent the variable of restraint vs. lack
of restraint. The major distinction seems to be between the factor
loadings for time spent working $(+.45)$ vs. time spent hanging around
coffee shops, bars, etc. $(-.76)$; neither of these is appreciably loaded on
the assertiveness factor. Of the activities loading high on assertiveness,
only amount of liquor consumed on an average occasion has a substantial loading on this factor—namely, $-.59$ indicating lack of
restraint. Though the Activity Inhibition score correlates negatively
with a number of activities loading negatively on this factor, indicating
low restraint as one would expect, its overall negative correlation with
the factor scale score does not reach an acceptable level of significance.
Once again, the reason appears to be the fact that the positive or
restraint end of this factor is not well represented, even though it is still
possible to find assertive activities with modest positive loadings like
office holding, and reading "sporty" magazines.

Factor III loads heavily on all the sports variables except current
participation in non-contact sports. It is also of interest to note that
beer drinking loads appreciably here, as it does not on the assertiveness
factor. We have labeled the factor gregariousness, because it appears to
represent a kind of convivial interest in sports and beer drinking
quite separate from the assertiveness or power dimension. It is also
associated with lack of restraint, as indicated by the nearly significant
negative correlation of the Factor III scale score with the Activity
Inhibition score.

Figure 8.1 has been prepared to display some of the same findings
in a graphic, more easily comprehensible form. In this instance the
n Power and Activity Inhibition fantasy codes were included in the
factor analysis to show where they would load in relation to various
assertive activities. This of course changes the loadings for the activities
themselves as shown in Table 8.4 but only slightly. What is particularly
interesting about this form of presentation is that it parallels in many
ways the factor structure for the analysis of folk-tale themes shown in
Figure 4.2. Here as there, independent power and inhibition dimensions
organize the factor space.

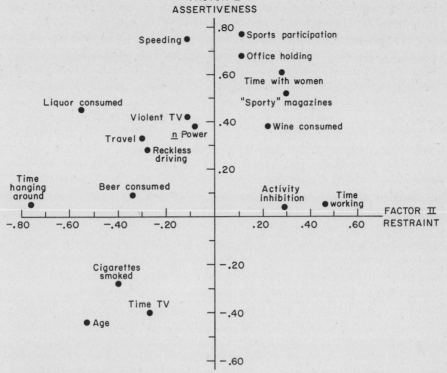

Figure 8.1 Plot of drinking and other activities variables on Assertiveness and Restraint factor dimensions.

There is another parallel as well. The Vigorous Activities tag (*run, jump,* etc.) in the folk-tale study loads highest on the assertiveness factor, and current participation in informal sports loads highest on the same factor in the individual analysis. This similarity suggests that people who think a lot about vigorous activities are likely to be those who engage in them. The study of individual participation in activities supports the inference drawn from the cross-cultural study of folk tales that one of the major defining aspects of assertiveness is vigorous physical activity. Furthermore the study of individuals shows specifically that these assertive activities are closely associated with n Power—an inference only indirectly confirmed in the cross-cultural study.

Unfortunately, few of the other tags in the folk-tale study have such readily identifiable counterparts in the present study of individual activities. The only other similar variable is drinking, which is associated with cultures having folk tales scoring high on the assertiveness factor and low on Activity Inhibition, corresponding in Figure 8.1 to the upper lefthand quadrant. What the study of individuals adds to the study of cultures is that only heavy liquor drinking, at least at the individual level, belongs in the upper lefthand quadrant. Wine drinking, for this sample of individuals in our society, is located in the upper righthand quadrant representing high assertiveness and high control. Beer consumption, as already suggested by Table 8.4, loads low on the restraint factor but is not related to assertiveness; rather, it goes with some kind of conviviality syndrome (Factor III). It was this factor plot which convinced us, along with findings reported in Chapters 6 and 7, that beer drinking simply is not part of the assertiveness syndrome which lies behind liquor drinking and alcoholism.

This conclusion helped clarify a finding which had seemed to represent a flaw in the power theory of drinking—namely, the often-reported and significant association between cigarette smoking and drinking (cf. Cahalan, *et al.*, 1970, p. 181). Yet smoking appears to be a kind of passive sentient or oral activity, which in fact appears in the relaxed, unassertive quadrant in Figure 8.1. Why should it be related to drinking, if drinking is associated with assertiveness? The explanation lies in the distinction between the meaning of beer drinking and liquor drinking—a distinction not always drawn in other studies. In this sample, cigarette smoking is significantly correlated with beer drinking ($r = .41$, $p < .01$) but not at all with liquor drinking ($r = .05$, n.s.). Thus once more we must stress the suggestion inherent in our data: that the power theory of drinking applies in our studies of American men only to liquor drinking, and that beer drinking is engaged in for different reasons, perhaps as part of some kind of convivial gregariousness syndrome.

Figure 8.1 also underlines another fact already mentioned—that outside of liquor and wine consumption there are very few activities to show up at the extremes of the upper lefthand or upper righthand quadrants representing the presumed two faces of power. Nevertheless it was necessary to do the best we could with what we had to see which method of partitioning the power coding system would best discriminate participation in activities from these two quadrants.

What was finally done was to take all the variables that loaded at least $+.27$ on the assertiveness factor and classify them either as indicating *restrained* assertiveness if they loaded positively on Factor II (even at a very low level) or as indicating *unrestrained* assertiveness if they loaded negatively on Factor II even at a low level. Then each of the power sub-scores was correlated with the activities variables so classified. The results are shown in Table 8.5. In the upper half of the table the columns of *b* correlations should be larger than the *a* correlations, whereas in the lower half of the table the reverse should be true.

Let us first consider the Weak vs. Strong partitioning of the power categories. It does fairly well in the upper half of the table. For five out of the six types of restrained assertiveness, the Strong Power correlations are larger than the Weak Power correlations. But unfortunately this appears to be the case simply because the Strong Power score is a better predictor of all assertive activities, for it also predicts unrestrained assertive activities better on the whole. Thus in the lower half of the table only one Weak Power correlation is slightly larger. Most serious of all, the Weak Power score does not correlate more highly with average liquor consumed than does the Strong Power score. Thus it must be concluded that the Weak vs. Strong Power method of partitioning the power coding categories does not succeed in capturing the distinction between participating in restrained vs. unrestrained assertive activities.

A comparison of the Id with the Other Power correlations for the two types of activities yields no better results. On the whole the differences in size of the pairs of correlations are small; where big, they are in the wrong direction. For instance, it was certainly not expected that imagery associated with Sex and Aggression Power would be significantly correlated with the number of clubs a person belonged to—something we have considered a measure of a person's interest in "organizational" power. And once again we failed to come up with a type of power imagery which correlated significantly with liquor consumption. Since we had demonstrated in Chapters 1, 2 and 6 that drinking increased Sex and Aggression imagery, we had expected that the Id Power score would also predict average liquor consumed better than the Other Power score would. If anything the reverse is true. The Id Power score correlates only .09 with the amount of liquor consumed on an average occasion, while the Other Power score correlates .25 with the same measure.

It was the failure of these two methods in obtaining measures of the two faces of power that led us to develop the p Power and s Power scores. The latter two sub-scores behaved much more according to expectation. The Socialized Power score correlated more highly than the Personalized Power score with all six types of restrained assertive activities in the upper half of Table 8.5. Three of the correlations are significant, though two of them refer to essentially the same phenomenon. Joining clubs and holding offices in them are highly correlated ($r = .95$, $p < .01$, in this sample). Both could represent an interest in organized power; that is, even a member of a club presumably feels somewhat more influential by belonging to a group larger than himself. Office holding, on the other hand, seems more clearly to represent an interest in having a position of influence; thus to avoid duplication it will be used in future discussions as the variable representing "organization power."

The performance of the p Power score in predicting participation

Table 8.5—Correlations of n Power sub-scores with restrained and unrestrained assertive activities Bar Study I, N = 50

Activity	Loading on		Correlations with					
	Factor I Assertive-ness	Factor II Restraint	a Weak Power	b Strong Power	a Id Power	b Other Power	a Pers. Power	b Soc. Power
A. Restrained Assertiveness								
Time with women	.61	.25	.06	.29*	.16	.16	.10	.20
"Sporty" magazines[1]	.51	.28	.39*	.27+	.28*	.34*	.20	.38**
Ave. wine consumed	.41	.22	.07	.12	.21	.09	−.23	.08
Club memberships	.80	.12	.23	.25+	.37*	.10	.07	.38**
Office holding	.68	.10	.09	.12	.18	.05	.07	.29*
Sports participation	.77	.08	.24+	.30*	.25+	.27+	−.05	.22
No. b correlations > a			5/6		2/6		6/6	
B. Unrestrained Assertiveness								
Ave. liquor consumed	.43	−.59	.14			.25	.24+	.00
Speeding[2]	.75	−.12	.14			*	.10	.20
"Violent" TV	.42	−.14	.0d				.08	.18
Money for travel[3]	.34	−.34					−.17	.03
Reckless driving[4]	.27	−.28					.21	.04
No. a correlations > b							2/5	

+p < .10 *p < .05 **p < .10
[1] Reading Playboy, Sports Illustrated, etc.
[2] Fastest speed driven.
[3] If $10,000 available, mentioned travel as use for it.
[4] Number of traffic tickets for moving violations.

ɪ unrestrained assertive activities is less satisfactory; in only two out f five instances is its correlation with a given activity larger than the ₅ Power correlation. Yet it does match expectation in one critical respect; it correlates with liquor consumed on an average occasion at very near the .10 level of significance, whereas the s Power score does not correlate at all with liquor consumption. Thus while the distinction obtained through p and s Power scoring is not perfect, it does a better job of predicting participation in the two types of assertive activities than the other two attempts to partition the power concerns expressed in fantasy.

Having decided that the distinction had some promise, we next checked to see whether the pattern of correlations just noted could be cross-validated on a new sample of subjects in Bar Study II. As any personality researcher knows, finding a pattern of interpretable relationships is hard enough; replicating it under somewhat different conditions is far more difficult. The first set of relationships may in fact be partly attributable to chance variations, with the researcher capitalizing on error in searching through a large matrix for significant correlations. For instance, in Bar Study I, where there were some 45 "outside" variables correlated with two fantasy sub-scores, one might well expect a number of significant correlations obtained in the last two columns in Table 8.5 to arise by chance out of 90 correlations. To be sure many of these "outside" variables were practically duplications (fastest speed ridden, for example, vs. fastest speed driven) so that the "real" number of different variables was much smaller. (See Appendix III.) Nevertheless, it is highly desirable to check the findings of Table 8.5 on a different sample to make certain that they hold up in general.

Bar Study II was not, however, a simple replication of Bar Study I. Though the pictures in the TAT were the same, they were administered under different conditions. In the first study, the men told the stories in the bar to an examiner who wrote down what was said. In the second study, the men *wrote* their own stories in an employment agency during the daytime in a session quite unrelated to drinking in the bar. The men in the second bar study, moreover, were about seven years older on the average than those in the first, and came more often from a blue-collar working-class background. (See Table 7.1.) Finally, the Activities Questionnaire itself was changed in a number of ways. Some items were omitted and some added, and certain questions were asked in slightly different ways. For instance, in Bar Study I queries about current and past participation in sports were separated; in Bar Study II they were combined. This was a mistake, as Table 8.4 makes clear, because the two variables load on quite different factors. At the time the changes were made in the questionnaire for Bar Study II, however, this analysis had not been made, and it seemed reasonable to put together all current and past sports activities.

The first step was to factor analyze the response variables obtained to the revised Activities Questionnaire used in Bar Study II. Our purpose was to see if once again we could locate fairly clear-cut factors of assertiveness and restraint on which the same activity variables would load in the same way as in Bar Study I. It was not difficult to locate the assertiveness factor; in fact it came out as the first principal component factor in the analysis. There were 15 activity variables based on questions asked in the same way in Bar Study II as in Bar Study I. All but two of them loaded positively on the factor labelled Assertiveness in Bar Study I. All 15 of the same variables loaded positively on the first principal component factor in Bar II. Since nowhere near as close a correspondence in loadings was found for any other factor (including rotated factors), it was decided to consider this factor the equivalent of the assertiveness factor in Bar Study I and to use the saturations on it in classifying all activities variables in Bar II as to degree of assertiveness.

It was far more difficult to locate a restraint factor in Bar Study II. None of the factors did a very good job of classifying the 15 comparable activities variables in the same way as in Bar Study I. One possible reason is that one of the main questions which identified this dimension in the first bar study was omitted in the second—namely, the question about how much time a man spent working, hanging around with women, etc. (see Figure 8.1.). In the end it was decided to pick that factor as indicating restraint which differentiated satisfactorily the two variables of most theoretical importance—office holding and drinking. Ever since the study reported in Chapter 5, we had assumed that drinking is most typical of the impulsive, personalized face of power and office holding most representative of organized or socialized power. Hence they would seem the best choices for "marker" variables to locate the restraint factor. And they indicated that the third principal component factor could most probably be considered the restraint factor, since they loaded on opposite ends of it. Parenthetically the second principal component factor loaded substantially a number of the same variables which appeared in the "sports gregariousness" factor III indentified in Bar Study I (see Table 8.4).

The decision to consider the third principal component factor as a measure of the restraint dimension not only leads to a proper classification of office holding and drinking; it also gives reasonably good results for other variables as well. Owning a large number of prestige supplies turns out to be indicative of restrained assertiveness, and watching violent TV shows as indicative of unrestrained assertiveness, both as also classified in Bar Study I. Reading "sporty" magazines, the driving variables and the sports variables must be classified differently, but the latter might be considered of little importance in this analysis. Aside from current participation in informal sports, which was not questioned in Bar Study II, they do not load high on the assertiveness factor in either study. So while the comparability of the two factors in the second bar study to those in the first leaves something to be desired, particularly so far as identifying the restraint factor is concerned, enough similarity appears to have been established to enable us to go about the task of seeing how the p Power and s Power scores correlate with assertive activities classified as restrained or unrestrained.

Table 8.6 shows the correlations of various power scores with assertive activities classified as *restrained* in either or both of the two bar studies. Two variables—office holding and prestige supplied owned— were consistently classified by both factor analyses. As predicted, the s Power score correlates significantly with office holding in both studies, and the p Power score does not. This is a most important cross-validation of the hypothesis that s Power represents a concern for wielding socialized power which leads a person into seeking and holding office in organizations. For prestige supplies owned, on the other hand, the correlations are the reverse of expectation. In both samples it is the p Power score which correlates significantly with owning items like a colored television set, a tailor-made suit, a Playboy Club key, a rifle or a pistol, a convertible, etc. The factor analyses determine that owning such things indicates restraint, as well it may in the sense that a person must at least work and save to get the money to buy them. Yet it also makes sense to find that prestige supplies are more likely owned by people whose power concerns are focused towards personal rather than social goals. The most likely explanation for this deviation from prediction appears to be that the dimensions of restraint and socialized power are not identical, even though the socialized power score was derived by studying the power themes of restrained people. Nevertheless it can still be true that while most restrained assertive activities are organized to gain *social* influence, not all of them need be. The ownership of prestige supplies can indicate restraint but at the same time an interest in personalized rather than socialized influence.

Three other variables in Bar Study I are classified as restrained assertive activities with no information available on them in Bar Study II. In all instances the correlations are higher with s Power as predicted, particularly when the p-s Power score is used as the overall index. In other words, men whose s Power score is higher than their p Power score tend to spend more time with women (playing the assertive male

Table 8.6—Correlations of personal and social power scores with restrained assertive activities in two bar studies. Bar I, N = 50; Bar II, N = 108

	Bar Study	Factor loadings Assertiveness	Restraint	p Power	s Power	Correlations with n Power scores p–s Power[1]	n Power
Office holding	I	.68	.10	.07	.29*	−.20	.14
	II	.04	.31	.04	.28**	−.20*	.19*
Prestige supplies owned	I	.07	.16	.32*	.24+	.07	.25
	II	.16	.33	.20*	.03	.14	.15
Time with women	I	.61	.25	−.02	.20	−.20	.18
Ave. wine consumed	I	.41	.22	−.23	.08	−.30*	−.10
Sports participation	I	.77	.08	−.05	.22	−.26+	.12
Credit cards	II	.23	.30	.17+	.06	.09	.21*

+p < .10,   *p < .05,   **p < .01
[1]Difference between standard scores for p and s Powers.

role), to drink wine, and to participate regularly in informal sports. In Bar Study II, the men were asked how many credit cards they had in their wallets "right now." The number they reported was classified as a restrained assertive characteristic by the factor scores but correlated more with the p Power score than the s Power score, just as in the case of prestige supplies. In fact, credit cards for all practical purposes might be considered a prestige item.

Table 8.7 presents similar data for assertive activities classified as unrestrained in the two bar studies. Of greatest theoretical interest is the way the power measures relate to consumption of liquor. The correlation of the p Power score with amount of liquor consumed on an average occasion is disappointingly low and insignificant in Bar Study II. As noted in Chapter 7, however, the crucial measure of heavy drinking is a quantity-frequency index which takes into account not only how much a person drinks but how often he takes large amounts. Using this index, the p Power score does much better, and the p-s Power score predicts heavy consumption significantly in both studies. As in the case of the item on office holding in the previous table, this result is of major importance for the whole study, since it confirms the fact that our laboriously derived method of partitioning power concerns successfully predicts heavy drinking if it is oriented one way, and office holding if it is oriented the other.

At the bottom of Table 8.7 some correlations are also given for liquor consumption during the course of the evening at the bar in the experiment proper. Strictly speaking, the two measures are not comparable. The amount of liquor consumed was used in Bar Study I because it was obviously a more sensitive measure than the simple dichotomy of liquor drinkers versus beer drinkers. This same measure, however, could not fairly be used in the second bar study, because the men had been subjected to different treatments before they entered the bar, and one treatment produced significantly heavier drinking (see Chapter 12). Nevertheless it was thought that whether or not the person chose to drink liquor rather than beer might be less influenced by the specific experimental treatment and more by the person's stable level of p-s Power concerns. In any case it is interesting to note that the p-s Power score in both studies is positively associated with liquor drinking at the bar during the experiments when measured in these somewhat different ways.

The remaining findings in Table 8.7 for other variables are more scattered and only suggestive. Reckless driving is associated as expected with the p Power score but at an insignificant level in Bar Study I. Technically speaking, spending some of a gift of $10,000 for travel classifies as an unrestrained assertive activity, although intuitively it is not readily apparent why it is assertive. In any case it correlates

Table 8.7—Correlations of personal and social power scores with unrestrained assertive activities in two bar studies. Bar I, N = 50; Bar II, N = 108

	Bar Study	Factor Loadings Assertiveness	Restraint	p Power	Correlations with n Power scores		n Power
					s Power	p–s Power	
Ave. liquor consumed	I	.43	−.59	.24+	.00	.22	.24
	II	.48	−.14	.03	−.06	.08	.07
QF index, liquor	I	1		.44**	.10	.32*	.30*
	II	1		.14	−.14	.24*	.10
TV violence	I	.42	−.14	.08	.18	−.10	.09
	II	.13	−.22	−.02	−.05	.02	−.14
Reckless driving[2]	I	.27	−.28	.21	.04	.16	.21
Money for travel[3]	I	.34	−.34	−.17	.03	−.19	.08
Freq. gambling	II	.18	−.46	.12	−.11	.19+	−.03
Fist fights	II	.49	−.05	−.02	−.08	.04	−.08
Amount of liquor consumed at bar (N = 39)	I			.03	−.20	.19	.01
Liquor chosen at bar[4] (N = 82)	II			.09	−.30**	.33**	−.02

+p < .10, *p < .05, **p < .01

[1]High QF vs. all others. See footnotes to Table 7.5. Not in factor analyses but since both frequency and quantity measures are in this quadrant in both studies, the QF index clearly belongs here.
[2]Number of traffic tickets for moving violations.
[3]Mentioning travel as one of the ways we would spend a gift of $10,000. See Appendix II for complete wording.
[4]Used instead of amount consumed because presumably less influenced by experimental treatments than amount consumed. Same measure unavailable in Bar I.

negatively instead of positively with p Power score, at a very low level of significance. In the second bar study, of the two additional activities classified as unrestrained assertive actions—gambling and number of fist fights—the former correlates more highly with p Power than s Power and the latter correlates with neither. On the whole the harvest of findings outside the drinking area is slight.

For the sake of completeness Table 8.8 reports correlations of the power scores with activities that were either inconsistently classified in the two studies or unclassified because they were not part of the factor analyses. While speeding and reading "sporty" magazines are both significantly correlated with the overall *n* Power score in Bar Study I, they are not in Bar Study II. They also switched classifications on the restraint variable. One possible explanation that comes to mind lies in the fact that both of these activities are significantly negatively associated with age in both studies, and it should be remembered that the men in the second bar study were significantly older. It may well be that for the younger group reading *Playboy* may be a relatively restrained activity compared with actually going out and chasing women, whereas in an older group of presumably more settled men continuing to read *Playboy* might indicate lack of restraint. Similarly, speeding in the younger group may indicate "wildness" or lack of restraint; but among older men, a continuation of such behavior may indicate a genuine interest in driving fast as a hobby or as a means of getting somewhere in a hurry. There are no significant correlations with attending college sports events in either study, though again the switch in classification on the restraint dimension may well be due to the different significance of attending such events among older and younger people. The lesson of these inconsistent findings is either that significant results can in fact arise by chance or that the meaning of a given activity as expressive of a power concern changes significantly with age.

There is only one new and interesting positive result in Table 8.8. In the second bar study the men were given a list of various impulsive aggressive acts like yelling at someone in traffic, throwing books or magazines around the room, destroying furniture or glassware, making insulting remarks to storekeepers, clerks, etc., walking off leaving one's wife or girl to fend for herself the rest of the evening, etc. They were to check whether they had done such things often, once or twice, "haven't but would like to," or "never considered doing" them. An overall score was obtained labelled in Table 8.8 "average frequency committed" by giving a weighting of 4, 3, 2, or 1 for each of the alternatives just listed. Another score was simply the number out of the 11 activities which the person listed as something that he had not done but would like to. This measure we will refer to later as the "aggressive-impulses"

Table 8.8—Relations of personal and social power scores with miscellaneous assertive activities
Bar I, N = 50; Bar II, N = 108

(A) Inconsistently classified in two studies

	Bar Study	Factor Loadings Assertiveness	Restraint	r with age	p Power	Correlations with n Power scores s Power	p–s Power[1]	n Power
Reading "sporty" magazines	I	.51	.28	−.34*	.20	.38**	−.18+	.29*
	II	.39	−.28	−.19*	−.06	−.06	−.10	−.11
Fastest speed driven	I	.75	−.12	−.35	.10	.20	−.10	.30*
	II	.69	.28	−.24*	−.09	−.02	−.06	.00
Attend college sports	I	.21	.17	−.32*	.07	.13	−.05	.03
	II	.18	−.31	.01	.07	−.07	.13	.02

(B) Unclassified aggressive acts (Bar II)

	p Power	s Power	p–s Power	n Power
Ave. frequency committed	−.04	.04	−.07	.10
Ave. "liked to have committed"	.22*	.03	.16	.18+

+p < .10,   *p < .05,   **p < .01
[1]Difference between standard scores for p and s Power.

score. As Table 8.8 shows, it is significantly correlated with the p Power score, while actually committing aggressive actions is in no way associated with any of the fantasy power scores.

DRINKING AND THE PERSONAL POWER SYNDROME

This completes the review of relationships between the various fantasy power scores and assertive activities. What have we learned? In particular have we learned anything more about the relation of power concerns to drinking? In Chapter 7 we showed that in both bar studies classifying individuals both by their *n* Power and their Activity Inhibition scores enabled us to pick out a high percentage of the heavy drinkers. We then went to great trouble to develop a p Power score representing the heavy drinking classification (high power, low inhibition) and an s Power score representing a low drinking classification (high power, high inhibition). One very simple question is whether these new scoring systems improve our ability to pick out the heavy drinkers as compared with a two-way classification on *n* Power and Activity Inhibition. Table 8.9 provides the answer.

Table 8.9—Percentages of heavy and light drinkers scoring high on various indexes of power concern

	High n Power[1] Low Inhibition[2]	High p Power[3]	p > s Power[4]
Bar Study I			
Heavy drinkers (*N* = 16)[5]	56%	50%	63%
Light drinkers (*N* = 20)[6]	15%	25%	40%
Bar Study II			
Heavy drinkers (*N* = 18)[3]	61%	50%	61%
Light drinkers (*N* = 58)[4]	31%	31%	33%
Combined χ^2 =	10.5, *p* < .01	4.4, *p* < .05	7.1, *p* < .01

[1]Score of 4 or more.
[2]Score of 2 or less in Bar I; 1 or less in Bar II.
[3]Score of 2 or more.
[4]Difference between standard scores for p and s Power.
[5,6]For method of classification, see notes to Table 7.5.

It compares the percentages of men with heavy and light drinking histories identified by the various fantasy coding schemes. Obviously the double classification by high *n* Power/low Activity Inhibition discriminates very well between the two types of drinkers in both studies. A high p Power score also discriminates but at a lower level of efficiency. Finally the p-s Power score discriminates well in both studies. Heavy drinkers are much more likely to have a p Power standard score which is higher than their s Power standard score as contrasted with men who have a history of not drinking very much. The p and s Power codes do almost as good a job of picking out the heavy drinkers as does the double classification by n Power and Activity Inhibition. What then has been gained if the new system is as good as but certainly no better than the old one?

The gain does not lie in diagnosis or selection of men who are likely to be or become heavy drinkers. Rather it lies in the area of understanding the dynamics of heavy drinking and its associated activities. At the simplest level we have learned that heavy drinking is not associated with all types of power concerns but with one particular type, namely, the concern for personalized as contrasted with socialized power. As noted earlier, a man with a high p Power score tends to think of the world as made up of protagonists who are fighting active opponents for personal power, glory or influence. They are not concerned to use their power for the good of others nor do they have the doubts about themselves or the ultimate triumph of power which characterize the men with a high s Power score. This fact helps us understand precisely what the heavy drinker has on his mind— personal aggrandizement; but also a knowledge of the other actions a high p Power score leads to helps us to set drinking in its context.

Table 8.10—Intercorrelations of alternative manifestations of personal power concerns (before drinking) Bar I, N = 50; Bar II, N = 108

Bar study:	Prestige supplies		Gambling	Aggressive impulses	p Power	
	I	II	II	II	I	II
Heavy liquor drinking[1]	.06	.11	.19	−.08	.44**	.14
Prestige supplies	—	—	.04	−.00	.32*	.20*
Gambling frequency			—	−.05		.12
Aggressive impulses[2]				—		.22*

[1]Those individuals reporting they had three–five or more drinks of liquor two–three times a week or more often vs. all others.
[2]Aggressive acts not committed but "would like to."

What is most striking about the action correlates of p Power is that they are unrelated to each other. Table 8.10, which has been prepared to illustrate this point, shows the intercorrelations of four action correlates of p Power—two from both bar studies, and two from the second study only. All the intercorrelations are low and some— especially with aggressive impulses—are negative. In other words, people who gamble are not likely to collect prestige supplies nor are those with lots of prestige supplies likely to drink a lot. Yet all of these things are independently related to the p Power score. The result is surprising, because ordinarily one would expect that activities all related to some outside variable would also be related to each other.

It is precisely to handle such situations in personality study that the motive concept is ordinarily invoked. As McClelland (1951) pointed out long ago, when a cluster of activities are all interrelated, it is convenient to speak of them as representing a *trait*. But when they are unrelated to each other, yet are all related to some apparently underlying disposition, the *motive* concept is customarily employed. One can conceive of such unrelated actions as *alternative manifestations* of the need for power. If a man expresses his personal power concern in gambling, he does not need to drink. Or if he accumulates prestige supplies, that may satisfy his personal power drive, and he does not gamble or drink.

It is useful to contrast this cluster of assertive activities with another cluster made up of highly intercorrelated activities—namely, speeding, fighting, acting aggressively in various ways, and reading "sporty" magazines. These acts are not only highly related to each other; they are also related to heavy drinking. In other words, a man who speeds is likely to fight and drink. We might think of him as having a consistent trait or style of aggressively "acting out." Paradoxically, none of the components of this acting out syndrome correlate with the p Power score, except for drinking.

The figures have been arranged in Table 8.11 in a way to make these various points clear. The correlations are shown only for the second bar study in order to simplify the presentation and make the theoretical argument as clear as possible. At the top have been listed the alternative power manifestations, all of which have been shown to relate positively to p Power, but not to each other.

Unfortunately in this analysis we could not use the measure of heavy liquor consumption employed previously and shown to be at least moderately related to p Power, because it is a simple dichotomy and in the subsequent analysis we needed a wider variation in standard scores than a dichotomy provides. So we chose what seemed to be the best alternative—a total alcohol consumption score which combined amounts and frequencies of both liquor and beer consumed. The fact that p Power is not as closely related to this measure of heavy drinking should make it less likely that the results to be reported in a moment would be obtained.

At the bottom of Table 8.11 are listed the elements of the aggressive "acting out" syndrome which intercorrelate but do not relate to p Power. In the upper righthand corner are the figures indicating that heavy drinking is related consistently to aggressive acting out; and this is just as true also in Bar Study I. For instance, in Bar I heavy liquor drinking (the quantity-frequency dichotomy) correlates .47, $p < .01$ with speeding. What are we to make of the apparent contradiction in the fact that p Power is related to drinking (Table 8.10), but not to the things to which drinking is related?

Table 8.11—Intercorrelations of p Power score, alternative power manifestations, and acting out Bar II, N = 108

	p Power	ALTERNATIVE POWER MANIFESTATIONS				ACTING OUT			
		Heavy drinking	Prestige supplies	Gambling	Aggr. impulses	Speeding	Fights	Aggr. Acts	"Sporty" mags.
Alternative manifestations									
Heavy drinking[1]	.05	—				.25*	.52**	.27**	.14
Prestige supplies	.20*	-.03	—			.17	.01	.14	.03
Gambling frequency	.12	.09	.04	—		-.11	-.11	.14	.14
Aggr. impulses[2]	.22*	-.12	.00	-.05	—	.02	-.04	.00	.11
Alternate power manifestations									
Maximum score[3]	.35**					.28**	.30**	.20*	.28**
Mean score[4]	.29**					.16	.19*	.27**	.21*
"Acting out" syndrome									
Speeding[5]	-.09					—	.35**	.43**	.23*
Fights	-.02						—	.19	.14
Aggressive acts[6]	-.04							—	.20*
Reading "sporty" mags.	-.06								—

[1] Sum of beer, quantity times frequency, and liquor, quantity times frequency.
[2] Number of 11 aggressive acts, not committed but "would like to."
[3] Maximum standard score on any one of four alternative power manifestations just above.
[4] Mean standard score on four alternative power manifestations.
[5] Fastest speed driven.
[6] Average frequency of having committed eleven different types of aggressive acts, where 1 = never considered, 2 = haven't but would like to, 3 = done once or twice, 4 = have done often.

The scores for alternative power manifestation in the center of the table help clarify the matter a little. If it is true that a personalized power drive can be satisfied in one of several alternative ways, it stands to reason that the correlation of the p Power score across individuals with any one of these outlets might be low. Some individuals with high p Power scores will not pick a particular outlet (and therefore will get a zero score on it, just like the people with low p Power), because they are finding their outlet in another channel. The way to handle this problem appears to be to get some kind of summary score across the possibilities for alternative manifestation. And theoretically a mean score for all these alternatives might not be as good as a maximum score, because a person might satisfy his personal power drive, let us say, wholly by gambling, receiving zero scores for the other three alternatives and lowering his average below the mean for all subjects. More diagnostic would appear to be the maximum standard score a man receives on any of the four power manifestation alternatives. That is, the stronger a man's personal power concern, the more likely it would be that he would engage in at least one of these four alternative activities in a more extreme fashion than that which is typical for his group. As the correlations in the center of Table 8.11 show, this is exactly what happens. The correlation of p Power with the maximum score obtained on any of the four alternatives is substantial (.35, $p < .01$) and considerably higher than it is with any of its individual components, suggesting that the hypothesis of alternative manifestations is correct. It is further buttressed by the fact that the mean standard score on all four alternative manifestations correlates *less* with the p Power score than the maximum score, even though the former should be a more stable indicator of the strength of personalized power concerns. Apparently there is a real tendency for men to express their personalized power concerns in *alternative* pathways rather than an appreciable amount in all of them. It is worth noting that Adler and Goleman (1969) report a similar finding in a cross-cultural study. Tribes that gamble a lot do not drink, and vice versa. Both appear to be alternative outlets for the power drive.

What is particularly interesting is that the maximum score for alternative power manifestations in turn *correlates significantly with every one of the components of the aggressive acting-out syndrome.* One might suspect that these correlations result from the fact that the alternative manifestation scores include drinking which, as Table 8.11 also shows, is significantly correlated with each of the components of the acting-out syndrome. But note that in the maximum summary score, the components are all standardized so that only about a quarter of the individuals score highest in drinking.

As a matter of fact, it is possible to estimate how much those who score highest on the drinking alternative ($N = 23$) are contributing to the correlations of the maximum summary score with the components of the acting-out syndrome. The method involves determining whether, compared to those who score highest on other alternatives, they are more likely to speed, fight, etc. For the most part, they are not. The biserial correlation, for instance, between being highest in drinking vs. highest on one of the other three alternatives and speeding, is only .04. Thus excessive drinking does not appear to be the primary reason for the .28, $p < .01$ correlation between being high on *some* manifestation of personal power and speeding. All the biserial correlations between being high on a particular power manifestation and the components of the acting-out syndrome are insignificant—except one, namely that between being highest on drinking and fighting ($r = .30$, $p < .01$). With this exception, it may be concluded that it is being high on *some* action manifestation of a personalized power concern, *not any particular manifestation*, that leads to acting out in one of the four ways listed.

The same point is made by the fact that the *mean* alternative manifestation scores correlate on the whole less strongly with the components of the acting-out syndrome, despite the fact that drinking enters into *every one* of these scores. What this fact suggests is that not all of the relationship between the alternative power manifestation scores and acting out can be attributed to drinking. Rather, some of it must be attributed to a generalized power orientation which is better picked up by the alternative manifestation summary scores than by the p Power scores themselves.

How are we to interpret these somewhat confusing results? How is it that p Power, for example, is related to aggressive impulses but not to aggressive acts, whereas drinking is related to p Power and aggressive acts? One assumption makes sense out of this tangle of relationships. It is simply that there is a *regular sequence* in the action effects of a personalized power concern. One may conceive of primary action symptoms followed by secondary symptoms which are reactions to the primary ones. Figure 8.2 outlines the way the pattern of interrelationships fits into a sequence. It starts with the assumption that an individual has a characteristic level of concern with personalized power, which expresses itself in one or more of four alternative actions identified in these studies; the inner concern or thought pattern is thus conceived as preceding or leading to actions of various types. Of course there is nothing in a correlation matrix to indicate the direction of causality: accumulating a large number of prestige supplies might lead to an increase in p Power concerns as easily as the reverse. The fact is, as we shall see in a moment, that probably the lines of influence work in both directions in some kind of mutually reinforcing cycle. But for the sake of

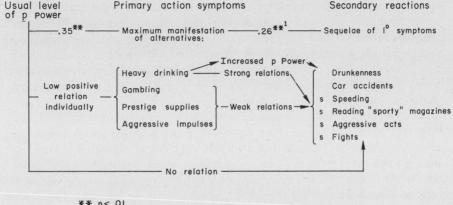

[1]Median intercorrelation of maximum alternative power manifestation score with individual secondary symptoms (marked s). See Table 8.11.

Figure 8.2   Scheme for relating action consequences of personal power concerns.

simplicity of analysis, we must break into the cycle at some point; and in the scheme presented in Figure 8.2, we have started with the inner level of personalized power concern as measured on the first TAT. The usual level of p Power correlates .35, $p < .01$ with the maximum manifestation of any of the alternative ways of expressing power in action, although it correlates with any particular one of these alternatives at a much lower level. These primary action expressions of the personalized power drive are assumed to have secondary action consequences, since the maximum score on any one of them correlates significantly with each of a set of "acting-out" symptoms (median $r = .28, p < .01$).

While we have just argued that not all of these consequences can be attributed to drinking, the theoretical argument can be outlined most clearly for drinking. Heavy drinking has strong correlations with secondary action consequences like speeding, fights and other types of aggressive acts—scarcely a surprising finding, either in terms of common knowledge or theory. We know, in short, that drinking increases personalized power concerns (see Chapter 6) and that it decreases such reality restraints as Time Concern. The result should be more un-inhibited assertive action such as speeding and fighting. The argument requires, however, that the usual level of p Power not produce fighting and speeding independently of drinking (or whatever other primary power manifestation is maximized). It should lead first to drinking, which then in turn leads to fighting and speeding. Drinking also leads to reading "sporty" magazines which deal with the sex and aggression themes that we found in earlier chapters to be more prominent in men after drinking, as a special way of expressing a personalized power concern. Heavy liquor drinking also leads more commonly to drunkenness ($r = .28$, $p < .05$, Bar Study I) and to accidents ($r = .18$, n.s.).

The link may be the increased p Power produced by drinking itself. Table 8.12 shows how p Power scores, measured before and after drinking, correlate with a series of actions which, we have argued, result from the primary action expressions of p Power, such as drinking. Note that in every case a correlation with the p Power score obtained after drinking (the primary symptom) is greater with the secondary action consequence than it is when the p Power score was obtained before drinking. Put very simply, the usual level of p Power will not predict speeding. It will predict drinking. Drinking in turn produces a p Power score which will predict speeding, accidents and frequency of drunkenness.

Table 8.12—Correlations of p Power scores with secondary reactions to primary power expressions before and after drinking Bar study I (N = 50)

"Consequences"	p POWER SCORE	
	Before drinking	After drinking
Speeding[1]	.10	.28 *
Car accidents	.21	.34 *
Frequency of drunkenness	.20	.28 *
Reading "sporty" magazines	.20	.22

*p < .05
[1]Fastest speed driven.

The easiest way to make sense out of all these relationships seems to be to assume that p Power has some primary action effects, one of which in particular—drinking—has secondary effects such as momentarily increasing p Power and decreasing restraint, a combination which leads to drunkenness, car accidents, speeding, fighting, and so forth. Although it may be that the other primary effects, like gambling or collecting prestige supplies, also have secondary effects, this study was not designed particularly to pick them up. So far as the fourth primary effect of p Power is concerned—aggressive impulses—it is easy to imagine how they would be converted into aggressive acts and fights especially in combination with that other primary effect, drinking, which increases p Power and decreases restraints. Yet normally it must be stressed that there is no significant relationship between the ordinary level of p Power and fighting. p Power may prepare the ground for fighting by increasing aggressive impulses, but it requires the intervention of some other factor to covert them into acts.

VALUES, POWER NEEDS, AND DRINKING

The analysis so far purports to give a picture of how heavy drinking and some of its consequences are related to personalized power concerns. But our measures have all been indirect, based on the thoughts and actions reported by the men participating in the bar studies. To what extent are they aware of the processes just described? What do the heavy drinkers consciously want? What are the seekers of personalized power after? The men living through the sequences shown in Figure 8.2 must have some view of what is going on, and this view is important; it will at the very least help us to understand the various theories of alcoholism which have been developed largely from interviews with alcoholics. There have been many studies of self-descriptions of alcoholics which are reviewed elsewhere in this book. But the unique opportunity provided here is to study the pattern of interrelationships among such self-descriptions, power needs, drinking, and associated assertive activities.

The instrument used to measure conscious values and attitudes was a questionnaire devised by Jessor and others (1968) to get at factors associated with heavy drinking in a Southwestern community. Their theoretical orientation was, to oversimplify it considerably, that drinking like any form of social deviance is produced by lack of fulfillment of personal goals on the one hand and lack of real opportunities in life on the other. One measure of lack of opportunity—low socioeconomic status—they found to be significantly associated with heavy drinking (1968, p. 338). In our two bar studies the association was not nearly so marked. Low (blue-collar) occupational status was not associated with any of the drinking measures in either of our two bar studies. To choose the measures most similar to theirs, occupational status was correlated .03 with frequency of drunkenness in Bar Study I and .01 with the combined beer and liquor drinking index in Bar Study II. Years of eduction, also a measure of opportunity, shows a negative correlation, as expected, with the same two drinking measures, the values being $-.09$ in Bar Study I and $-.23$, $p < .05$ in Bar Study II. In other words, there is some evidence to suggest that the more educated people are, the less likely they are to drink heavily—perhaps, as Jessor *et al.* argue (1968), because they are less frustrated and better able to fulfill their expectations.

A direct measure of the lack of fulfillment of personal goals obtained from the questionnaire did not correlate significantly with any of the drinking indexes. The relevant correlation ($r = .08$) is shown in the first line of Table 8.13, wherein are also assembled other pertinent data from the responses of the men in Bar Study II who were

Table 8.13—Correlations among personal power needs, value expectations, drinking and acting out. Bar II, N = 108

	p Power	Heavy drinking[1]	Speeding	Aggressive acts
Personal disjunctions[2]	−.15	.08	−.11	.27 **
Expect recognition[3]	.13	−.16	−.10	−.26 **
Expect help[3]	.18 +	−.24 *	−.11	−.14
Expect affection[3]	.23 *	−.09	−.09	−.17
Expect independence[3]	.06	.06	.30 **	.20 *
Expect a lot from family[4]	−.24 *	.19 +	.14	.18 +

+p < .10,   *p < .05,   **p < .01

[1]Sum of beer, frequency times amount, and liquor, frequency times amount.
[2]Disjunctions between importance of four values and expectations of getting them in general, at work, from family, and friends. (Jessor *et al.*, 1968.) See Appendix II.
[3]Sum of items asking about expectations of getting deserved values in general, at work, from family and friends.
[4]Sum of expectations of getting all values from family.

given the questionnaire. First they were asked to rate the importance to them of such things as "the good opinion of the family for the things you do well" (part of the Recognition score), or "having somebody in the family you can count on to help you" (part of the Dependency score). We have re-labeled this the Help score because it suggests the questions more accurately. Items like these were asked in two additional value areas (Independence and Affection), and were repeated five times in all in slightly different form to get at the importance of such values in general, at work, from family, and from friends. Then the whole procedure was repeated, except that now the respondent was asked how strongly he *expected* each of these things to happen—"to be able to count on the family for help when you need it" (expect help), or "to get affection from others in the family" (expect affection), etc. A personal disjunctions score (indicating lack of personal fulfillment) was calculated by summing the major discrepancies between how important a person thought something was and how confidently he expected to get it across all value areas. (See Appendix II.) The result has no relation to drinking here, as in fact it did not to any great degree in the Jessor study (Jessor *et al.*, p. 345).

Scores in the different value areas, however, yielded an interesting pattern of correlations. To simplify the presentation, only those for the "expect" scores are given in Table 8.13. The pattern of correlations for the "want" or "importance" scores is similar. In discussing this study later in Chapter 11, we find it particularly noteworthy that only on the "expect recognition" scale did the Indians score significantly lower than either the Spanish Americans or the Anglo-Americans in the sample; we suggest that this may explain why the Indians have a much higher drinking rate than the other two groups (see Jessor *et al.*, p. 296). That is, it seems consistent with the personalized power theory of drinking to expect that men who want recognition (or want to be considered impressive, or powerful), but do not expect it, should turn to drinking as a means of enhancing their sense of power.

The same relationship appears in Table 8.13. The less recognition the men said they expected, the more they tended to drink ($r = -.16$, $p \sim .10$). The drinking index used here is the one that combines beer and liquor, because it is most comparable to those used by Jessor *et al.* (1968), who made no distinction between beer and liquor. The findings are the same for the quantity-frequency index used earlier in the chapter for discriminating heavy drinkers from all other drinkers, although the relationships are somewhat attenuated because the variable is dichotomous. The finding is difficult to interpret for several reasons. First, Jessor *et al.* do not report the relationship for the area concerned with recognition separately for individuals, but only for the comparison among the three ethnic groups, as will be noted in Chapter 11. Second, it is impossible to be sure in either study whether the expectation of little recognition is a cause or a consequence of drinking. It is as reasonable to assume that drunks realistically expect less recognition because they know drinking is disapproved as it is to argue that they drink because they don't get enough respect.

Furthermore in this study, as contrasted with theirs, the negative relationship with drinking is even larger with the score for "expect help." Here, those who say they expect the least help drink the most ($r = -.24$, $p < .05$). One might suppose that they are drinking because they fail to get the help they want, as dependency theorists would argue, but heavy drinkers also rate help as not very important ($r = -.18$, $p < .10$ for the quantity/frequency index of liquor drinking or $-.08$ for the index used in Table 8.13). It makes a little more sense to take the correlations at their face value and simply note that heavy drinkers expect not to get much recognition and help from others because they know they are deviant. The pattern is if anything even more striking for the assertive activities generally associated with heavy drinking. Men who drive fast and commit a large number of aggressive acts also tend to say they expect to be left alone and not to be afforded much recognition, help or affection from others. (See the two righthand columns in Table 8.13.)

But then what are we to make of the fact that the p Power score correlates in the opposite direction with all the conscious expectation variables? If p Power is associated with heavy drinking, then one would certainly expect that it would correlate negatively with the "expect help" score, just as heavy drinking does. But the reverse is true. Men high in p Power say they expect *more* recognition, help and affection than men low in p Power. What is to be made of this apparent paradox?

Once again to resolve it, it is helpful to think in terms of primary and secondary reactions, or of unconscious and conscious motives. Let us be explicit about what is going on. Men who fill their fantasies with thoughts of striking out against opponents in order to gain personal power are also saying that they expect help and affection from others, at the conscious level. They have dreams of grandeur, and like all "king-emperors" they expect more recognition, help, and affection from others. The one exception is that they expect to get less from their families—perhaps because they know they will not get help there, perhaps because they want recognition from a wider audience. Now as we have just shown, such people express their personalized power concerns in several alternative ways, one of which is heavy drinking. Those who drink, then, say that they do not expect much recognition, help, or affection, and this may be seen as a realistic appraisal of what is happening to them as a result of their drinking.[4] Or it may be seen as a kind of defensive denial that these matters are of importance to them, since they are doubtless well aware that heavy drinking is disapproved by many in the world outside. Once again the only exception to this pattern is what is expected from the family. Here the interpretation appears to be somewhat similar to the one made earlier: such men expect more from their families, because their drinking has forced them to retreat in their expectations of recognition and help from the outside world in general.

Put in this way, the analysis shows that drinking is a self-defeating process so far as the man with high p Power is concerned. He wants recognition and support, but drinking is one manifestation of his power drive which denies him the very things that he desires. And he seems to know it. Just as in the case of interpreting the pattern of events in Figure 8.2, it is useful here to think of drinking as a primary effect of the personalized power drive leading in turn to secondary effects which are quite frustrating or at least unrelated to that personalized power drive. If we accept the fact that heavy drinkers really want and expect respect and affection (because they are high in p Power), and if we accept the fact that they know that they are not getting it because they are drinkers, then we may conclude that they turn to drinking even more in order to increase directly their sense of personal power, saying in effect: "To hell with recognition from others that I am powerful! I *feel* powerful." Thus the basis for a vicious cycle in which drinking

---

[4]As a matter of fact only the 23 whose maximum alternative manifestation score is for drinking say they expect less help ($r = -.23$, $p < .05$, between the Expect Help score and these 23, scored 1, vs. the remaining 83, scored 0). For those who choose one of the other three alternatives maximally there is no negative relation to the Expect Recognition Score. In fact for those who choose gambling, the correlation is even positive ($r = .16$, $p \sim .10$), as it is for those with a high p Power score in general. Gamblers expect recognition, drinkers do not—which seems to *reflect* rather than to determine their action role.

leads to more drinking is clearly evident in the pattern of correlations displayed in Table 8.13. As Davis points out in Chapter 9, failure to gain social power, or recognition, may turn a man to drinking in order to gain a primitive and narcissistically gratifying sense of personal power. The action is self-defeating because it makes even less likely the support and recognition he needs, which again turns him to alcohol as a means of giving himself at least a temporary boost in his feeling of potency.

Can the vicious cycle be reversed? How? Here our laborious efforts to develop two power coding systems might yield an unexpected bonus. For our analysis suggests that therapy involves not the destruction of the personal power drive or merely attaining insight into it, but its redirection and socializing. Certain methods of expressing the personalized power drive—such as accumulating prestige supplies— are not in themselves especially self-defeating in terms of their consequences, certainly as compared to drinking heavily. But a drinker's power drive could also be shifted in a more distinctly social direction. He could be taught to find ways of joining organizations, running for office, or participating in sports, so that his power needs would be met but in socially acceptable ways. The problem appears to be more one of switching the mode of gaining satisfaction for the power drive rather than destroying it completely. In Chapter 14 we report a pilot attempt to develop a therapeutic program for alcoholics based on this theoretical understanding of why they drink and how their power drives could be satisfied in other ways.

One final word: the p and s Power scoring systems were developed to provide a better understanding of heavy drinking. But the patterns of correlations in Tables 8.6, 8.7 and 8.8 suggest that we may have hit on a distinction that has a much wider applicability. Personalized power concerns appear to express themselves not only in drinking but in other types of deviant acts like fighting and perhaps crime, which are badly in need of further explication in motivational terms. The social face of power, furthermore, should provide insight into political and military activity, in which power relationships are carefully controlled and exercised, presumably on behalf of the whole organization. As so often in research, a persistent effort to solve one problem leads on to a whole new series of problems that cry out for investigation. The fact that the power motive system has two faces and that they appear to be organized along the personalized versus socialized dimension may turn out in the long run to be a more important discovery than the explication of their role in drinking.

Chapter 9

Drinking: A Search
for Power or Nurturance?

by William N. Davis

Earlier chapters have developed the thesis that a man's concern with power plays a crucial role in determining how much he is likely to drink. In contrast, many researchers in the field have concluded that dependency needs or desires for nurturance are the most important psychological antecedents of drinking (e.g., Knight, 1937; Lisansky, 1960; McCord & McCord, 1960; Bacon, Barry, & Child, 1965; Tähkä, 1966). This possibility was mentioned in Chapters 3 and 8 and will be discussed at length in Chapter 13. The data that have been presented point to the conclusion that experiences involving dependency and nurturance are not nearly so significant in producing drinking as those involving power. It is important to remember, however, what sort of findings are reported in previous chapters. On the one hand, clinical and correlational data have been gathered which connect power experiences and drinking; on the other hand, studies on the effects of drinking have shown that liquor consumption increases the drinker's sense of power. Thus, the evidence for a relationship between power—particularly as measured by the TAT—and drinking is fairly strong, whereas dependency and nurturance seem both unrelated to drinking and unaffected by it.

Still, if power concerns are truly the most important antecedent of drinking, then additional evidence needs to be accumulated. It must be shown that power experiences are not only correlates of drinking, but also that they stimulate drinking. Thus far, it has not been established experimentally that this is actually the case; nor has it been shown that dependency and nurturance do not stimulate or otherwise directly affect drinking. To demonstrate a direct, causal relationship between power and drinking (or between nurturance and drinking) what is required is an experimental study in which feelings of power or nurturance are aroused in various forms, in a setting where the effects of these experimental manipulations on drinking can be determined. The study to be described in this chapter was designed to do just this. Its purpose was to explore, by experimental means, the effects of power-related feelings and nurturance-related feelings on subsequent drinking.

An experimental game, called the Blind Man Game, was chosen as the general setting in which to manipulate feelings of power and of nurturance. The game is played in pairs. One member of each pair is blindfolded, and the other who is not blindfolded serves as his partner's guide. The Blind Man Game is played out by requiring that the pairs interact to complete certain tasks, or simply to get from one place to another.

The Blind Man Game was selected for three reasons. First, past experience has shown that playing this game naturally—that is, without any special experimental intervention—tends to arouse feelings related to power and nurturance (Kolb & Rubin, 1967). In general, blind-foldees report feeling helpless or taken care of, while their partners and the guides tend to report feeling powerful or somewhat frustrated by the fact that they have to be so considerate of their pairmates. Second, because of the kinds of reactions stimulated naturally, it seemed that experimental manipulations related to power or to nurturance could be introduced with real credibility. Third, the Blind Man Game provides a practical, reasonably simple method of testing whether experiences related to power or nurturance have immediate effects on subsequent drinking.

Two experimental conditions were created. In the "power" treatment, the subjects were led to perceive the game primarily in power-related terms; in the "nurturance" treatment they were led to perceive it in nurturance-related terms. Within the power treatment it was emphasized to blindfoldees that they would be very helpless or power-less while playing the game because they would be unable to do anything for themselves. The guides, on the other hand, were told they would be very powerful, because they would be in complete control of and have great influence over their partners. In the nurturance treatment blindfoldees were told that they would be secure and well taken care of since it would be the guides' job to assist them constantly; whereas it was emphasized to the guides that they would be alone and somewhat deprived because they would have to give a great deal to their blindfolded pairmates without getting anything in return (Davis, 1969).

Thus, in the power treatment, the experimental manipulations were intended to enhance a feeling of power among guides, and a feeling of powerlessness among blindfoldees. In the nurturance treatment, the manipulations were designed to make blindfoldees feel nurtured, and the guides deprived of nurturance.

To participate in this study a total of 108 men were recruited by placing an advertisement for part-time work in a local newspaper (see Chapter 7 for procedure). Sixty-four of the 108 actually played the Blind Man Game. Their characteristics are summarized in Table 9.2. Most of the subjects were between 30 and 49 years of age, with an average of a little over 13 years of education. The sample was just about evenly divided between professionals (or white-collar workers) and blue-collar workers (including the unemployed). A little more than one quarter of the sample was single, about one half was married, and the other quarter was either separated or divorced.

When a potential subject answered the newspaper advertisement, he was given a brief description of the purpose and procedure of the study. In essence, potential subjects were told the experimenter was interested in investigating how certain feelings were affected by a barroom atmosphere.

If a caller indicated he would like to participate, an appointment was made for him to meet with the experimenter for a preliminary session. The purpose of these preliminary sessions, which were held in the evening at a local employment agency, was to gather background information on potential subjects, particularly in regard to their self-reported drinking history. About 15 men were invited to each session, and between six and 10 usually showed up. There were 14 preliminary sessions altogether. At the end of each preliminary session the experimenter explained the Blind Man Game in detail. At this time the experimenter specified that he was particularly interested in how the feelings generated by the Blind Man Game would be changed by spending more time in a bar. By doing so, the real purpose of the study —to discover how the Blind Man Game affected amounts of drinking— was concealed from subjects. Finally, everyone who participated was paid five dollars, and information was gathered regarding the future availability of potential subjects.

Following each preliminary session the drinking history of the men who participated was examined. If a potential subject was an admitted alcoholic, or a member of Alcoholics Anonymous, or had a medical problem which could be aggravated by drinking, or if he was an abstainer, he was not allowed to participate any further.

Those subjects who were eligible to continue were divided into several groups on the basis of their self-reported history of drinking. Light drinkers were defined as those who said they drank two drinks or less on an average occasion; moderate drinkers were those who reported drinking three to five drinks on an average occasion; and heavy drinkers were those who said they drink six to eight or more drinks on an average occasion.

Once subjects were grouped in this way they were further divided into matched pairs on the basis of a common drinking history. Each pair was then assigned to an experimental session. This was done in a systematic way such that each session had about the same number of light, moderate, and heavy drinkers. Within each pair subjects were randomly assigned the role of blindfoldee or guide.

There were eight experimental sessions altogether—four power sessions and four nurturance ones. An average of eight subjects or four pairs participated in each of them. Power sessions were alternated with nurturance ones until the series of eight had been completed.

Every experimental session was conducted in exactly the same way. First, the experimenter went over the rules of the Blind Man Game. Then the experimenter introduced an assistant, explaining that the latter was an expert on the Blind Man Game since he had played both roles a number of times. The experimenter went on to say that he had asked his assistant to speak briefly about the game in order to give subjects the benefit of his experience. This "expert testimony" given by the experimenter's assistant was designed to influence subjects' thoughts and feelings about the Blind Man Game (see Davis, 1969). For a power session the assistant's comments emphasized that blindfoldees usually feel powerless and guides usually feel powerful when they play the game. For a nurturance session his comments emphasized that blindfoldees usually feel nurtured and guides usually feel deprived of nurturance when they play the game.

Immediately after the "expert testimony," roles were assigned and the game began. Each of the four subject pairs who participated in an experimental session was required to walk from the employment agency where the preliminary sessions were held to a bar that was located about eight blocks away. The blindfolds worn by one member of each pair were actually large blacked-out, wrap around sunglasses. Two pairs started at once, one of them walking down the near side of the street, and the other down the far side. In general, it took subject pairs about 15 minutes to walk from the employment agency to the bar.

Table 9.1—Adjectives used in check lists classified by mood theme

MOOD THEMES

	Powerful	Powerless	Nurtured	Deprived of Nurturance	Inhibited	Impulsive
Form A	powerful persuasive respected competent	weak dominated unimportant inadequate	take care of befriended helped comforted	ignored disliked disregarded isolated	cautious serious attentive restrained	hasty happy-go-lucky careless impulsive
Form B	dominant influential important capable	helpless powerless insignificant incompetent	protected liked provided for reassured	neglected friendless slighted alone	careful in earnest alert inhibited	rash frivolous reckless spontaneous

Note: Half the subjects checked Form A at the end of the game, Form B in the bar at the end of the evening; the other half checked Form B followed by Form A. Adjectives were listed in a scrambled order.

The barroom which was their objective was a neighborhood tavern—neither a cocktail lounge nor a "dive." As subjects arrived there, they were met by the experimenter's assistant, who gave each subject a "Game Questionnaire" and asked him to sit by himself for a few minutes in order to fill it out.

The Game Questionnaire was designed to get a brief measure of the way subjects reacted to the Blind Man Game. It consisted of five questions that concerned overall reactions to the game and an adjective check list, containing 24 words, from which they were to pick the four adjectives most descriptive of how they felt while playing the game, and then the four that were least descriptive. Four adjectives were included on a theoretical basis to represent each of six psychological moods, or themes—Powerful, Powerless, Nurtured, Deprived of Nurturance, Inhibited, and Impulsive. (See Table 9.1.) About half of the subjects received Form A of the adjective check list, and the other half a parallel Form B. The adjectives that appeared on each form were randomly ordered with regard to the themes they represented, rather than classified by theme as in Table 9.1.

After subjects had completed the Game Questionnaire, they were given an hour and one-half of free time, during which they could have some drinks if they wanted to, at the experimenter's expense. Alcohol consumption for each subject was recorded by a waitress who took all the orders. During the free time subjects usually talked together in groups of three or four. Just before an hour and a half had elapsed, a last call was taken and thereafter no more drinks were allowed any of the subjects. At this point the subjects were separated again in order to fill out a "Bar Questionnaire," designed to give a brief indication of how each subject felt at the moment, or in other words at the end of the free-time period.

The Bar Questionnaire was constructed in exactly the same way as the Game Questionnaire. It contained the same five general questions as the Game Questionnaire, although the wording for each was slightly different. Then subjects who had filled out Form A of the adjective check list were given Form B to fill out as it applied to their current feelings, and vice versa.

Following the completion of the Bar Questionnaire subjects were given ten dollars for their participation, and several taxis were called to take them all home. At this point the experimental sessions were over.

RESULTS

Table 9.2 compares the four experimental groups by age, years of education, occupation, marital status, and drinking history. Aside

Table 9.2—Numbers of men with various background characteristics in the four treatment conditions

Treatment:	POWER INSTRUCTIONS		NURTURANCE INSTRUCTIONS	
Role:	N = 16 Guides	N = 16 Blindfoldees	N = 16 Guides	N = 16 Blindfoldees
Age, mean years	40.2	39.1	38.9	37.1
SD	6.8	9.0	7.2	8.1
	↑————————— p diff. < .01 —————————↑			
Education, mean years	14.0	13.4	13.8	13.1
SD	2.3	2.0	2.2	2.0
Occupation				
white collar	6	10	8	6
blue collar (including unemployed)	10	6	8	10
Married	10	8	8	8
Single, divorced, separated	6	8	8	8
Liquor drinking history, Matched pairs				
Both average 6 or more drinks		4		4
Both average 3–5 drinks		8		8
Both average 2 or less drinks		4		4
Total pairs		16		16
Pairs matched by drinking history for beverage chosen at bar				
6 or more drinks		5		5
3–5 drinks		7		6
2 or less drinks		2		2
Total pairs		14		13

from the difference in age between power guides and nurturance blindfoldees, there were no statistically significant differences among the groups on any of these variables. The fact that power guides tended to be about three years older than nurturance blindfoldees does not seem important, because it is hard to think of a really important change that occurs in a man's life between the ages of 37 and 40. Since, with this slight exception, the four groups were matched statistically for age, education, occupation, and marital status, it is unlikely that any of these background variables could have been responsible for the significant differences in responses that occurred among the groups during the experiment.

Table 9.2 also shows the success with which subjects were paired on the basis of their self-reported drinking history. So far as liquor-drinking history is concerned, subjects were matched perfectly within pairs and across treatments. They were not nearly so well matched within pairs and across treatment on beer-drinking history (see Davis, 1969), the reason being that it was assumed they would choose to drink liquor rather than beer if given the opportunity. As it turned out, however, a number of subjects did drink beer during the experimental sessions, creating the possibility that the members of certain pairs, although matched on liquor-drinking history, were *not* matched in terms of the type of beverage they chose to order at the bar. Thus within pairs differences in amount consumed might be due not only to differential experiences in the Blind Man Game but also to differences in habitual level of consumption of the beverage chosen.

There were in this way two unmatched pairs in the power condition and three in the nurturance condition, in the sense that the two members of a pair reported different drinking histories for the beverage they consumed. Since it is impossible to determine how these differences in drinking history might have affected differences in alcoholic consumption between the members of each unmatched pair, all five were excluded from the analysis of the effects of the Blind Man Game on drinking. Table 9.2 shows the distribution of the remaining 27 pairs, across drinking history and treatment. All of these were matched in that the two members of each pair reported similar drinking histories for the type of beverage they consumed in the bar.

Table 9.3—Mean adjectives checked by mood theme and alcohol consumed for various conditions

Mean adjectives Checked by theme	POWER INSTRUCTIONS			NURTURANCE INSTRUCTIONS			All
	Guides (G) $N = 16$	Blindfoldees (BF) $N = 16$	G — BF diff.	Guides (G) $N = 16$	Blindfoldees (BF) $N = 16$	G — BF diff.	G — BF[1] diff.
Powerful	3.38	.99	2.38**	2.19	1.00	1.19*	1.78**
	↑————— p diff. $< .01$ ————↑						
Nurtured	1.13	2.06	− .83+	1.63	2.38	− .75+	− .84**
Inhibited	2.75	2.50	.25	3.44	2.00	1.44**	.84*
Alcohol consumed	$N=14$	$N=14$		$N=13$	$N=13$		
No. of drinks	7.07	5.57	1.50**	5.31	5.15	.16	.85*
	↑————— p diff. $< .10$ ————↑						
Oz. of 86-proof alcohol consumed	9.37	6.44	2.93*	8.70	8.00	.70	1.86*

[1] Based on sum of the discrepancies between guide and blindfoldee in each of the pairs.
+$p < .10$; *$p < .05$; **$p < .01$, two-tailed tests.

Table 9.3 summarizes the effects of instructions and of role in the game on mood themes and on drinking. Only the data for the positive mood themes are included, because the number of adjectives checked in their negative equivalent—Powerless, Deprived of Nurturance and Impulsive—was generally lower, and the results less reliable, though always in the same direction as for Powerful, Nurtured and Inhibited.

Clearly role in the game had an effect on feelings: guides under both sets of instructions felt significantly more powerful than blindfoldees, less nurtured, and more inhibited. See the last column of Table 9.3.

Instructions also had some effect, though it was less marked. The guides receiving power instructions reported feeling significantly more powerful than the guides receiving nurturance instructions. Also, under nurturance instructions, the guides felt significantly more inhibited than their blindfoldees (who had been instructed to feel relaxed), whereas there was no significant difference on this dimension under power instructions.

So far as drinking is concerned, once again the role in the game had a larger effect than instructions. The guides drank more in both treatments, both in terms of number of drinks and ounces of 86-proof alcohol consumed. But really the effect was significant only for the pairs operating under power instructions; there the guides subsequently drank significantly more on the average than the men they had been guiding. While the results are given only for the 27 pairs matched for drinking history, they are essentially the same if all pairs run are included, the mean number of drinks being 7.11 and 5.68 for the power guides and blindfoldees respectively, and 5.38 and 4.76 for the nurturance guides and blindfoldees. In other words, those who felt most powerful during the game drank the most, whether one looks at role in the game (guides vs. blindfoldees) or role combined with instructions (power guides vs. nurturance guides).

Table 9.4—Correlations between mood themes on game questionnaire and alcohol consumed subsequently in the bar ($N = 64$)

Mood Check list theme	Total number of drinks consumed	Ounces of 86-proof alcohol consumed
Powerful	.17	.25*
Powerless	−.07	−.10
Nurtured	−.09	−.03
Deprived of nurturance	.03	−.03
Inhibited	−.09	−.14
Impulsive	.13	.17

* $p < .05.$

A similar finding shows up if one ignores role and treatment, and simply correlates reactions of the subjects on the check list with what they drank subsequently. That is, one could argue that what is important here is not what the experimenters thought they were doing to the subjects, but how in fact the subjects felt, regardless of the treatment that was intended. Table 9.4 reports these correlations for all the mood themes checked on the questionnaire given them on their arrival in the bar after participating in the game. The only correlation reaching significance is that between reported feelings of being powerful, respected, dominant, important, etc. and amount of alcohol subsequently consumed. Of further importance is the fact that all correlations between feeling nurtured, helped, liked, etc. or ignored, alone, friendless, etc. and drinking are close to zero. Once again there is no support here for the hypothesis that either positive or negative feelings in the nurturance area are related to drinking. The correlations in the inhibited-impulsive area are in the expected direction—that people feeling rash and happy-go-lucky drink more—but they do not reach significance.

Finally Table 9.5 brings together the data on feelings after the game and later on in the evening after drinking. Changes within treatment groups have to be interpreted with caution; scores often start out at very different levels, and changes may represent simply regression toward the mean. There are, however, some points of interest in the

Table 9.5—Mean adjectives checked by theme After Game (AG) before drinking, and later After Drinking (AD) in the bar

Mean adjectives checked by theme	All subjects	GUIDES		BLINDFOLDEES	
		Power	Nurturance	Power	Nurturance
Powerful, AG	1.85	3.38	2.15	.94	1.00
AD	2.33	2.94	2.00	2.44	1.88
diff.	.48 +	−.44	−.15	1.50 **	.88 *
Nurtured, AG	1.82	1.13	1.69	2.06	2.38
AD	1.98	1.88	2.15	1.81	2.13
diff.	.16	.75 +	.46	−.25	−.25
Inhibited, AG	2.62	2.75	3.38	2.50	2.00
AD	1.95	1.81	2.31	2.19	1.56
diff.	−.67 **	−.94 +	−1.07 **	−.31	−.44

$+ p < .10$, $* p < .05$, $** p < .01$, two-tailed tests.

table. To begin with, the over-all shifts after drinking, regardless of treatment, are consistent with other findings reported in this book. Consumption of alcohol produces an increase in reported feelings of powerfulness, no change in feelings of nurturance, and a decrease in feelings of inhibition (first column, Table 9.5). It is obviously the blindfoldees who increase in feelings of power (as they started out low on this variable) and the guides who decrease in feelings of inhibition (as they started out high on this variable). Before one infers that the opposite effects do not occur, it is worth noting that they often cannot really occur: for instance the power guides are already so high on the power check list (3.38 out of a possible 4.00) that they cannot really show an increase. Furthermore, they are so low on the nurturance theme that even random variations would produce the increase that occurs.

DISCUSSION

Two major conclusions are suggested by the analysis of the psychological conditions which affect drinking behavior. First, experience of nurturance does not seem to have any effect at all on drinking; but second, and more important, feeling powerful does seem to precipitate a desire to drink. The results indicate that the power guides felt more powerful than any other group during the Blind Man Game, and that they drank more than any other group at the bar. The question of course is, why was this the case?

A better understanding of the findings can be obtained by examining more closely the check list theme, Inhibited. With the benefit of hindsight it seems that the words making up this theme have varying connotations, some of which are less related than others to the psychological state of inhibition. The eight words that compose this theme, four in each form are listed below.

Form A	Form B
restrained	inhibited
attentive	alert
cautious	careful
serious	in earnest

The words "restrained" and "inhibited" are directly related to the concept of inhibition; both suggest a certain amount of blocking of ongoing activity. "Attentive" and "alert" both suggest generalized awareness, while both "cautious" and "careful" reflect a kind of watchfulness. The words of most interest here are "serious" and "in earnest," which seem the least related to a state of inhibition. Instead they suggest a concerted effort, or a quality of involvement and commitment.

"Serious" and "in earnest" were used differently by the power guides than by any of the other experimental groups on the Game Questionnaire check list. Seven of the eight power guides who received Form A listed "serious" as most descriptive of how they felt during the game; six of the eight power guides who received Form B did the same for "in earnest". In contrast, only four of the 16 nurturance guides said that "serious" or "in earnest" was most descriptive of how they felt during the Blind Man Game; one even said that "in earnest" was least descriptive of how he felt. If the percentage of power guides who said they felt most serious or most in earnest (82 percent) is compared with the proportion of the nurturance guides who said they felt this way (25 percent), the difference is highly significant ($X^2 = 8.03$, $p < .01$). On the other hand, the proportions of nurturance guides, nurturance blindfoldees, and power blindfoldees using these words did not differ significantly. Therefore, the power guides described themselves more often as serious or in earnest than any other experimental group. Since these words seem to reflect a quality of commitment or involvement, it seems likely that the power guides felt most involved and most committed while they were playing the Blind Man Game. The job, or task, that each power guide had, it will be remembered, was to lead his partner from the employment agency to the bar, and this, therefore, is what the power guides were so serious or in earnest about—the job of getting their blindfoldees to the bar.

Added support for the notion that the power guides felt particularly committed or responsible while playing the Blind Man Game comes from one of the five general questions on the Game Questionnaire. Before responding to the adjective check list all subjects were asked to write down the one word that would best describe how they felt while playing the game. On this free choice item 10 of the 16 power guides, or 62 percent, thought of words like "fatherly," "helpful," or "responsible," words which convey the same sense of task involvement that is suggested by "serious" and "in earnest," but with a connotation of interpersonal concern. In contrast, significantly fewer subjects in the other three conditions freely chose such words. Table 9.6 summarizes

Table 9.6—Proportions of men in various conditions describing themselves as predominantly personally committed or relaxed

	PERSONALLY COMMITTED DURING GAME[1]				
	Power instructions N		Nurturance instructions N		
Guides	16	62%	16	19%	$\chi^2 = 4.7, p < .05$
Blindfoldees	15	7%	16	6%	
	$\chi^2 = 9.6, p < .01$				
	RELAXED, COMFORTABLE, PLEASANT[2] AFTER DRINKING				
Guides	16	75%	14	22%	$\chi^2 = 8.6, p < .01$
Blindfoldees	15	27%	16	25%	
	$\chi^2 = 7.0, p < .01$				

[1] Adjectives indicating task involvement or personal concern.
[2] More active positive mood words not included, like "good," "fine," and "cheerful."

these findings. The table also presents a contrast between these and the free responses given after drinking. Later in the evening the power guides differed significantly from the other three groups in the frequency with which they thought of words like "relaxed," "comfortable," "pleasant" as best to describe the way they felt at that moment. Since at most one person in each group had used such an adjective to describe his state of mind during the game, one must conclude that this tendency for the power guides to feel uniquely relaxed could not be attributed to a generally greater preference for such adjectives among them, as indicated in the earlier test. The power guides also decreased significantly in the frequency with which they checked the words "in earnest" or "serious," while the other groups did not. But this result could be ascribed to the fact that they were higher to start with in checking these words and had a greater opportunity to show a drop than the other groups did.

It is therefore particularly important to note that the greater use after drinking of words indicating relaxation among the power guides cannot be explained away as being the direct outcome of a decrease in the use of words like "serious" or "responsible." The men could have thought of a variety of other words like "good," "fine," "cheerful" at the end of the evening, as in fact subjects in the other groups were likely to do. What is *unique* about the power guides is that they said they felt more relaxed after drinking, just as they had said they felt more involved and responsible during the game, than any of the other groups of subjects. It is as if the power guides went from being extremely concerned about their task to feeling completely at ease with themselves and their surroundings. How can we understand what drinking did for them?

Recall that basically the power guides did not change significantly on the theme of Power as a result of drinking. Table 9.5 shows that they dropped slightly on this theme from the Game Questionnaire check list to the Bar Questionnaire check list; but the decrease was not significant, and the power guides continued to have the highest score on this theme as compared to the other experimental groups. Moreover, as mentioned before, since they were already nearly at the top of this scale, any random variations would be likely to produce a downward shift. The point is that the power guides continued to feel powerful while they were in the bar; they maintained their feelings of power at the same time they relaxed and felt a diminished sense of responsibility. Put in another way, it would seem as if drinking enabled them to feel powerful without having to feel responsible—without feeling the need to express and therefore experience their power in a socially responsible manner.

In this connection, it is worth recalling the data on the psychological effects of alcohol reported elsewhere in this book. In general, it has been shown that light drinking increases fantasies of socialized, instrumental power, whereas heavier drinking leads to fantasies of more personal, narcissistically gratifying power (Chapters 6 and 8). Now, it is highly likely that during the Blind Man Game the power guides felt powerful in a controlled and instrumental way; their strong concern over being socially responsible certainly suggests such a finding. On the other hand, it seems unlikely that they experienced very many feelings of primitive, personally enhancing power while they were leading their partners from the employment agency to the bar. Indeed, they may actually have felt a certain lack of this particular kind of power, since almost all their energy was devoted to expressing themselves in a socially constructive fashion. All this leads to the possibility that the power guides entered the bar feeling themselves very powerful in an instrumental, socialized way, but wishing they could be more powerful in a personally enhancing way. Since relatively heavy drinking tends to induce fantasies of personal, narcissistically gratifying power (Chapter 6), perhaps the power guides drank more because they wanted to induce precisely these kinds of feelings—to forget about exercising instrumental power and the feelings of concomitant responsibility in favor of increasing power feelings that were more ego-enhancing and personally satisfying.

Thus, it seems possible that the power guides drank more heavily not only to reduce their stronger feelings of responsibility, and not only to maintain their feelings of power without having to feel responsible, but because they wanted *both* to dissipate their feelings of responsibility *and* experience a qualitative shift in their feelings of power. The essence of what is being suggested is captured nicely in the distinction between socialized power and personalized power. Socialized power is involved when someone exhibits an interest in controlled, responsibly expressed power such as is usually carried out in the interest of others. Personalized power is expressed when someone shows an interest in more impulsive power thoughts and activities which directly make a person feel big and strong. Because the power guides experienced a greater sense of socialized power while playing the Blind Man Game, according to this explanation, they drank more than the other experimental groups to exchange some of their burdensome feelings of socialized power for more narcissistically gratifying feelings of personalized power.

While the findings of this study may not unequivocally support so detailed an explanation of what is happening, they do make real difficulties for alternative theories of drinking. There is, as already noted, hardly a shred of evidence to support the idea that drinking is resorted to by people who are ambivalent about or in any way concerned about nurturance. The nurturance instructions practically wiped out the difference in subsequent drinking between those who were guides or blindfoldees—presumably because it weakened the difference in the sense of being powerful between them. Neither those who felt deprived of nurturance nor those who felt nurtured drank more than anyone else. The only way the nurturance theory can be maintained in the face of such evidence is to argue that people like the power guides both feel more powerful and also feel less nurtured (see Table 9.5). So they drink more for that reason. But such a claim is out of line with the correlational data reported in Table 9.4.

Nor is there support in these data for those theorists who feel that drinking is the resort of men who want to reduce their anxiety. Those who felt more inhibited, subsequently drank *less*, not more (Table 9.4). Or, if one chooses a more direct, less ambiguous measure of anxiety by coding the free descriptive adjectives, the results are the same. After the game, 48 percent of the blindfoldees wrote down words suggesting anxiety—e.g., "weird," "darkness," "uneasy," "nervous"—as contrasted with only 12 percent of the guides, a difference which is highly significant ($X^2 = 9.8$, p < .01). Yet the more nervous blindfoldees drank significantly less than the guides (Table 9.3).

Finally, one of our own theories as to why men with power needs drink more seems not to be supported by these findings. In Chapter 3 we put forward the notion that men who were concerned about power but *deprived of it* would be likely to drink more because they could find substitute satisfaction for their power needs in alcohol-induced fantasies of glory. According to this line of reasoning, the power-blindfoldees should have consumed the most alcohol because power was made salient for them in the instructions and yet they were clearly deprived of it and felt powerless (Table 9.3). Yet they did not drink more. Does this mean that our theorizing on this point is wrong, that depriving a man of a sense of power has nothing to do with leading him to drink or creating an alcoholic?

Not necessarily. It is more likely that we failed to simulate in the Blind Man Game the conditions which in Chapters 3 and 4 we thought would be most likely to lead to heavy drinking. In its simplest terms our theory was that the power drive is most likely to be accentuated in societies where power is both required of the individual but not dependably achievable. We used this as an explanation of why the power drive is higher in the folk tales of socio-economically simple societies (see Table 4.7). The higher power drive then leads people to drink more not because drinking provides a substitute satisfaction for lack of power in reality, but because power cues are simply more present in such a situation and therefore the individual drinks more.

An analogy with the hunger drive may help explain the situation. A man may eat more because he is deprived of food or because he sees or smells things which arouse his appetite to experience the pleasures of eating. In the latter instance, it is proper to speak of a food *motive* in the sense of an increased disposition to search out food and eat. In the former instance, we ought to distinguish between the food *need* (in the sense of objective absence of food) and the food *motive*, which is usually dependably aroused by internal cues resulting from food deprivation.

So far as the power motive is concerned, we were arguing that heightening the importance of power and making it uncertain of attainment should normally over time strengthen the power motive which in turn should lead people to drink more.

Simulating this condition, however, for 20 minutes during the Blind Man Game simply failed to arouse power concerns in the blindfoldees in the power condition (see Table 9.3). Therefore there is no reason to expect them to drink more. By this interpretation, the hypothesis as to the role of power deprivation in drinking is not tested by the present experiment because the procedures were not adequate to raise the power motive in the blindfoldees deprived of power. This is not surprising, since the blindfoldees were scarcely in the position of hunters who are expected to show their prowess by making a kill, but who experience considerable variability in their success in doing so.

IV

EXPLAINING ALCOHOLISM

The final section of the book turns to applying what has been learned about the reasons for drinking to the problem of explaining excessive drinking. Chapter 10 demonstrates that the self-portraits of college problem drinkers, many of whom later become alcoholics, already show the characteristics one would expect if the personal power theory of drinking is correct. Chapters 11 and 12 provide two case studies of excessive drinking in other cultural settings. In both instances, drinking can be seen as a response to a need for greater personalized power, although the interpretation Maccoby gives of the Mexican case has elements which are more in line with the usual psychodynamic explanation of alcoholism.

How does the new theory square with the facts and theories of alcoholism as found by other investigators? Chapter 13 attempts to show that the power theory accounts for the known facts as well as alternative theories do.

As a final application of the new theory, a pilot project is reported in Chapter 14 in which brief retraining of alcoholics was attempted along lines suggested by the power theory of drinking. While the results are no more than suggestive, they do indicate that therapy based on the theory of drinking developed here may prove more successful than other therapies based on less well-supported explanations of why men drink to excess.

Chapter 10

Self-Descriptions
of College
Problem Drinkers

by Rudolf Kalin

The purpose of the study reported in this chapter was to explore the relationship between self-descriptions and heavy drinking among college students. As in the other studies reported in this volume, it is assumed that there is a personality syndrome common among heavy drinkers and that heavy drinking is dynamically related to this syndrome. The assumption of an "alcoholic personality" is the subject of considerable controversy. It has been argued, for example, that there are no general characteristics among heavy drinkers, but that many different types of people can become alcoholics (Bowman, 1956). Other investigators have proposed that social, as opposed to personal factors are primarily responsible for excessive drinking (e.g. Ullman, 1952). Still others, while not denying the possible influence of personal factors, have looked for the reasons behind excessive drinking in the cultural context (e.g. Bales, 1946).

A primary reason why many investigators doubt the existence of an alcoholic personality is the fact that its discovery is subject to a number of difficulties. Although a frequent strategy has been to describe the personalities of full-fledged alcoholics, a major problem with such an approach is the confounding of those personality attributes that predispose a person to alcoholism with characteristics that are outcomes of a long history of excessive drinking. A strategem for overcoming this difficulty is to study "pre-alcoholic" heavy drinkers and compare them with alcoholics. The "pre-alcoholics" in the present study were heavy-drinking college students. Of course heavy drinkers can be regarded as pre-alcoholics only in a statistical sense, but a sample of heavy drinkers is likely to contain a greater proportion of future alcoholics than a sample of light drinkers or abstainers. It is generally assumed that a person becomes an alcoholic after a prolonged period of heavy drinking and not suddenly after taking his first drink at the age of 40. To call heavy-drinking college students pre-alcoholics does not imply that all or even most heavy drinkers are doomed to become alcoholics.

In the present investigation, personality characteristics are defined in terms of self-descriptive statements typically found in personality inventories. Rather than relying on existing personality scales or dimensions, however, we decided to work with individual items and organize them into empirically related clusters. Such a decision was prompted by several considerations, one being the fact that an initial attempt to find correlations between various standard personality scales and measures of drinking yielded meager results. Either there are no personality correlates of drinking or the personality dimensions commonly used are inadequate in differentiating between heavy and light drinkers. Hence the use of individual items might reveal personality characteristics that are obscured by the findings of existing personality dimensions.

A second consideration had to do with the possibility of comparing the results of the present study with those of other investigations. A comparison of the various descriptions of the alcoholic personality is generally a difficult task because of the abstract clinical concepts that are typically used. With the presentation of basic facts, however, such as answers to self-descriptive statements, detailed comparisons become possible. Directly relevant in this context is a report by MacAndrew (1965) with 51 self-descriptive items in terms of which alcoholics can be differentiated from non-alcoholics.

One of the major disadvantages of working with individual items, on the other hand, is that the meaning of a given item is frequently unclear. It is also difficult to summarize succinctly the content of a long list of such terms. In this difficulty, factor analysis both provides a way of indicating the meaning of any one item by showing its covariance with a cluster of others, and constitutes a convenient way of encoding a large list into a limited number of categories.

In the present investigation, the search for personality characteristics of heavy-drinking college students was accomplished in three stages. In stage I a list of self-descriptive statements was collected on empirical and theoretical grounds. In stage II the purpose was three-fold: (1) to determine which of the list of items assembled in the preceding stage were reliably related to drinking in a new sample of subjects; (2) to determine the factor structure of these items; and (3) to build scales reflecting the factor structure and to correlate these scales with the measure of drinking. Stage III was designed to cross-validate the correlations between drinking and the empirically derived scales in new samples of subjects.

Personality characteristics discovered in this fashion can then be compared with personality descriptions of alcoholics available in the literature. Insofar as we can establish that pre-alcoholic heavy drinkers differ from light drinkers in personality characteristics that are similar to those in terms of which alcoholics differ from nonalcoholics, we can justifiably speak of an alcoholism-prone personality. It should be clear that this point of view does not presuppose that no differences exist between heavy drinkers and alcoholics.

THE COLLECTION OF SELF-DESCRIPTIVE STATEMENTS

Information on drinking behavior was available from two samples of subjects who had previously taken various personality tests. One sample (sample A) consisted of 106 subjects who had participated in the experiment described in Chapter 2, and in addition had taken the femininity scale from the CPI, the extraversion-introversion scales from Eysenck's Maudsley Personality Inventory, and subscale 5 of the Terman Miles masculinity test. The drinking measure of this sample consisted of the self-reported amount of beer consumed at a typical sitting.

The other sample (sample B) consisted of 149 undergraduates from fraternities at a Western state university who completed the femininity scale of the CPI and the Yeasaying scale of Couch and Keniston (1960). A sub-sample of 72 subjects from sample B had also taken the Omnibus Personality Inventory while they were freshmen. Another sub-sample of 41 subjects had similarly taken the California Psychological Inventory. Information concerning the drinking behavior of these subjects was obtained through peer rating. Each subject was categorized by his fraternity brothers as a "hard," a "moderate," or a "light" drinker. A subject's drinking score consisted of the difference between the percentage of "hard" ratings and the percentage of "light" ratings.

Each self-descriptive item from the different personality measures was then correlated with the measures of drinking in samples A and B, and the ones that correlated significantly with drinking, or seemed theoretically relevant to drinking behavior, were retained for further study. These items, together with the 51 items from the MMPI found by MacAndrew (1965) to discriminate between alcoholics and non-alcoholic psychiatric outpatients, were collected in a new inventory consisting of 310 items called the Personal Reaction Inventory (PRI-310). All items were of the true-false variety; those not in this form originally (e.g. items from the Maudsley Personality Inventory) were rephrased.

THE CONSTRUCTION OF PERSONALITY SCALES

Subjects

The personality inventory PRI-310 was administered to 118 male undergraduate fraternity members (sample C) at a Western state university who volunteered for a study of personality. The major reason for using fraternity members was the fact that students who live together in a fraternity house get to know each other's drinking habits, and thus it is possible to obtain a drinking measure from mutual ratings. Although many of the subjects were under the legal drinking age of 21, alcoholic beverages could be obtained and consumed quite easily.

Drinking Measure

A list was obtained of the names of all the members of a fraternity. Several days after the completion of the personality inventory, the list was presented to the fraternity men who were in attendance at a meal, with the request that they indicate against each name whether the person was a "hard," "moderate," "light" drinker, or an abstainer. The number 3 was assigned to a "hard" drinker, 2 to an "average" drinker, 1 to a "light" drinker, and 0 to an abstainer. Raters were further told to leave blank those persons whom they did not know well enough to rate. A subject's drinking score consisted of the average of all ratings received. Although scores could theoretically vary between 0 and 3, in fact they varied between .04 and 3.0. Since drinking ratings were available for all the members of a given fraternity, a check was possible as to whether the subjects who had volunteered to take the personality questionnaires were in any way atypical of the fraternity as a whole. The average score of the volunteers from each of the fraternities did not differ significantly from the average drinking scores of their respective fraternities.

Scale construction

When each of the 310 items was correlated with the drinking rating, those items were retained for further analysis that met the following criteria: (1) items that were significantly ($p < .05$) correlated with the drinking measure in sample C, and related to drinking in the same direction, though not necessarily significantly, in the earlier samples; (2) items that correlated significantly with a drinking measure in at least one of the earlier samples (A and B) and that related to the drinking rating in the same direction in sample C; or (3) items that were found by MacAndrew to discriminate between alcoholics and non-alcoholics and that showed a significant or near significant relationship in sample C. Eighty-eight items met one of these criteria.

In order to examine the internal structure of these 88 self-descriptive items, they were factor analyzed according to the principal components method. When factors were extracted until the last factor reached 10 percent of the communality, six factors were obtained. Three of these six were rotated by the Varimax method in order to obtain simple structure.

The personality scales were constructed on the basis of the three rotated factors. A given item was included in that scale that corresponded to the factor on which the item had the highest loading. Another criterion for inclusion of an item in a scale was a factor loading of at least $\pm .400$. Each item had a weight of $(+/-)1$, and contributed to the scale score in the direction of the factor loading.

A fourth scale was built from those items that had factor loadings of less than $\pm .400$ on the three rotated factors. Although these items are drinking-related, they did not meet the criteria for inclusion in the three scales. The sign of each item was based on the direction of the correlation with drinking.

As a final step in this part of the investigation, the personality scale scores were correlated with each other and with the drinking ratings.

CROSS VALIDATION OF SCALES

Students in two psychology classes at the same Western state university participated in a "study to discover patterns among various interests and activities of people." That alcohol was a major focus of the study was not mentioned. Eighty-three of the subjects were male (sample D male) and 177 female (sample D female).

Subjects filled out a shortened version of the "Personal Reaction Inventory" and an "Activity Questionnaire" during a regularly scheduled class hour. Anonymity was guaranteed and the subjects were specifically told to omit their names. The Personal Reaction Inventory (PRI-100) contained the 88 self-descriptive statements previously found to correlate with drinking, and 12 buffer items. The inventory could be scored for the scales developed in the previous section. The "Activities Questionnaire" dealt with participation in various extracurricular and leisure activities. Answers to these questions are not analyzed in the present report. The questionnaire also contained several questions on drinking which provided the basis for the drinking measure.

A quantity frequency index based on self-report by the subjects was constructed. The following questions were asked to elicit relevant information. "How often do you typically consume alcoholic beverages? 4–7 times a week (5), 1–3 times a week (4), 1–3 times a month (3), a few times a year (2), once or twice before (1), never (0)." The numbers in parentheses here and below refer to the scale score for the index. "On an average occasion, how much do you drink? (Check one for each of three types of beverages: beer, hard liquor, and wine.)" Subjects were asked to check their answers for each beverage on the following scale: nine or more (cans for beer, drinks for hard liquor, and glasses for wine) (5); 6–8 (4); 3–5 (3); 1–2 (2); less than one (1); do not drink (0). The quantity-frequency index was then obtained by multiplying the frequency score by the maximum of the three quantity scores. The resulting index has been criticized as not reflecting accurately a person's drinking pattern (e.g., Knupfer, 1964); more specifically, that it fails to distinguish between frequent light and occasional heavy drinkers. For several reasons, nevertheless, the combination index was used in the present study. Because of the youth of the subjects, it was unlikely that adult, stable drinking patterns had already been established. Empirically, it was found that the quantity measure correlated .69 with frequency in the male and .73 in the female sample. Finally, a different drinking measure, "frequency of drunkenness," yielded virtually the same correlations with the personality scale scores.

RESULTS

The 88 self-descriptive statements found to relate to heavy drinking and selected for further analysis in samples C, DM, DF can be found in Tables 10.1–3 and in Appendix VI. Items appear in the order of their factor loadings. Also presented are the correlation coefficients of the items with the drinking measure obtained in sample C. A positive correlation indicates that a "true" answer to the item predicts drinking positively, and a negative correlation that a "false" answer is associated with heavy drinking.

In general, the labels given to the factors appearing in Tables 10.1–3 represent our interpretations of the factors.

Table 10.1—Self-descriptive statements grouped in Factor I: Assertive antisocial behavior

Source of Statement[a]	Statement	Factor Loading	N = 190 r with drinking
1. OPI-D-184	As a youngster in school I used to give the teachers a lot of trouble.	.644	.34**
2. OPI-D-27	During one period when I was a youngster I engaged in petty thievery.	.588	.32**
3. Gough-Fem-29 OPI-D-349 CPI-214 MMPI-118	In school I was sometimes sent to the principal for cutting up. (A)[b]	.526	.40**
4. CPI-420	I used to steal sometimes when I was a youngster.	.526	.35**
5. CPI-393 MMPI-215	I have used alcohol excessively. (A)	.507	.46**
6. OPI-D-228	I have often either broken rules (school, club, etc.,) or inwardly rebelled against them.	.483	.24**
7. CPI-262	There have been a few times when I have been very mean to another person.	.442	.23**
8. Yea-Nay 17	Let us eat, drink, and be merry, for tomorrow we die.	.428	.35**
9. CPI-189	In school my marks in deportment were quite regularly bad.	.426	.25**
10. OPI-D-416 CPI-143 Gough Fem-21	I like to be with a crowd who play jokes on one another.	.421	.31**
11. MMPI-419 CPI-36	I played hooky from school quite often as a youngster. (A)	.420	.37**
12. OPI-D-404	I crave excitement.	.414	.14
13. OPI-D-57	I have always hated regulations.	.413	.27**
14. EYS N-48	I like to play pranks upon others.	.411	.23**
15. CPI-323 OPI-D-338	I have never done any heavy drinking.	−.426	−.42**
16. OPI-D-333	I have never indulged in any unusual sex practices.	−.445	−.39**
17. MMPI-460	I have used alcohol moderately (or not at all). (A)	−.490	−.55**

"Notes to Table 10.1."

* $p < .05$ (two-tailed).
** $p < .01$ (two-tailed).
[a]Abbreviations refer to the following sources:
  OPI-D, Omnibus Personality Inventory, Form D
  CPI, California Psychological Inventory
  Gough-Fem, Femininity Scale of CPI administered by itself
  MMPI, Minnesota Multiphasic Personality Inventory
  Yea-Nay, Yea-Naysaying Scale (Couch and Keniston, 1960)
  EYS-E-N, Extraversion and Neuroticism Scales from Eysenck:
    Maudsley Personality Inventory
  T-M, Terman Miles Masculinity Subscale 5
[b](A) indicated item is endorsed in same direction by alcoholics (Cf. MacAndrew, 1965).

The first factor, "Assertive Antisocial Behavior," contains statements dealing with behavior that can get a person into trouble. To label these behaviors antisocial may be somewhat strong; a better description might be petty "acting out" behavior.

The second factor, "Lively Social Presence," is composed of items dealing, on one pole, with social outgoingness—carefree lively sociability with a flavor of exhibitionism—and on the other pole, with social reticence, awkwardness, shyness, or more generally a negative self-concept.

The third factor consists of items that are negatively correlated with drinking; that is, endorsement of these statements is associated with low drinking. The third factor is less homogeneous than the first two. Instead of calling it "Adherence to Order" we might better have

Table 10.2—Self-descriptive statements grouped in Factor II :
Lively social presence

	Source of Statement[a]	Statement	Factor Loading	N = 190 r with drinking
1.	MMPI-57 CPI-242	I am a good mixer. (A)	.741	.20*
2.	EYS-E-N-8	I would rate myself as a lively individual.	.598	.25**
3.	EYS-E-N-44	Other people regard me as a lively individual.	.571	.22**
4.	MMPI-309 OPI-180	I seem to make friends about as quickly as others do. (A)	.519	.11
5.	EYS-E-N-34	I would rate myself as a happy-go-lucky individual.	.503	.28**
6.	EYS-E-N-38	I can usually let myself go and have a hilariously good time at a gay party.	.499	.37**
7.	CPI-251	I like large, noisy parties.	.458	.33**
8.	CPI-163 T-M-I-13	I like parties and socials.	.437	.18*
9.	MMPI-445	I was fond of excitement when I was young (or in childhood). (A)	.429	.17*
10.	Gough Fem- OPI-D-63 CPI-208	I like to go to parties and other affairs where there is lots of loud fun.	.404	.31**
11.	Yea-Nay-31	I really enjoy plenty of excitement.	.405	.18*
12.	OPI-409 Yea-Nay-13	Little things upset me.	−.420	−.13
13.	CPI-272 Gough Fem-36	I must admit I feel sort of scared when I move to a strange place.	−.441	−.15
14.	CPI-279	I often get disgusted with myself.	−.463	−.17*
15.	Gough Fem-5 CPI-38	It is hard for me to start a conversation with strangers.	−.563	−.13
16.	EYS-E-N-14	I am inclined to keep in the background on social occasions.	−.610	−.32
17.	CPI-111	When in a group of people I have trouble thinking of the right things to talk about.	−.636	−.17

Note : See "Notes to Table 10.1."

Table 10.3—Self-descriptive statements grouped in Factor III: Adherence to order

Source of Statement[a]	Statement	Factor Loading	N = 190 r with drinking
1. CPI-380	I am known as a hard and steady worker.	.632	−.28**
2. OPI-D-48	I have been inspired to a way of life based on duty which I have carefully followed.	.617	−.20*
3. CPI-112	I set a high standard for myself and I feel others should do the same.	.608	−.38**
4. OPI-D-361	I do not like to see people carelessly dressed.	.571	−.23**
5. OPI-D-7 CPI-361	I like to have a place for everything and everything in its place.	.557	−.39**
6. CPI-123 CPI-400 Gough Fem-19	I think I am stricter about right and wrong than most people.	.542	−.40**
7. CPI-24	I always like to keep my things neat and tidy and in good order.	.526	−.44**
8. CPI-14	I always follow the rule: business before pleasure.	.504	−.25**
9. CPI-204	I like to plan a home study schedule and then follow it.	.495	−.17*
10. OPI-D-97	The surest way to a peaceful world is to improve people's morals.	.476	−.15
11. OPI-D-28	The trouble with many people is that they don't take things seriously enough.	.470	−.25**
12. CPI-376	I enjoy planning things, and deciding what each person should do.	.459	−.22**
13. CPI-371 CPI-230	I would rather be a steady and dependable worker than a brilliant but unstable one.	.449	−.20*
14. CPI-260	I always try to do at least a little better than what is expected of me.	.417	−.18*

Note: See "Notes to Table 10.1."

called it "Order and Conscience." The "order" side of the dimension contains statements dealing with order, steadiness, planning—for example, "I am known as a hard and steady worker," "I like to have a place for everything and everything in its place." Examples of items indicating a strong conscience are: "I have been inspired to a way of life based on duty which I have carefully followed," and "I set a high standard for myself and I feel others should do the same."

Those statements with factor loading of less than ±.400 on the three factors are presented in Appendix VI. Even though these items did not meet the criteria for scale inclusion, they nevertheless covary with drinking, and among them are several items that are endorsed in the same way by alcoholics (cf. MacAndrew, 1965). A cutting point of .400 for scale inclusion is, of course, arbitrary, and many of these ungrouped items may actually belong to one of the three clusters previously described.

The correlations of the scales based on the three factors and on the rest of the items are presented in Table 10.4. Note that the direction of the scale based on factor III is reversed in the direction of Lack of Order to yield positive correlations with drinking. The correlation of each of the scales with drinking is highly significant in the original (Sample C) as well as in the cross-validation samples (Samples DM and DF). From the intercorrelations of the scales it can be seen that they are not completely independent, as might be expected from factors obtained through orthogonal rotation. In sample C all intercorrelations are positive and significant. The greatest independence exists between Lively Social Presence and Lack of Order, as the correlations between these scales are low and nonsignificant in the two cross-validation samples. This result suggests that heavy drinkers describe themselves in terms of two somewhat different clusters of characteristics, that is, Assertive Antisocial Behavior and Lively Social Presence or Lack of Order. Of further interest in Table 10.4 is the fact that the scale built on the ungrouped items shows the highest correlations, after Assertive Antisocial Behavior, with drinking. It is apparent that the aggregate of these items contains valid covariance with drinking, even though the meaning of the components is not perfectly clear.

DISCUSSION

The characterization of heavy drinkers as having tendencies for antisocial behavior and a lively social presence, and as lacking order receives support from other studies of heavy drinkers and alcoholics. Williams (1967) obtained self-descriptions of problem drinkers of college age through the adjective check list scored for the Heilbrun needs. Problem drinkers were found to be high in aggression and autonomy and low in succorance, deference and self-control. Jones (1965) found that those adult subjects from the Oakland Growth Study who were classified as problem drinkers were higher in TAT aggression than moderate drinkers. Further support for the conclusion that heavy drinking is associated with a tendency for antisocial behavior comes from a study not primarily concerned with drinking. Siegman (1966) studied the effects of father absence during early childhood on antisocial behavior among medical students. He administered an anonymous questionnaire asking about various behaviors such as truancy, the damaging or destruction of private or public property, having premarital and extramarital sex relations, and theft. One of the

Table 10.4—Means, standard deviations and intercorrelations of drinking measures and personality scale scores in three samples

Variable	Sample		AASB	LSP	LO	Ungrouped items
Mean	C	(N = 118)	6.82	10.96	7.36	18.91
	D	males (N = 83)	6.71	9.83	8.92	19.27
	D	females (N = 177)	4.08	10.03	8.24	15.74
SD	C	males	4.05	4.13	3.68	5.71
	D	males	3.20	4.43	3.06	4.51
	D	females	2.73	4.03	3.03	5.09
Drinking measure (Drink)	C		.64**	.40**	.49**	.69**
	D	males	.69**	.31**	.21**	.42**
	D	females	.43**	.22**	.30**	.43**
Assertive Antisocial Behavior (AASB)	C			.26**	.41**	.75**
	D	males		.41**	.34**	.65**
	D	females		.19**	.35**	.62**
Lively Social Presence (LSP)	C				.25**	.25**
	D	males			−.09	.43**
	D	females			.05	.23**
Lack of Order (LO)	C					.61**
	D	males				.55**
	D	females				.57**

** *p* < .01.

behaviors considered antisocial was drinking, and Siegman found that the drinking score loaded highly on the antisocial factor.

That alcoholics, as well as heavy social drinkers, are characterized by a tendency toward antisocial behavior is indicated in several reports. MacAndrew and Geertsma (1963) concluded on the basis of a review of the literature that the Pd scale of MMPI was the only consistent personality correlate of alcoholism. A factor analysis of the responses of alcoholics to the items of the Pd scale established six factors, one of which, called social deviance, is similar to our factor of antisocial behavior. This factor was one of the only two that discriminated between alcoholics and nonalcoholics.

Another defining feature of the heavy drinkers in the present study was lively social presence. Jones (1965) found that the sociability scale of the CPI was positively associated with heavy drinking. She also found, however, that heavy drinkers scored *lower* than moderate drinkers in the need for affiliation measured through the TAT. A close look at the self-descriptive statements of heavy drinkers reveals the kind of sociability that is involved; the heavy drinker, in short, is more of a wild, narcissistic social show-off than a person who simply longs for the company of others. This impression is further strengthened when we look at those aspects of sociability that are *not* related to drinking. The kind of social relations that requires social commitment and long-term social involvement shows no relationship with drinking. There were several items in the original inventory dealing with such things as "being a good leader," "belonging to clubs," etc., that were not systematically related to drinking.

Our characterization of the sociability of the heavy drinker as being narcissistic, short-term, exhibitionistic and wild rather than oriented toward long-term social commitment also seems to hold for alcoholics. Blane (1960) noted that although alcoholics were frequently engaging individuals who enjoyed the company of convivial groups, and could be charming companions, their sociability often paradoxically coexisted with an inability to maintain a long-term relationship based on mutual give-and-take.

A similar picture is presented by Shulman (1951) who describes the alcoholic as having a "salesman type of personality," yet rarely belonging to groups and being indeed somewhat isolated. Force (1958) comes to similar conclusions. He describes the alcoholic as an emotional, sympathetic extrovert, gregarious and exhibitionistic, as a person who likes to be with people largely to be looked at, who favors exploitative, selling contacts, but who does not have close emotional ties. Machover and Puzzo (1959) consider the alcoholic "schizoid," characterized on the one hand by superficial, inconstant and self-centered participation in interpersonal relationships and, on the other, as basically isolated and narcissistic.

Antisocial behavior and lively social presence describe the interpersonal behavior of heavy drinkers. Lack of order indicates their intrapsychic functioning. Other studies of heavy drinkers and alcoholics have also found disorganization and lack of order. Williams (1967) showed problem drinkers to be higher than nonproblem drinkers in change and lability and lower in endurance and order. Jones (1965) came to picture the problem drinker in a similar way, but only in a roundabout way. She discovered that problem drinkers scored higher than moderate drinkers on the flexibility scale of the CPI, a scale that is supposed to "indicate the degree of flexibility and adaptability of a person's thinking and social behavior" (Gough, 1957, p. 11). Apparently concerned that problem drinkers should be described as "flexible," a favorable attribute, Jones reasoned that "it is highly probable that impulsivity is what we are measuring" (p. 5). The present results bear out her reasoning. Items such as "having a place for everything," "being a hard and steady worker," "being stricter about right and wrong," all from the flexibility scale of the CPI, in our study appear in Factor three which we called lack of order.

Impulsivity, or lack of order, seems to be characteristic of alcoholics as well as heavy social drinkers. Lentz *et al.* (1943) concluded, on the basis of a questionnaire study, that alcoholics were more impulsive that controls. Force (1958) described alcoholics as having low perseverance and discharging energy openly, thus not allowing prolonged endeavor, long periods of preparation toward a constant goal, immediate self-denial, or postponed satisfaction. Similar conclusions were reached by Halpern (1946), Buhler and Lefever (1947), and Quaranta (1947).

A DIRECT COMPARISON OF HEAVY DRINKERS WITH ALCOHOLICS

Similarities between heavy drinkers and alcoholics in terms of major personality dimensions found in this study have already been pointed out. The general similarity is further evident in the similarity of responses by the two groups to the 51 items from the MMPI found by MacAndrew (1965) to discriminate between alcoholics and nonalcoholics. Thirty-seven of the 51 items were answered in the same direction as alcoholics by heavy-drinking college students ($p < .01$, sign test), indicating a greater correspondence than would be expected by chance.

Because both the studies by MacAndrew and Geertsma (1963) and MacAndrew (1965) employed methods similar to the one used in this investigation, a detailed search for possible differences between heavy normal drinkers and alcoholics becomes possible. The former researchers found that a factor indicating remorseful intropunitiveness discriminated between alcoholics and nonalcoholics. The items contained in this factor such as "I know who is responsible for most of my troubles," or "Much of the time I feel as if I have done something wrong or evil," cannot be found among the items included in Tables 10.1–3 and in Appendix VI. Several items like these, however, had been included in PRI-310 and failed to differentiate between heavy and light drinkers. The most likely explanation is the possibility that remorseful intropunitiveness is a consequence of a history of prolonged drinking, and is especially likely to be admitted by a person who seeks treatment as an alcoholic.

A further difference between heavy social drinkers and alcoholics seems to be the readiness to report symptoms. The MacAndrew study, for example, shows that alcoholics are more likely than nonalcoholics to endorse such items as, "I have had blank spells in which my activities were interrupted and I did not know what was going on around me," "I have a cough most of the time," and "I frequently notice my hand shakes when I try to do something." These items do not discriminate heavy from moderate social drinkers, probably because the latter have not had a sufficiently long period of excessive drinking to produce these symptoms. Another possible difference is that only alcoholics who seek treatment admit such symptoms.

The conclusion that heavy-drinking college students are similar to alcoholics in some personality attributes is extremely significant with regard to establishing the etiology of alcoholism. Studies of alcoholics alone say little about the "alcoholic personality," if by this term we mean personality characteristics that *lead to* excessive drinking, for any attribute that distinguishes an alcoholic from a nonalcoholic could be the result of excessive drinking as well as its cause. When we find personality attributes that are similarly characteristic of the pre-alcoholic (i.e., the heavy social drinker) and the alcoholic, we can be more certain that we are dealing with personality dimensions antecedent to alcoholism.

HEAVY DRINKING, POWER, AND INHIBITION

How do the present results fit the theory proposed in this volume, that heavy drinking is a response to a strong need for power, coupled with a lack of inhibition? Antisocial behavior, the social aggressiveness inherent in playing pranks, and the excitement to be found in wild parties indicate aggressive ascendancy and can be considered as ways of behaving potently. By engaging in this behavior, a person demonstrates to himself and to the world that he is strong. Such an interpretation is similar to Siegman's (1966) conception of antisocial behavior as a masculine protest in response to a basic feminine identity, or simply a lack of masculine identity. Siegman's results, as well as his theory, could easily be translated into the present conception. The boy whose father is absent, because he identifies with his mother or fails to identify with his father, develops a basic feeling of weakness but also a need for potency. In response to this need, he displays aggressive ascendancy and drinks heavily.

Lively social presence represents a response to potency needs because it can be thought of as a short-term, inconsequential quest and display of potency. The narcissistic, center-of-stage, exhibitionistic type of sociability is both a way of telling the world that one is not weak, and at the same time of receiving social reinforcement that can provide a sense of potency. After all, who does not like and react favorably to the life-of-the-party?

Finally, the cluster of self-descriptive statements grouped in Factor 3, Lack of Order, seem to fit the concept of lack of inhibition, or impulsivity. Heavy drinkers describe themselves in terms suggesting rapid action, little or no planning, and a lack of long-term values.

On the basis of these results, as well as those of other investigations of heavy drinkers and alcoholics, the following conclusions seem warranted. Heavy drinkers display interpersonal relationships characterized by aggressive ascendancy and narcissistic sociability, and their intrapsychic functioning shows lack of order. Such conclusions support the theory of drinking proposed in this volume. Aggressive ascendancy and narcissistic sociability can be considered a manifestation of the need for power, whereas a lack of order can be subsumed under the concept of lack of inhibition.

Chapter **11**

Alcoholism
in a
Mexican Village

by Michael Maccoby

Prefatory Note to Chapter 11—The following chapter was written in 1965 in the midst of our research. The ideas in it, as ably expounded to us by Dr. Maccoby, had a considerable influence on our thinking at the time. In fact they shaped an earlier version of Chapter 13 which explained alcoholism as defense, as a compensation for felt weakness, as a reaction against being overly protected and dominated by wives and mothers.

As subsequent research findings came in, we were gradually forced, we thought, to revise our views, to take account of the fact, for instance, that men drink more not when they are made to feel helpless, but when they are made to feel powerful (Chapter 9). Alcoholism began to appear to us as an assertive as much as a defensive strategy, and the responses of wives and mothers as consequences, rather than exclusively as causes of drinking. Yet we have reproduced the chapter as it was initially written because, as noted in the Introduction, we are not certain that we have interpreted the facts correctly and we feel the reader should be given the same chance as we had to interpret them in any way he likes.

It might be useful to indicate briefly how our current interpretation differs from the stance taken by Dr. Maccoby in this chapter. As explained in Chapter 13, since we have been unable to find any direct evidence for passive receptiveness—

the wish to be comfortable, warmed and treated like an infant—we have come to believe the signs usually taken to signify this desire, by Dr. Maccoby as well as others, should be reinterpreted. Some oral signs appear simply to reflect the obvious fact that alcoholics abuse their gastrointestinal systems. They need not be interpreted as signifying a deep personality trend "causing" drinking, but may be just a consequence of drinking too much.

Other signs of a receptive character in alcoholics—such as the greater tendency to go to magic healers (curanderos) *or to marry dominating wives—we interpret below as strategies aimed at increasing the feeling of personal power by borrowing strength from others. To be sure, this is a kind of receptivity, but it is a little different from wanting to be fed, warmed and infantilized. Although it is clear that alcoholics have disturbed relations with women, as Dr. Maccoby's findings make abundantly clear, we tend to see these as consequences of their personal power drives, rather than as consequences of what women have done to them. The mother fixation he reports for alcoholics characterizes moderate drinkers to the same degree. Here as elsewhere in his analysis it is the abstainers who are deviant. Thus it is their* lack *of mother fixation that needs explanation in Mexican culture rather than the mother fixation of alcoholics. In general we have avoided comparing abstainers with alcoholics because both groups deviate from the norm in our culture; if they differ from each other, it is hard to know whether it is the psychodynamics of the one or the other which is responsible.*

Aside from the reinterpretation of what is meant by Receptive Character, the rest of Dr. Maccoby's report strengthens our current interpretation of the reasons for excessive drinking—particularly his findings of greater machismo, *and narcissistic sadism in alcoholics. In our terms this is practically a definition of what we mean by p Power—the need for personalized power.*

But whatever their final interpretation, the facts in this study of a Mexican village are fascinating in themselves and make an important introduction to an understanding of the cultural, economic, psychosocial and psychological factors that contribute to alcoholism.

T his study of alcoholism in a Mexican village is part of a five-year investigation of emotional disturbances that block the human and material development of peasant villagers.[1] The project, conceived and directed by Erich Fromm, has focussed on both the character structure of the peasant and his social reality, on the motivation for behavior and the socioeconomic forces—mode of work, family relations, and cultural institutions—which mold and reinforce

[1]The investigation has been supported by the Foundations Fund for Research in Psychiatry. For the statistical analyses, the study owes much to Ing. Sergio Beltran who made available the facilities of the Centro de Calculo of the National University of Mexico, and to Sra. Gloria U. de Beltran. I am especially grateful to Dr. Erich Fromm for his suggestions and criticism during all phases of the investigation.

character structure. The project has set out first to delineate social problems, second to relate these problems to social conditions and character structure, and third to understand the sociopsychological forces which determine character. The methods used have been participant observation combined with projective questionnaires administered to each of the adult villagers. These methods have eliminated sampling bias and have made it possible to chart the character structure of the villagers and relate social variables to motivational syndromes.

Alcoholism is a critical problem for the village. Drinking plays a part in most fights and murders.[2] Those who drink neglect families and work. The alcoholics, including 18 percent of the male population over 20, abandon responsibility as farmers, husbands, fathers, and members of the community. By abandoning his land, renting it or selling it and drinking up the proceeds, the alcoholic damages the *ejidal* system which was meant to free him from exploitation by *hacendados* and *caciques*. In other words, alcoholism results not only in violence and broken families, but also in the undermining of those institutions that might improve the villager's life.

Before probing into the causes of alcoholism, it is worth considering the village in the context of Mexico as a whole. This demands a critical examination of definitions of alcoholism, estimates of its prevalence, and methods generally used for its study.

The village is a mestizo agricultural community of 850 inhabitants in the state of Morelos. Before the revolution of 1910, the village was part of a hacienda, built in the late 16th or early 17th century, which depended on the sugar cane crop. In the center of Zapata's struggle for land reform, village life was shattered by the revolution. Afterwards, in the 1920's, immigrants from Guerrero and the state of Mexico swelled the population, so that only a third of the inhabitants are descended from families that lived under the hacienda. This pattern is common to the surrounding villages. The immigrants to the village brought with them a reformist spirit. They sought to do away with traditional and costly fiestas which they blamed for drinking, violence, and poverty. Indeed, by its neighbors the villagers are considered peaceful and progressive, more than the average, an impression confirmed by the municipal court records of the *municipio*, including neighboring villages.

In 1926, most of the farm land was partitioned to the villagers as *ejidos*, unalienable and indivisible plots averaging five acres that belong to the peasant as long as he works it, and can be inherited by his family. Ideally, each peasant was to have an ejido, but since 1926 the continued rise in population, through immigration and high birth rate, has been

[2]According to a report by Dr. Miguel Silva Martinez (1963), the sale of alcoholic drinks and the crime rate are highly correlated throughout Mexico. In the city of Mexico, 66 percent of the acts of violence, including fights and accidents, involve people who have been drinking.

such that only 27 percent of the men are *ejiditarios*, the rest earning their living mainly as day-laborers. The major crop of the village is still cane, accounting for 54 percent of the land in use, with rice (22 percent) the second most important crop.

With respect to patterns of work, the village is representative of the area. In terms of alcoholism and violence, the village is known as less troublesome and less alcoholic than its neighbors. However, the state of Morelos, according to statistics published by the Sociedad Mexicana de Higiene, has the third highest per capita expenditure for alcohol in the Republic, exceeded only by the bordering states of Mexico and Puebla (Martinez, 1963). Such data serve only for crude comparison, since they lump together nonequivalent types of drinks, and they do not include unregistered alcohol which makes up a high percentage of alcoholic drink in areas where *pulque* or cane alcohol is produced (*Seminario Latinoamericano Sobre Alcoholismo*, 1961). Indeed, it is common in peasant villages to drink a type of *aguardiente* made from pure distilled cane, mixed with water or soft drinks.

Other comparative statistics are also of doubtful validity. The best indirect estimate of prevalence, the Jellinek formula based on number of deaths due to cirrhosis of the liver, may underestimate the number of alcoholics. Jellinek's equation, which depends on the constancy of the relation between deaths due to cirrhosis and alcoholism, assumes reliable data from autopsies, which cannot be counted on in a peasant society. Even if autopsies were accurate, the formula assumes without reason that the percentage of cirrhosis cases that are fatal does not vary from one culture to another. A report by the Pan American Sanitary Office of the World Health Organization shows that in Chile, prevalence estimates based on the Jellinek formula were consistently smaller than those based on field studies.[3]

Even field studies run the risk of undestimating the problem. Our data are based on the findings of Dr. Felipe Sanchez who lived in the village five years as participant observer and physician to the villagers. Although the villagers, in answering interview questions, were frank about many intimate details, the alcoholics underestimated or misrepresented their drinking habits. Clinical experience confirms the impression that alcoholics either consciously or unconsciously distort the extent of their drinking. Dr. Sanchez' ratings of alcoholism result from observation and not from interview. The method used to rate all of the village men in terms of drinking habits was thus more exhaustive than studies based on estimates, and a reliable comparison of prevalence in other areas would demand equivalent methods and controls.

[3]*Seminario Latinoamericano Sobre Alcoholismo*, 1961. In a 1958 study in Chile, the Jellinek formula gave an estimate of 3.4 percent while the interview study indicated a percentage of 5.1.

With these problems of accuracy in mind, it is still interesting to report that the Jellinek formula gives an estimate for male alcoholism in the City of Mexico which is similar to that observed in the village. Using the Jellinek equation, Dr. Miguel Silva Martinez estimates that 8.7 percent of the population over age 20 are alcoholic, with or without complications. Since the Pan American Sanitary Organization (1961) calculates the ratio of male to female alcoholics in Mexico as 5.3 to 1,[4] it would appear that about 15 percent of adult men in Mexico City as compared to 18 percent of the villagers 20 or older are alcoholics.

According to the report of the Pan American Sanitary Organization, the prevalence of alcoholism in Mexico is one of the highest in the world. Whatever the exact comparison between prevalence in this village and in the rest of the country, the study of alcoholism in this village is relevant to understanding a national and not merely a local problem.

To explore the causes of alcoholism, it will be necessary first to define alcoholism and then to describe the methods of studying characterological and socioeconomic variables.

METHOD OF STUDY

In defining degree of alcoholism, either the physiological aspects of the disease or its social results can be emphasized. Since the purpose of this study is to focus on social pathology, the social effects of drinking are primary. Degree of alcoholism was determined by the extent of failure, due to repeated drinking, to meet social obligations. This definition does not take into account the amount of alcohol consumed nor the injury to the drinker's health. Yet, it is consistent with Keller's carefully analyzed definition of alcoholism as "a chronic disease manifested by repeated implicative drinking so as to cause injury to the drinker's health or to his social and economic functioning" (Keller, 1962). Although the operational definition used in this study is based on social and economic functioning, all of the villagers whose health has suffered due to drinking are included in the classification of alcoholism.

The 208 men of the village were divided into four major categories: alcoholics, excessive drinkers, moderate drinkers, and abstainers.[5] The alcoholics are defined as men who drink whenever they get the chance, without regard for their responsibilities. While some alcoholics work

[4]However, the report notes that the field studies in Chile show a much higher proportion of male to female alcoholics than is indicated by studying deaths by cirrhosis. The same may be true for Mexico.

[5]No female alcoholics were discovered in the village. These four categories correspond to those suggested by the *Seminario Latinoamericano Sobre Alcoholismo*, see Footnote 3.

some of the time, their drinking invariably makes them lose working days each week. On the basis of Dr. Sanchez' observations, confirmed by interviews with older villagers including the owner of a *cantina*, 30 men or 14.4 percent of the male villagers age 16 or older were judged to be alcoholic.

The excessive drinkers differ from the alcoholics only in degree. Excessive drinking during the weekend is not considered abnormal in the village, but the excessive drinker exceeds the cultural norm by losing Mondays and sometimes other workdays because of his drinking. Twenty-seven men, 13 percent of the adult males, were judged to be excessive drinkers.

The moderate drinkers, including 109 (52.3 percent) men are villagers whose drinking does not conflict with their responsibilities. The moderate drinkers may occasionally get drunk during the weekend or at a fiesta, but this is the exception rather than the rule.

The fourth group of 34 men (16.3 percent) are the abstainers. These are men who never drink in public; if they drink at all, it is at a family reunion or fiesta, and they stop after one or two drinks. The final category, including 8 persons or 4 percent of the adult men, includes men who have stopped drinking. This category is too small for statistically meaningful comparisons, but it will be useful for illustrating the importance of psychosocial factors.

On the average the alcoholics and excessive drinkers are older than the moderate drinkers and abstainers (Table 11.1). Of the alcoholics,

Table 11.1—Percentages of alcoholic and other males in various age groups

Age	Alcoholics (N=30)	Excessive Drinkers (N=27)	Moderate Drinkers (N=109)	Abstainers (N=34)	Total Male Population (N=208)
16–30	26.7	33.3	69.9	52.9	54.3
30–40	13.3	33.3	13.7	23.5	18.8
40–50	33.3	7.4	2.7	11.8	10.0
50–60	20.0	22.2	11.0	5.9	12.9
60–70*	6.7	3.8	2.7	5.9	3.9
Total	100.0	100.0	100.0	100.0	99.9

Correlation: Alcoholism with age = .287, $p < .01$.

60 percent are over 40, compared to 33.4 percent of the excessive drinkers, 23.6 percent of the abstainers and only 16.4 percent of the moderate drinkers. Indeed, of the male population over 40, 32 percent are alcoholics and 16 percent heavy drinkers, so that almost one-half of the older men suffer problems of alcoholism. These data reflect the observation that many villagers become alcoholics or excessive drinkers later in life and that the majority of young men start out as moderate

drinkers. In the United States, Pittman and Gordon (1958) have found that the percentage of inebriates over 40 in their sample of police cases is greater than the percentage under 40.[6] They offer the explanation that these are working-class men whose livelihood depends on manual skills, and they become more susceptible to drink as their working capacity declines. In the village, sociopsychological more than economic vulnerability to alcoholism increases with age, even though character structure remains invariant.

There is no significant difference in the marital status of alcoholics, excessive drinkers, and abstainers, with married men predominating in all three groups. A higher percentage of moderate drinkers are unmarried, reflecting the predominance of young men in this group. (Table 11.2.)

Table 11.2—Percentages of alcoholic and other males in various marital categories

Marital status	Alcoholics (N=30)	Excessive Drinkers (N=27)	Moderate Drinkers (N=109)	Abstainers (N=34)	Total Male Population (N=208)
Unmarried	26.7	18.5	37.4	23.5	29.6
Free union	6.6	3.7	22.4	11.8	15.5
Married (by church or civil law)	60.0	77.8	27.1	61.8	46.6
Widowed or divorced	6.7	0.0	13.1	2.9	8.3
Total	100.0	100.0	100.0	100.0	100.0

Two questionnaires were used. One about age, marital status, schooling, income, church attendance and work habits was administered to all the villagers (208 men and 207 women) of age 16 and over. The second questionnaire, which was used to interpret character structure, was based on a projective questionnaire developed by Fromm and used in an unpublished study of German workers and employees, undertaken at the Institute of Social Research of the University of Frankfurt. The projective questionnaire, which takes from two to four hours to administer, was given to all the adult villagers with the exception of a few who refused to cooperate. Of the 208 men, 191 were interviewed, including 28 of the 30 alcoholics, 26 of the 27 heavy drinkers, 107 of the 109 moderate drinkers, and 30 of the 34 abstainers.

The scoring of character traits was based on answers to open-ended questions and projective questions about attitudes to work, leisure and love, relations with parents, wife and children. Some of the questions call for the subject to report his feelings, likes, and dislikes directly. Other questions pose hypothetical situations, and the subject is asked

[6]David J. Pittman and C. Wayne Gordon, *Revolving Door*, New Haven, Conn.: Yale Center of Alcohol Studies, 1958, p. 43.

how he or another person would act. The interview is scored according to both manifest responses and by an interpretive, psychoanalytic method. The subject's direct statements are not taken at face value, but studied for their emotional charge, doubt or conviction, internal contradictions, underlying beliefs and expectations. What is sought is the basic motivation, which may be unconscious, hidden under rationalizations and denials. A man may claim to be gentle and loving, but if he reveals in his responses to hypothetical situations that a father would brutally punish a child who disobeys, the interview is studied carefully for other signs of an underlying sadism covered over by idealistic rationalizations. The goal of the analysis is to chart character structure, the relatively permanent way in which energy is channeled and directed, in which a person assimilates and relates.

The three basic scales employed in this analysis are the mode of relation, the mode of assimilation, and the scale of productivity or activity which modifies the first two scales. The mode of relation includes those traits which are the result of the socialization process and which describe how a person relates himself to others for work, for defense, for sexual satisfaction, for play, and for child rearing. The mode of assimilation expresses the way a person habitually assimilates and acquires things in order to satisfy his needs. He may produce things through his own effort, or he may depend fundamentally on the effort of others. The mode of assimilation is also related to a person's underlying feelings of what he can expect from the world, what types of experience he feels as good and satisfying, and what is experienced as unsatisfying.[7]

As a check on the validity of the interpretive scoring of the interview, the modes of relation, assimilation and productivity have been independently scored from a sample of Rorschachs. Both Schachtel (1950) and Schafer (1954) have discussed the basis for determining character traits from the content of the Rorschach. Schafer employs a classification based on libido theory which in most cases can be modified in terms of Fromm's characterology which shares with libido theory the expectation that unconscious motivation is revealed by expressive imagery. Furthermore, although Fromm's receptive character, for example, is not determined by libidinal factors, the clinical description of this character type from the point of view of humanistic psychoanalysis is the same as in libido theory. Similarly, Freud's anal character is the starting point for the concept of the hoarding mode of assimilation, and the oral-sadistic character is at the core of the exploitative mode. As the results of the interpretive scoring are reported, the Rorschach evidence supporting this scoring will be described.

[7]For a fuller analysis of these scales and their theoretical basis see Erich Fromm, *Man for Himself*, New York, Holt, Rinehart, and Winston, 1947.

What causes alcoholism in the village? As many studies have shown, it is not possible to pick out a single trait which invariably causes alcoholism. Rather, as Jellinek (1960) suggests, there are "vulnerabilities" to alcoholism, social and psychological syndromes that increase the likelihood of excessive drinking. Vulnerability in the village is a combination, as in other societies, of cultural, psychological, and socioeconomic factors. There are primitive societies in which the cultural vulnerability is so great that alcoholism is institutionalized. In such societies, it is likely that even those people who are free from psychological vulnerability would become heavy drinkers. In other cultures, the opposite happens, and only those individuals with intense characterological vulnerability become alcoholics.

Four types of vulnerability emerge from the investigation. The first is cultural vulnerability, including institutions that encourage drinking, interests which involve drinking, and lack of interests which make drinking more attractive. Second is psychological vulnerability, the unconscious motivation that characterizes the alcoholic. Third is psychosocial vulnerability, the interpersonal patterns, the conflicts, particularly between the sexes, which reinforce or trigger the impulse to drink. And fourth is economic vulnerability, the economic pressures which interact with character structure and increase the likelihood of alcoholism.

CULTURAL VULNERABILITY

Almost without exception, the villagers consider drinking a harmful vice. Even the alcoholics state that alcohol is a great danger to health, and that it is likely to lead to violence and enmity between friends. One villager who drinks rarely sums up the feeling of the majority. "The vice of drinking makes a man lose his chance to gain money for his family. If he is a worker, he does not earn money. He harms his body and his family. If he is a peasant, it is the same, and he also neglects his crops." Yet this man adds that drink makes him feel happiness, great pleasure, and the desire to communicate with others. Some of the alcoholics say that drinking is the only thing that gives them the joy of being alive, the desire to sing and shout.

The attractions of drinking increase when contrasted to the boredom of peasant life. There are seven *cantinas* in the village, and when men congregate in the plaza in the afternoon, they often find themselves drawn to a *cantina* for want of anything else to do. Drinking also is traditionally associated with the few special events in the village, *fiestas*, *jaripeos*, dances, and weddings. Sometimes, men drink only out of politeness, since it is unfriendly to abstain when friends are drinking.

Although most village men begin as beer drinkers, the alcoholics end up drinking pure cane alcohol, which is stronger and cheaper (about 50 centavos for two ounces). Sometimes the alcohol is mixed with a soft drink and called *teporocha*. Only a few villagers drink *tequila*. Invariably a drinker sticks to one type of alcohol. Brandy is drunk by the richer non-alcoholic peasants at fiestas only.

For many villagers drinking is the most attractive activity the village has to offer. They have no other interests. Agricultural work, which has changed little in the past centuries, is monotonous and routinized; the peasant has neither the land nor the capital to make farming more interesting. Under these conditions, those who work harder gain but little more, and some men who are able to support themselves with little work spend their time loitering and drinking.

Those who do not drink, the abstainers, have forceably broken away from the old cultural patterns to support new institutions. Many of them either play on the town basketball team or did so when younger. The team was formed 25 years ago by a progressive schoolmaster who with a group of the villagers campaigned against the *jaripeos* and *fiestas* that reinforced patterns of alcoholism. The abstainers avoid many of the old traditions, preferring modern sports such as basketball and soccer football to bullfights. Their concept of manliness is not the hard drinking, touchy and violent "macho" figure, but the well-trained, disciplined athlete. In every way they can, they seek cultural stimulation to make their lives more interesting and less monotonous. When our

Table 11.3—Percentages of alcoholic and other males attending Mass and cultural events

CHURCH ATTENDANCE

Attendance	Alcoholics (N=30)	Excessive Drinkers (N=26)	Moderate Drinkers (N=107)	Abstainers (N=33)	Total Male Population (N=208)
Frequent	6.7	26.9	36.4	48.5	33.3
Infrequent	26.7	19.2	27.2	33.3	26.5
Never	66.7	53.9	36.4	18.2	39.2
Total	100.0	100.0	100.0	100.0	100.0

Correlations: Alcoholism with church attendance $= -.315, p < .01$
Church attendance with age $= -.041$, insignificant

ATTENDANCE AT MOVIES, CONCERTS, READINGS

Attendance	Alcoholics	Excessive Drinkers	Moderate Drinkers	Abstainers	Total Male Population
Frequent	6.7	23.1	19.0	36.4	21.4
Infrequent	0.0	3.8	17.0	24.2	14.3
Never	93.3	73.1	64.0	39.4	64.3
Total	100.0	100.0	100.0	100.0	100.0

Correlations: Alcoholism with attendance $= -.316, p < .01$
Attendance with age $= -.058$, insignificant

project brought movies, musical performances, and readings from good literature to the village, 60 percent of the abstainers, 36 percent of the moderate drinkers, 27 percent of the excessive drinkers, and only 6.7 percent of the alcoholics attended at least one of these events. (Table 11.3.) The chi-square of alcoholics vs. abstainers is 20.1, significant at the .001 level. The correlation between age and attendance is $-.058$ showing that the difference is not due to the youth of the abstainers. Neither is the difference due to educational level, since approximately half of both alcoholics and abstainers have had no schooling (Table 11.4). There is also a clear-cut relationship between church attendance and sobriety; 67 percent of the alcoholics compared to only 18 percent of the abstainers never attend mass (chi-square = 15.2, significant at the .001 level). Again, the rank order of mean church attendance corresponds exactly to degree of alcoholism. (See Table 11.3.) It is not that the alcoholics do not consider themselves good Catholics; possibly,

Table 11.4—Percentages of alcoholic and other males attaining various levels of education

Educational leve	Alcoholics (N=28)	Excessive Drinkers (N=26)	Moderate Drinkers (N=97)	Abstainers (N=34)	Total Male Population (N=193)
No Schooling	50.0	34.6	15.5	44.1	28.5
1–6 years of primary	42.9	61.5	63.9	35.3	55.4
Graduated primary	7.1	3.9	20.6	20.6	16.1

Correlations: Alcoholism with education = $-.146$, insignificant
Age and education   = $-.180$, $p < .05$

some of them seek to avoid the moralizing of the priest. But in general they take no part in activities that do not involve drinking. In a culture with few cultural stimuli, they have become dependent on drinking as their sole diversion.[8] The only alcoholics who have any interest outside of the *cantinas* are members of the village band, where the traditional reward for services is free drinks.

PSYCHOLOGICAL VULNERABILITY

Clinical studies in the United States have produced broad agreement as to the psychological traits that characterize the alcoholic.

[8]Lack of interest in cultural stimuli also characterizes alcoholics in other parts of the world. Jellinek writes of the Swiss alcoholic that he is a "primitive hedonist," a person "with an extremely narrow field of interests and a veritable inability to take interest in anything else but himself and a narrow circle around him. There is also, generally, an inability to respond adequately to the finer stimuli of life. The narrowness of interests constitutes a psychological vulnerability which is the source of the 'mere habit' of heavy drinking." (See Jellinek, 1960, p. 387.)

These include oral receptive dependency, deep mother fixation, narcissism, extremely aggressive impulses, and the wish to escape the anxiety of aloneness. (Zwerling and Rosenbaum, 1959.) Despite this agreement, it cannot be said that these traits constitute an "alcoholic character," since they also characterize people who do not become alcoholics but develop other serious personality disorders. What these character traits appear to represent is a syndrome of psychological vulnerability.

Knight (1937) has described this character syndrome in more dynamic terms. The alcoholic's childhood experiences with a characteristically overprotective mother tend to produce excessive demands for indulgence. Disappointment and frustration of these oral needs trigger rage, but the individual feels guilty about his hostile impulses and punishes himself masochistically. He needs excessive indulgence to pacify his guilt, thus stimulating a vicious cycle. Alcohol, which smothers the rage and disappointment, is a symbolic substitute for affection; but it serves also to spite those who withhold affection and results in masochistic debasement.

To some extent, Knight's dynamic description of the alcoholic, based on clinical observation in the United States, agrees with what we have observed in the village. The Mexican peasant mother is extremely overprotective. Many village mothers refuse to let their children play outside of the limits of their houses. They make their children feel that the world is dangerous, and that they will be safe only at home and close to the mother. Such overprotectiveness was once a rational impulse to protect children from the real dangers of the *hacienda*, where peasants lacked rights and where the best way to avoid trouble was by keeping close to the family group. Furthermore, there is a strong emphasis on oral gratification. The average weaning period in the village is 18 months, a period which is cut short only by the birth of a new child. Boys more than girls are especially indulged, not only orally, but also because little responsibility is expected from them, at least until the age of six. Girls are raised more severely, being expected at an early age to be cleaner, more responsible, and to share in the housework and the tending of younger siblings. By the age of six, when boys just begin to take on small work assignments, the little girls are already experienced workers. Indeed, the attitude of greater indulgence of male irresponsibility and impulsiveness is widespread in Mexico, while women are expected to be *abnegada*, to bear greater burdens without complaints. This difference between the sexes may help to explain why male vulnerability to alcoholism is much greater than female vulnerability.

On two points observation of village alcoholics points to interpretations different from Knight's. The alcoholics in the village are usually not guilty about their hostile impulses, but are frightened that their rage will make other people abandon them and refuse to satisfy their receptive needs.[9] The renewed need for excessive indulgence is not to pacify guilt but to reassure the alcoholic that his symbiotic ties have not been severed, and he may drink in order to show that he can satisfy himself magically, as well as to spite those who withhold affection.

The second point is that although some of the alcoholics drink when they are frustrated in their oral needs, such an interpretation is overgeneralized. There is another type of alcoholic whose impulse to drink is determined mainly by frustration of his sense of manliness. These alcoholics are the men who only start to drink later in life, after marriage. Although they share the receptive, passive traits of the more mother-fixated alcoholic, their needs for oral indulgence in themselves are not great enough to cause alcoholism. The determining stimulus for drinking is rooted in their psychosocial vulnerability.

The dynamic analysis of alcoholism serves as a basis for the investigation of the prevalence of the characterological vulnerability syndrome in the alcoholics as contrasted with the abstainers.

Receptive Character

Although the presence of a receptive character trait is general among the village men (see Table 11.5), the trait is more pronounced in those who drink more. Over 80 percent of the alcoholics, 60 percent of the heavy drinkers, 47 percent of the moderate drinkers, and only 37 percent of the abstainers were scored as dominantly receptive in their mode of assimilation. The comparison between alcoholics and abstainers produces a chi-square of 12.3 significant at the .001 level. The correlation of alcoholism and the receptive trait is .186 significant at the .01 level. The scoring of a dominant receptive mode of assimilation indicates that the alcoholics feel the source of all good is outside of themselves, that the only way to get what they want, be it affection, food, love, or pleasure, is by receiving it from others. They feel incapable of producing it for themselves. They also are particularly sensitive to rejection by others, since they feel lost and paralyzed when they must act alone, when they must make decisions or take responsibility. Although they often express a genuine warmth, an enjoyment and optimism, especially when satisfied, and wish to help others, nevertheless the process of doing things for others also assumes the function of securing favor. The receptive person is also characterized by his tendency to overcome anxiety and depression by eating and drinking.

A check on the interview scoring of receptiveness was based on an

[9]One alcoholic frankly admits that drinking leads him into arguments or fights with his wife which is dangerous because she then refuses to feed him.

analysis of nine Rorschachs of alcoholics and 11 of abstainers, which were scored independently (without knowledge of the alcoholism classification) according to Schafer's (1954, p. 131) thematic indications of the oral-receptive orientation. The individual was scored as receptive if there was an emphasis on: perceptions of food, food sources (breasts, udders, nipples), food objects (cups, pots), food providers (cooks, waiters), passive food receivers (bird waitings to be fed), food organs (mouth, lips, stomach), nurturers and protectors (cow, mother hen, protective angel), givers (Santa Claus, the Three Kings), and oral eroticism (figures kissing). On this basis, 67 percent of the alcoholics compared to 27 percent of the abstainers were scored as receptive, producing a Fisher's exact probability of .097.

Table 11.5—Percentages of alcoholic and other males classified as possessing certain character traits based on their answers to projective questions

Character Trait	Alcoholics (N=28)	Excessive Drinkers (N=25)	Moderate Drinkers (N=107)	Abstainers (N=30)	Total Male Population (N=208)	Correlation with Alcoholism
Sadistic	42.9	36.0	17.4	26.7	29.8	.167 *
Dominant receptive	82.1	60.0	47.0	36.7	51.4	.186 **
Receptive	92.9	84.0	77.8	70.0	79.3	.083
Dominant hoarding	10.7	16.0	22.2	36.7	22.4	−.189 **
Hoarding	17.9	48.0	46.2	60.0	45.2	−.262 **
Aggressive	67.0	68.0	36.0	26.7	42.6	.276 **
Strong "machismo"	63.0	60.0	30.6	34.6	38.6	.253 **

* $p < .05$ ** $p < .01$

The receptive-passive orientation of the alcoholics can also be inferred from their answers to the interview question: "What are the forces that determine the destiny of man?" Of the alcoholics, 68 percent saw man as passive, dependent on God's will or on accidents of birth. Of the abstainers 45 percent took this view, while more than half felt that man's decision and energy are factors in determining his destiny. The difference between alcoholics and abstainers results in a chi-square of 4.6, significant at the 5 percent level.

The receptive person also seeks "magic helpers." If this is so, it might be expected that the alcoholic would turn to curanderos rather than medical doctors when he is sick. The curandero, more than the doctor, is likely to take seriously the peasant's fears and depressions rather than tell him that there is "nothing wrong with him." He presents an image of magic authority and concern for even those ailments which appear to have no physical basis. On the basis of the villagers' statements, 76 percent of the alcoholics as compared to 39 percent of the abstainers seek help from curanderos. (Table 11.6.) The chi-square of this difference is 8.4, significant at the 1 percent level. Although using curanderos is also correlated with age, 60 percent of the alcoholics under 40 compared to only 28 percent of the younger abstainers employ curanderos (chi-square is 3.76, with one tail probability less than .05).

Narcissism and Sadism

The village alcoholic's narcissism is expressed not only in his lack of interest and activity, but also in his need to present himself as invulnerable, irresistible to women, without sentiment, yet always capable of defending his honor by force if necessary. These traits as they show up on the responses to the interview are the basis of scoring a four-point scale of "machismo," including extreme machismo, marked machismo, few or no indications of machismo. Machismo is inversely correlated to ratings of responsibility, cooperation, satisfaction in work, and productivity. It is directly correlated to aggressiveness and belligerency. The

Table 11.6—Percentages of alcoholic and other males using curanderos and modern medicine

	Alcoholics (N=29)	Excessive Drinkers (N=26)	Moderate Drinkers (N=107)	Abstainers (N=33)	Total Male Population (N=203)
Modern medicine only	24.1	38.5	66.4	60.6	54.7
Both curanderos and medicine	58.6	46.2	28.0	27.3	35.5
Curanderos only	17.3	15.3	5.6	12.1	9.8

Correlations: Alcoholism with use of curanderos = .223, $p < .01$
Age with use of curanderos = .892, $p < .01$

correlation with age is not significant (.077). Of the alcoholics, 63 percent were scored as extremely or markedly machistic, compared to 60 percent of the excessive drinkers, 31 percent of the moderate drinkers, and 35 percent of the abstainers. (Table 11.5.) The chi-square of the difference between alcoholics and abstainers is 4.3, significant at the 5 percent level. The correlation of alcoholism and machismo is .253, significant at the 1 percent level.

Machismo indicates an attitude of male superiority, a wish to control women and keep them in an inferior position. One of the interview questions concerned whether women should have the same rights as men. Of the alcoholics, 78.6 percent say no compared to 44.8 percent of the abstainers. The chi-square of the difference is 6.8, significant at the 1 percent level. In their explanations of why women should not have the same rights as men, the alcoholics express more a fear of women than a conviction of superiority. They imply that unless men are given an advantage, the women are likely to control them; in other words, the alcoholic's machismo is a reaction to his fear of women, a compensation for his feeling of weakness, dependence, and passivity.

If the alcoholic's machismo is contrasted to the reality of his relations with women, it becomes perfectly clear that his attitude of toughness is a facade for weakness. Dr. Sanchez together with Dr. and Mrs. T. Schwartz, two anthropologists who lived in the village for 14 months, rated all of the village families in terms of whether the husband or wife was the dominant one in the family. Their judgments were determined by observing which person deferred to the other in decisions about child-rearing and participating in activities. They also noted whether the husband or wife generally won arguments. Of the alcoholics, 15 of the 19 married men (78.9 percent) were judged to be dominated by their wives, while only 1 of 17 abstainers (5.9 percent) was dominated by his wife. The chi-square is 19.2, significant at the .001 level. Just as the married alcoholics are dominated by their wives, those who are unmarried are dependent on their mothers.

The particular sadism of the alcoholic must also be understood as a compensation for his receptiveness and weakness. Of the alcoholics, 43 percent were scored as sadistic, as compared to 36 percent of the excessive drinkers, 17 percent of the moderate drinkers and 27 percent of the abstainers. (The correlation of alcoholism and sadism is .167, significant at the 5 percent level.) The scoring of sadism implies a symbiotic mode of relating which has as its aim to avoid feeling alone and empty by absorbing another person, by forceably "swallowing" another. In the context of passive receptiveness, the sadistic trait is less a deep-rooted power drive than an attempt to force others to feed and care for the individual, and to overcome the feeling of impotence.

Passive and empty, the alcoholic tries to compensate by dominating others, especially women. Outside of his fantasies, he is seldom successful. But impotence and frustration may be ignited by a quarrel and the alcoholic will explode, lashing out against someone he feels has challenged the reality of the "macho" image. Most of the village violence, including murder, has resulted from sudden flare-ups in a cantina, sometimes caused by an imagined insult, magnified by self-doubts and by the fear of backing down and being shown up as a fraud, a "nobody."

The Mother Fixation

Dependence or fixation on the mother is consistent with the character syndrome of the passive receptive individual who never grows up. As long as the individual seeks mother's unconditional love, he does not become a man who produces actively; on the contrary, the continued fixation makes the task of developing his own powers even more difficult.

The measure of fixation to the mother was determined from the interview responses by considering: (1) whether or not the individual habitually sought advice from his mother, and when in "moral or economic" trouble first turned to her; (2) whether or not he had ever acted against his mother's wishes or thought that he might ever do so; (3) whether he described his mother in a realistic or an idealized manner; and (4) whether his responses to the hypothetical story of a mother becoming sick and dying after her son had married against her wishes indicated that the son was guilty and had done wrong. If the individual's responses were predominantly in the direction of dependence and idealization of the mother, he was scored as intensely fixated. Those with less actual dependence who still idealized the mother and felt guilty about being dependent were scored as moderately fixated. Only 4.3 percent of the men were neither intensely nor moderately fixated to their mothers (Table 11.7). This finding of course reflects the central position occupied by the mother in Mexican peasant society, a position reinforced by the idealization of motherhood in folklore, in the elaborate mother's day festival, and in the church which is dominated by the figure of the Virgin of Guadalupe.

Table 11.7—Percentages of alcoholic and other males judged to be fixated on the mother to various degrees

	Alcoholics (N=26)	Excessive Drinkers (N=25)	Moderate Drinkers (N=107)	Non- Alcoholics (N=30)	Total Male Population (N=208)
Intense fixation	57.6	44.0	56.4	33.3	51.0
Moderate fixation	38.8	48.0	41.8	60.0	44.7
Independent	3.6	8.0	1.8	6.7	4.3

Of the alcoholics 57 percent were scored as intensely fixated, compared to 44 percent of the excessive drinkers, 56 percent of the moderate drinkers, and 33 percent of the abstainers. The difference between alcoholics and abstainers calculates to a chi-square of 3.32, which is significant at the 5 percent level with a one-tailed test. Although the abstainers differ markedly from the other groups in the low percentage of intense mother fixation, the association between alcoholism and mother fixation is not so great as clinical evidence indicates. Furthermore, the alcoholics are no more intensely mother-fixated than the moderate drinkers. To explain this discrepancy between theory and data, it is necessary to refer to the different types of vulnerability to alcoholism.

The villagers most psychologically vulnerable to alcoholism are those with passive-receptive character traits, compensated by narcissism and machismo, and intensely fixated to their mothers. These villagers usually do not marry, but remain with their mothers, sometimes entering into unstable and brief liaisons with other women. There is another type of alcoholic, however, who begins to drink heavily later in life, after he has married. These are men whose psychological vulnerability is not so great, but when other factors intrude, especially conflict with their wives, they are driven to alcoholism. An indication of the greater dependence of the unmarried alcoholics is revealed by comparing the mother fixation of married vs. unmarried drinkers. Of the ten unmarried alcoholics eight are intensely mother-fixated, while of the 16 married alcoholics only seven were scored intensely mother-fixated. Similarly, of the unmarried excessive drinkers 5 of 6 are intensely mother-fixated while of the married group, the proportion is only 6 of 19. Combining the alcoholics and excessive drinkers, one finds that 81 percent of the bachelors are intensely mother-fixated, as compared to 37 percent of those married, producing a chi-square of 8.6, significant at the 1 percent level.[10]

The Abstainers

Just as the alcoholics are characterized by a vulnerability syndrome, the abstainers' resistance to cultural pressures calls for explanation, for the abstainer is as much a deviant from the village norm as is the alcoholic. Up to this point, the abstainer has been described mostly in contrast to the alcoholic. The abstainer is more interested in cultural stimulation, and he rejects those activities which reinforce patterns of drinking. Psychologically, he is less receptive, less "macho," less sadistic, and less mother-fixated. Describing the abstainer more positively, one would say that his underlying character structure is productive with a hoarding mode of assimilation.

This means that those men who drink the least are generally more interested than the drinkers in their work and in others. They seek to satisfy needs for food, security, and love by producing. As one of these men states, nothing grows correctly, neither one's children nor one's crops, without interest, concern and knowledge. A scale of productivity based on responses to the interview ranges from 1, implying active interest to 6, implying a rejecting attitude to life. The scale is significantly correlated with such independent measures as attendance at cultural activities and the percentage of land planted with intensive crops such as tomatoes or melons, that demand much care, as contrasted

---

[10]Of the abstainers the proportions of bachelors and married men intensely mother-fixated are the same, approximately one-third, which serves as a control to indicate that the lesser fixation of the married drinkers is not a result of marriage, *per se.*

to sugar cane which calls for little work or knowledge. The median score for the abstainers on the scale of productivity is 3 (mean = 3.23), indicating moderate interest and activity; for the moderate drinkers, the median is also 3 (mean = 3.67); for the excessive drinkers the median is 4 (mean = 3.73), indicating moderate interest with non-productive traits predominating; and for the alcoholics the median is 5 (mean = 4.75), indicating the passive-receptive, non-productive individual. The correlation between alcoholism and productivity is −.192, significant at the .01 level.

The abstainers are also characterized by traits of orderliness, conservatism, saving, and compulsive cleanliness that are lacking in the alcoholic. While the alcoholic seeks security by having others feed him, the abstainer seeks to build a protective wall around himself and his possessions. The abstainer's hoarding mode of assimilation makes him feel less dependent on others, since he guards against anxiety by accumulating supplies as well as people. In a peasant society where man is at the mercy of fluctuations in weather and in the market, where crop failure threatens the peasant with starvation, the hoarding orientation, combined with productivity, is a rational answer to life. The receptive orientation which tries to maintain the security of the suckling baby is less rational and less efficient.

Of the abstainers, 60 percent were scored as hoarding compared to 46 percent of the moderate drinkers, 48 percent of the excessive drinkers, and only 18 percent of the alcoholics. The difference between alcoholics and abstainers can be expressed in a chi-square of 10.7, significant at the .001 level. The correlation between alcoholism and the hoarding trait is −.262, significant at the 1 percent level.

An independent check of the interview scoring of the hoarding trait was made by analyzing the Rorschach responses for symbols which imply this mode of assimilation. The symbols used included Schafer's (1954, p. 132) themes of the anal orientation; direct anal reference, anal contact and perspective, dirt, and explosion. To these were added hoarding animals (rats, squirrels), plants and animals that protect themselves with a hard shell (cactus, snails, turtles). A final indication of the anal-hoarding character was a preoccupation with dead things (Fromm, 1964, p. 37ff.). On this basis, 73 percent of the abstainers as compared to 33 percent of the alcoholics were scored as hoarding, producing a Fisher's exact probability of .097.

PSYCHOSOCIAL VULNERABILITY

What is it that makes the men in this society so vulnerable to alcoholism? The conditions of life in the village, the boredom of work, and cultural barrenness, are not different from those of peasants in Italy or the Near East, where alcoholism is not a problem. Although drinking is a traditional part of fiestas, in other societies there is festive drinking without alcoholism; furthermore, the villagers disapprove of excessive drinking and consider it a disease. Neither is alcoholism explained by the fact that people profit from the sale of liquor or from the peasant's alcoholism, since there would be no profit if the villagers were not impelled to drink.

A clue to psychosocial vulnerability is found in a comparison of primitive societies where drinking to unconsciousness is common and often part of religious practice, with those in which drunkenness is either rare or prohibited. When drunkenness is institutionalized, the society chooses a regressive solution to life. Individuals seek to identify with animals and feel themselves less human and also less anxious by blotting out consciousness. In two distinct types of primitive societies male alcoholism is absent, either because it is psychologically unnecessary or forceably suppressed. These are societies characterized by either a strong matriarchal or patriarchal social structure (Field, 1962).

Based on the clinical evidence of psychological vulnerability to alcoholism, the lack of alcoholism in matriarchies can be understood in terms of the gratification of regressive yearnings. If men do not have to become fully responsible, if they can remain pampered and childlike, there is no reason for them to seek substitute gratifications.

In contrast, those societies with a patriarchal organization, where residence is patrilocal and male responsibility is based in male dominance, drinking is controlled, as though the men sense the need to maintain their position by resisting the seductive appeal of regression, offering as a substitute the promise of a superior status to those men who prove themselves mature.

The elders of the Bantu Tiriki, a patriarchal society, allow only initiated men to drink within male meetings, and there are severe penalties for drunkenness and disruptive behavior (Sangree, 1962). In the strongly patriarchal Aztec society, only old people or captured warriors about to be sacrificed could get drunk; otherwise, repeated drunkenness was punishable by death (Soustelle, 1964). Symbolically, the Aztecs saw alcoholism both as fixation to the mother and as a danger to a progressive solution to human existence. In the Fejerrary-Mayer Codex, Mayahuel, the goddess of pulque, is represented as a woman within a maguey plant, suckling a male child (Goncalves de Lima, 1956). In the Chimalpopoca Codex it is related that Quetzalcoatl, who sought to make men more civilized, to end human sacrifices, and to cultivate new arts, was destroyed by his enemies, the demons, who tricked him into getting drunk on pulque. Thus he shamed himself so that he "no longer served God." Clearly the Aztecs were vividly aware of the regressive dangers of pulque and rigidly guarded against them. The Spanish conquest destroyed the patriarchal authority of the Aztec male and rapidly led to the spread of alcoholism.[11]

A cross-cultural study of drunkenness in primitive societies by Field confirms the relationship between sobriety and social structure (Field, 1962). After showing that there is no consistent relationship between drunkenness and measures of anxiety, aggression, sexual problems, orality or any of the other traits that make up psychological vulner-ability, he concludes that "drunkenness increases markedly if the authority of the man in the household is lessened or diffused, and if the nuclear family is less integrated into larger kin structures through bilocal or neological residence." His conclusion does not explain the few matriarchal societies where alcoholism is also absent, but these can be understood in terms of a broader theory. Men remain sober either where patriarchal power is firm or their regressive impulses are satisfied by women. Men are especially vulnerable to alcoholism when they are undermined or frustrated by women.

This theory helps to explain both differences among societies and increased individual vulnerability within the village. The economy of the Mexican peasant village is similar to that of villages in Italy; the two societies share many psychological characteristics. The difference is that Italy has had centuries of unbroken patriarchal dominance, while the Mexican patriarchy has been undermined.[12] In Mexico, the battle of the sexes rages in full force, with the result that male prestige and self-esteem are shattered and compensated for by "machismo" and alco-holism.

In the village, 20 percent of the families are matriarchal, domi-nated by a mother, and sometimes a grandmother, with a series of weak men as consorts. In many families, over one-half, the husbands do succeed in dominating their wives, but they must win their positions. Male superiority is not supported by the social structure. The village war between men and women, which begins in the games of children,

[11]Concluding his study, *The Aztecs under Spanish Rule*, Charles Gibson writes: "What we have studied is the deterioration of a native empire and civilization. The empire collapsed first, and the civilization was fragmented in individual communities. . . . One of the earliest and most persistent individual responses was drink. If our sources may be believed, few peoples in the whole of history were more prone to drunkenness than the Indians of the Spanish colony." (Stanford University Press, 1964, p. 409.)

[12]The reasons for the undermining of the Mexican patriarchy are beyond the scope of this report. They appear related to the Conquest and the problems of *mestizaje*. For discussions of this problem, see Octavio Paz, *El Laberinto de Soledad*, Mexico: Fondo de Cultura Economica, 1959; Aniceto Arimoni, *Psico-analisis de la Dinamica de un Pueblo*, Mexico: Universidad Nacional Autonoma de Mexico, 1961; and Santiago Remirez, *El Mexicano*, Mexico: Paz-Mexicano, 1960.

may not be decided for many years.[13] In this battle the male tries to conquer by force and sexual dominance, while the woman fights back with coldness, ridicule, and an attitude of martyrdom which is meant to make the man feel guilty.

In the village, there are two types of alcoholics. One belongs essentially to a matriarchal sub-culture; the other attempts to live according to the patriarchal ideal, but his passivity and receptiveness lead to his defeat.

The matriarchal alcoholic is characterized by a most intense mother fixation. He remains unmarried, dependent on a mother who constantly frustrates his receptive needs, which he seeks to satisfy symbolically in drink. These mothers have raised their children by themselves. They too may have been brought up in fatherless families. With their sons, they are indulgent and sadistic, over-protective, and intolerant of independence or disobedience. Fiercely they defend their sons from the outside world, but they crush initiative and self-confidence. They demand unconditional loyalty, forbidding their sons to have anything to do with other women, and destroying any relationship that might develop. Although they complain constantly about having to feed and care for grown sons, they are satisfied only when these men remain at home with them. Thus they both smother the manliness of their sons and frustrate the receptive yearnings they have encouraged.

The second type of alcoholic attempts to carry on the patriarchal ideal, but he is ill-equipped for the battle between the sexes. Outwardly tough and aggressive, inside he lacks authority. If he is unfortunate enough to marry a sadistic or destructive woman, he is easily dominated and made to feel impotent and defeated. The impulse to drinks gains strength from his wish to get out of the house, to drink artificial courage, and to regain a joy in living. Sometimes an alcoholic will have the courage to beat his wife only when he is drunk, as appears the case in Bunzel's description of drinking in Chichicastenango and Chomula (Bunzel, 1940).

The character traits of the wives of alcoholics compared to those of the abstainers supports this interpretation. The dominant mode of relation of two-thirds of the alcoholics' wives and 60 percent of the heavy drinkers' wives is either sadomasochistic or destructive as compared to only 30 percent of the abstainers' wives. The chi-square comparing alcoholics and abstainers is 4.45, significant at the 5 percent level.

Another way of expressing the character traits of the wives is in

[13]See M. Maccoby, N. Modiano, and P. Lander, "Games and Social Character in a Mexican Village," *Psychiatry*, 27: 150–162. Soustelle comments on antagonism between the sexes even within Aztec society, but the men then had the advantage of a strong patriarchal system. See Fromm, 1964.

terms of the proportion whose dominant mode of relation with their husband and children is giving material care and affection. Of the alcoholics' wives, 27 percent were scored as dominantly relating in this way, compared to 36 percent of the excessive drinkers' wives and 60 percent of the abstainers' wives. The percentage whose main mode of relating is Material Care is even greater among the wives of those village men who are ex-alcoholics.

Of the six ex-drinkers who are married, none has a wife whose dominant mode of relating is sadomasochistic or destructive. One of these men stopped drinking after marrying a motherly and gentle woman ten years older than he. In another case, an alcoholic divorced his wife who was generally considered a sadistic and malicious woman and remarried, also to an older woman. Although the number of cases is small, it appears that despite psychological vulnerability, if a man can satisfy his receptive needs with a mothering wife, he is not likely to become an alcoholic.

But the only certain inoculation against alcoholism is the ability to enforce the patriarchal tradition. The alcoholics, either because they have lacked a father, because their own fathers were defeated, or because they themselves have been beaten down by destructive wives, are men without masculine strength. Indirect evidence for this statement can be observed in the responses of alcoholics and abstainers to Card IV of the Rorschach, which has been described by various investigators as the "father image," the symbol of paternal power and authority. Of the abstainers, 74 percent see integral images of force and firmness, (monkeys, men, elephants, bears, etc.) compared to 29 percent of the alcoholics. The alcoholic images are skeletons, lungs, a dead chicken, a spine, symbols of decay and defeat.[14] The chi-square of the difference is 4.29, significant at the 5 percent level.

ECONOMIC VULNERABILITY

The study of vulnerability to alcoholism would not be complete without taking into account economic factors, as they interact with cultural patterns and with individual character structure. The spectrum of economic variables relating to alcoholism in the village ranges from pressures of the alcohol industry to the influence of social class and forms of work on the individual's readiness to drink.

The major effect of the alcohol industry is to reinforce those cultural traits which are traditionally associated with drinking. In their publicity the breweries in particular identify themselves with bull fights

[14]This difference is not due to a general tendency of alcoholics to perceive destroyed figures, since there is no difference between the two groups on Card V.

and fiestas, by sponsoring broadcasts of the *corridas* and by sometimes donating musicians (*mariachis*) to enliven the fiestas. The breweries also capitalize *cantinas* and may help to make them more attractive by lending money to buy juke-boxes (*sinfonolas*). Thus by their efforts the breweries and the bar owners succeed in coloring the atmosphere of drinking with an illusion of excitement and gaiety missing in other village activities.

The economic interests of the liquor industry act on the peasant from the outside, capitalizing on the lack of interesting activities and the passivity of those men who do not seek other stimulation. But what is the effect of the villager's own economic situation on his drinking habits?

Socioeconomic class and alcoholism are not related in a simple way. The aim of the following discussion will be to present possible relationships in the light of the evidence, rather than to attempt a final conclusion.

Two variables must be considered in analyzing the village class structure: One is ownership of material goods as a measure of the standard of living; the other is possession of land. The second variable separates the population into two economic groups subject to distinct pressures and opportunities for earning income. The members of one group, the *ejiditarios*, have control or unalienable possession of a *parcela* (averaging about five acres) and therefore the means to make a minimum income, relative to variations in the weather, the market, and their own efforts. At the very least, by growing his own *maiz* and *frijol* the ejiditario avoids the landless peasant's worry over having enough to eat for himself and his family. But the *non-ejiditarios*, who include the 70 percent of the men who either arrived in the village after the partition of land or were sons who did not inherit the indivisible *ejido*, must live from day to day, mostly working as peons or day laborers (*jornaleros*). Only a few non-ejiditarios have managed to save enough to buy or rent land.

Since the economic reality of the ejiditario is basically different from that of the non-ejiditario, it is necessary to consider the two groups separately. For the non-ejiditarios, to begin with them, there is a direct relationship between degree of alcoholism and poverty. Poverty or affluence is measured by a scale of material possessions based on the value of capital goods (tractor, *nixtamel*), consumer goods (radio, electric iron), house type (ranging from concrete house with separate rooms for sleeping to a hut or *jacal* of straw with a dirt floor), and land under cultivation. Using the scores on this scale, the population was divided into three socioeconomic classes, each including close to one-third of the families. Of the alcoholic non-ejiditarios, 86 percent fall into the lowest class, compared to 47 percent of the heavy drinkers, 30 percent of the moderate drinkers, and 32 percent of the abstainers who are not ejiditarios. Among the non-ejiditarios, none of the alcoholics and only one heavy drinker scores in the highest class, compared to 27 percent of the moderate drinkers and 20 percent of the abstainers. These statistics are reported in Table 11.8. In other words, practically all of the alcoholic non-ejiditarios live on a subsistence level. The excessive drinkers are somewhat better off, but poorer than the moderate drinkers and the abstainers, who do not differ from each other.

These statistics raise as many questions as they answer. They do not indicate whether poverty causes drinking, whether drinking impoverishes the non-ejiditario, or whether the same passive receptiveness that leads to drinking also leads to poverty. It is hard to believe that the poorer non-ejiditario has more reason to escape from his misery by drinking than does his slightly richer neighbor. In absolute terms, all but the richest third of the population live on a level close to subsistence. Rooms are crowded, and the less poor might prefer the comparative gaiety of the cantina as much as the poorest. More likely, the poverty of the alcoholic non-ejiditario reflects his unproductive character structure, the result of losing work days, and of squandering too much of his income on drink. Even the most sober non-ejiditario, unless he is particularly fortunate and industrious, suffers a high likelihood of slipping into the lowest class. It is difficult to imagine how the alcoholic non-ejiditario can escape near starvation, unless there is someone else, his mother for instance, to support him. The hypothesis that best fits the facts is that the relationship between alcoholism and poverty is a resultant not a causal one, although it remains to be answered how much drinking leads to poverty and how much the poverty results from the same characterological unproductivity at the root of drinking.

Turning now to the ejiditario, it is surprising to discover that there is a higher percentage of alcoholics among the ejiditarios than among the non-ejiditarios. As Table 11.9 reports, 28 percent of the ejiditarios are alcoholics while only 9 percent of the non-ejiditarios are alcoholics. Furthermore, over half the alcoholics (53 percent) are ejiditarios, compared to 37 percent of the excessive drinkers, 20 percent of the moderate drinkers, and 20 percent of the abstainers. Considering the greater economic security of the ejiditario, it is puzzling why he should be more vulnerable to alcoholism. To understand the economic factors relative to alcoholism in the ejiditario, it will be necessary to analyze his mode of work in more detail.

Before undertaking this analysis, it should be noted that the same relationship between alcoholism and poverty observed for the non-ejiditario holds for the ejiditario, although the ejiditario on the average maintains a higher socioeconomic level. As Table 11.8 reports, the only ejiditarios who fall into the lowest class are alcoholics, and even among the alcoholic ejiditarios only 25 percent (compared to 85 percent of the

Table 11.8—*Percentages of alcoholic and other males by socioeconomic class and ejiditario status*

| Socioeconomic class | ALCOHOLICS | | EXCESSIVE DRINKERS | | MODERATE DRINKERS | | ABSTAINERS | | TOTAL MEN | |
	Ejid. (N=16)	Non-Ejid. (N=14)	Ejid. (N=10)	Non-Ejid. (N=17)	Ejid. (N=21)	Non-Ejid. (N=89)	Ejid. (N=7)	Non-Ejid. (N=25)	Ejid. (N=58)	Non-Ejid. (N=149)
Lowest	25.0	85.7	0	47.1	0	30.3	0	32.0	6.9	37.0
Middle	56.25	14.3	30.0	47.1	42.9	42.7	0	48.0	41.4	40.9
Highest	18.75	0	70.0	5.8	57.1	27.0	100.0	20.0	51.7	22.1

alcoholic non-ejiditarios) are to be found in this category. The excessive drinkers who are ejiditarios do not appear to suffer at all economically; 70 percent score in the highest class and none in the lowest class. Indeed, except for the alcoholic ejiditarios, none of the other ejiditarios falls into the lowest class.

Table 11.9—Percentages of ejiditarios and non-ejiditarios who drink at various levels

	Ejiditarios (N=58)	Non-Ejiditarios (N=149)
Alcoholics	27.5	9.4
Excessive drinkers	17.3	11.5
Moderate drinkers	36.3	58.3
Abstainers and ex-drinkers	18.9	20.8

In considering the relative poverty of the alcoholic ejiditarios, both logic and observation again indicate that poverty follows alcoholism rather than vice versa. The ejiditarios start out with similar economic opportunities. Even those excessive drinkers who prolong their weekends through Monday remain better off economically than many non-ejiditarios who are moderate drinkers or abstainers and whose failure to work is due to scarcity of jobs. Unlike the case of the non-ejiditario, excessive drinking does not penalize the ejiditario economically. Only the alcoholic ejiditario runs the risk of plummeting to the bottom of the society.

It remains to be explained why the ejiditario with his superior opportunity and his greater economic security is more likely than the non-ejiditario to become an alcoholic. To answer the question, we might begin by asking how the ejiditario differs from the non-ejiditario. Being an ejiditario has no effect on character, nor does it modify the relationship between the sexes. The major difference is that the ejiditario is able to make a living without working all of the time. Like those ejiditarios who are excessive drinkers, he may regularly absent himself from work for short periods without significantly losing income. In other words, the ejiditario has more time at his disposal and needs to work less than the non-ejiditario. The extent of his free time varies with the type of crop he plants and with the way he employs time not spent on his ejido. Some crops such as rice and garden vegetables demand a great deal of time and care. Sugar cane calls for much less work, but the profits are only a tenth as great as those from an equivalent rice harvest. The crop alone, however, does not determine the amount of free time. An ejiditario may plant cane because he wants the time to raise animals or to work at jobs that interest him more than farming.

For the ejiditario, the decision about what to plant and how to

employ free time are functions of character. It is true that the cooperative sugar refinery (*Ingenio*) near the village is interested in having the
peasant plant cane; to make this possibility more attractive, it offers
medical services, insurance, and a guaranteed minimum income to
those who plant cane. Furthermore, the Ingenio helps the peasant plow
his parcela and sends migrant workers to cut the zafra, thus making the
work of growing cane even easier for the ejiditario. By planting cane
exclusively, however, he sacrifices the possibility of much greater profits,
and it is possible to secure the social services of the Ingenio by planting
cane in part but not all of his parcela. Generally, the most passive,
inactive ejiditarios are satisfied to plant cane only; the product moment
correlation between the measure of psychological productivity and
percent of land in cane is $-.457$, which is significant at the one percent
level.

Thus, it turns out that the ejiditario with the most free time is likely
to be just the type of person who lacks productive interests, the villager
who has the least use for his time and who is most likely to loiter around
the plaza and be drawn into a cantina. By planting only cane, he has to
work less than half the year. If he lacks other occupations or interests—
as is likely the case for one who limits his planting to cane—he will be
idle most of the time. Since the same character traits that make him
idle also make him vulnerable to alcoholism, it is logical to suppose that
the prevalence of alcoholism would be greater among these ejiditarios
who plant cane only and who have no interest other than drinking.

Once the ejiditario becomes an alcoholic, he may not be capable of
working even half the year. He may fall into debt and be forced to rent
or sell his land, even though this is against the law. In fact, of the 16
alcoholics who are ejiditarios, eight rent their land and eight plant cane
exclusively.

The pattern of work of the excessive drinkers differs from that of
the alcoholics. Of the 10 ejiditarios who are excessive drinkers, only one
rents his land and only one plants cane exclusively. The other excessive
drinkers work at their ejidos when they are not drinking, which explains
their prosperity. Thus from the economic point of view, excessive
drinking, unlike alcoholism, does not imply a significant deviation from
the cultural norm for the ejiditario.

Of the 21 ejiditarios who are moderate drinkers, only one plants
cane exclusively. Of the seven abstainers who are ejiditarios, two plant
only cane, but both of these men employ the time they gain in productive activities.

It now becomes clearer why the ejiditario is more vulnerable to
alcoholism. It is not because his character structure is different from
that of the non-ejiditario, but because the economic system offers a bait
which appeals especially to those ejiditarios who are psychologically

vulnerable to alcoholism. This is the bait of limiting planting to cane, and the trap for men who have no interests other than drinking is idleness. The non-ejiditario with the same psychological vulnerability lacks this temptation. His psychological vulnerability must be stronger, if he is to become an alcoholic, since he ordinarily does not have so much idle time, and perhaps because the economic risks he faces are greater if he does not seek work every day.

In summary, alcoholism in the village is a widespread disease which both reflects the social pathology of the society and is, in itself, a cause of violence, abandonment of families, economic improductivity, and the undermining of the ejidal system. Of the men over 16, over one-quarter are alcoholics or heavy drinkers. Of those age 40 and over, almost one-half suffer from drinking. The roots of alcoholism are to be found in character structure, in cultural traditions, and in the psycho-social vulnerability of the whole society. The character traits which make a man most vulnerable to alcoholism are receptiveness, fixation to the mother, narcissism, aggressiveness, and the fragile masculine façade of "machismo." Depending on the strength of the mother fixation, there are two types of alcoholic, one who seeks to maintain the "symbiotic" ties with the mother, and another who drinks to repair the damaged image of male force and patriarchal power. What both types share is an inability to carry on the patriarchal tradition, due to their receptiveness and passivity, their fear of women, and their resignation to the hopelessness of peasant life. While it is true that the monotony of peasant farming, the lack of cultural stimulation, and the habit of drinking associated with the few festive occasions are factors which increase the temptations of alcoholism, the alcoholics are men who fall passively into the least effortful ways of life. Unlike the abstainers, they do not take advantage of such opportunities as do exist for cultural stimulation or more interesting and intensive work. Significantly, the villagers who do not drink have rejected traditional cultural patterns and have fought boredom in sports, in cultural activities, and in their work. These men have also rejected the exaggerated, compensated "machismo" pattern, with its implications of drinking and violence, for an image of manliness based on skill rather than aggression.

Chapter 12

The Sacred Water:
The Quest for Personal Power
Through Drinking
Among the Teton Sioux

by Gerald Mohatt

In his provocative book, *Custer Died for Your Sins* (1969), Deloria delineates the ways in which a Sioux gained prestige and power in the old days. To be a warrior one did not simply accomplish brave deeds for himself. Rather each deed brought glory—perhaps even food, horses, and land—to the tribe, for respect was more than a mere personal triumph. The young warrior's personal action certainly led to a sense of his own competence as a hunter and fighter, but, more than that, he knew that his deeds contributed to the life and vitality of the Indian nation. As the white man moved in, the deculturation process began to prevent the young warrior from acting in any way that would give him a sense of being effective for the community; yet he still wanted to become personally worthwhile and respected. For his difficulty liquor introduced a quasi-solution. He could drink until he was able to act in ways that proved to him and to others that he was indeed brave and to be respected; he could again feel the flow of strength in his veins. In this way tribal concerns were gradually overshadowed by the individual's desire for prestige and power. Such power was often not achieved by tribal mores and action, but through drinking large amounts of liquor.

In this chapter we will discuss the power of alcohol among the Teton Sioux and its relationship to the deculturation of their nation. Parallels with the old ways will be shown in the contemporary Sioux society through the case histories of three adolescents and an adult.

THE OLD WAY

In the days before their final defeat and containment in reservations, the Teton Lakota, commonly known as the Sioux, lived and fought for their common existence on the Western plains. Basically a nomadic hunting tribe, they became renowned as the greatest warriors, horsemen, and buffalo hunters of the Plains tribes, conquerors successively of the Iowas, Omahas, Kiowas, Cheyenne, the powerful Aridaras, the Crows, and the Pawnee. By 1830 they controlled the land in South Dakota including the Black Hills, parts of Nebraska, and North Dakota. In such a context the tribe developed male roles and identities tied closely to war, hunting, and horse stealing. The special importance of the horse—for war, hunting, and moving—made it a commodity associated with wealth and prestige. A man who stole an excellent gelding picketed close to an enemy's tepee was considered brave and worthy of honor (Hassrick, 1964).

The need both to defend one's horses and one's camp from enemies and to conquer new lands for food led to the high value placed on bravery. For a Lakota to ride against an enemy and strike him with his bow was to count coup—an action of great risk, since the Lakota did not shoot nor attempt to kill his enemy. The more coup counted, the greater his bravery. To bring back the horse of a fallen enemy or the scalp of an enemy who showed great bravery were other deeds of honor. In short, any number of acts demanding life-and-death risk brought respect from fellow tribesmen. To receive such respect the warriors boasted of their feats around the fires at their celebrations, as a consequence receiving an invitation to one of the warrior societies. This tie to older and respected warriors gave a younger tribesman the prestige associated with a powerful group, an overall reputation significant to younger members of the tribe who were beginning their careers as warriors. As his reputation for bravery grew, along with his wealth in horses, he had greater opportunities to marry into a prestigious family.

Hunting, fighting, and stealing horses gave the individual power through bravery; membership in warrior societies and a prestigious marriage added to his tribal fame. Beyond these, through the Hamblechea, or vision quest, the warrior won supernatural strength. Since the Sioux was bound so closely to the fluctuations of nature for survival, he sought to discover the gods' will for him through fasting, prayer, and purification. Following a sweat bath for purification, the individual went to a sacred hill, and fasted for four nights and days. During this time he lamented and cried for a vision. If he were successful, the holy ones sent winged creatures to talk to him of what he must do in his life. After the four days he returned to relate his vision to a holy man who helped interpret it.

Later, provided he was considered ready by the medicine man, he could take part in the Sun Dance. In this rite his chest was pierced, and leather skewers were attached to long pieces of leather and fastened under the skin. After the ends of the leather had been fastened to the sacred pole, he danced around the pole, leaning away from it, until he had ripped the skewers from his chest. The purpose of this all, as the medicine man Black Elk says, was that "strength would be given to the life of the nation through this great rite" (Neihardt, 1932). The visions gained, the scars on his chest from the Sun Dance, told the people of this man's selflessness and fortitude. As Hassrick says:

> In order to obtain the power essential to well-being, denial of self through the painful humiliation of torture was the accepted procedure. This was the price that men paid for mental and physical security, this was the most certain way to achieve success. (Hassrick, 1964.)

Though not all young men became renowned warriors whose advice was sought, most gained relative honor through their brave deeds and their quest for vision. The greatest of the warriors achieved wisdom, and the others mastered elements important for the survival of their people. Their boasting brought their deeds and visions into the public forum and gave them wider influence, respect, and subsequent power. Their personal prestige always grew into communal tribal power.

DESTRUCTION OF THE OLD WAY

As the white man arrived, he successively destroyed the Sioux male's channels for achieving central tribal values. The buffalo and other game were killed or driven miles away. Each tribe was put on reservation, and horse stealing punished. The invaders killed men, women, and children not only in battle, but by distributing blankets contaminated with smallpox or by bringing pneumonia. The Black Hills and the gold were taken and never paid for. The indomitable became the conquered, and the great expanse of their land shrunk to a handful of reservations.

Such destruction eliminated most channels of male expressiveness. No longer could a Sioux hunt, fight against the Crow or Pawnee and steal their horses. Though they won important battles, the massive strength of the enemy overcame them. Wounded Knee was the last great Indian battle with the U.S. Army. The Ghost Dance had promised invincibility for the Indians, the return of the buffalo, and the destruction of all white men, but when the soldiers at Wounded Knee opened fire, hundreds of Sioux died. After this final refutation of the Ghost Dance, the Sioux were conquered and humiliated. No longer could a man boast of brave deeds at the fire, except in the context of a distant past. Though he could seek a vision and fast for his people, the government outlawed the Sun Dance, while Episcopal and Catholic missionaries preached against the old religious ways. The Sioux were forced to send their children to white schools where their hair was cut and Lakota could not be spoken.

In such a context the pervasive feelings of power from the old ways were replaced by intense feelings of defeat, helplessness, and dependence. Attempts to make them farmers, an occupation detested by a hunting tribe, failed. An independent and powerful people found themselves fed rather than feeding themselves, and unable to achieve respect and prestige for themselves or for the tribe. As Black Elk said, "The white man has broken the sacred hoop" (Neihardt, 1932). The sacred circle had been broken by the squares of the white man: his square houses, churches, and whole bracketed way of living. Young Man Afraid spoke that which he felt after a meeting with Secretary Noble in 1892:

> The troubles spring from seed. The seed was sown long ago by the white man not attending truthfully to his treaties after a majority of our people had voted for them. When the white man speaks, the government and the army see that we obey. When the red man speaks, it goes in at one ear and out of the other. The Indian is for eternity interested in the subject, the white man only when he comes into office for two or three years. I am not yet an old man, but I have seen many Great Fathers and his headmen. (Utley, 1963.)

LIQUOR IN THE EARLY DAYS

Along with deculturation, the liquor trade grew and prospered. Liquor, which had come to the Teton in the 17th century, became more readily available as traders settled permanently. The Sioux named whiskey sacred water (*mni wakon*) in reference to its power to induce states of euphoria and to reduce pain and sadness. Liquor in general created a sense of strength similar to that associated with battle or the vision. Though before the coming of liquor the Teton were often embroiled in clan feuds that led at times to murder, their moral code prevented mass murders or brawls. Unfortunately, as Hyde explains, liquor reversed this situation:

The Oglalas had already been through a trade-war of this kind on the Upper Missouri about the year 1822, and had seen scores of their tribesmen killed in drunken brawls. These poor Indians knew that liquor was a bad thing, to their camps, but when it was pressed upon them they did not have the moral strength to refuse it. Beginning in 1840, this struggle among the traders kept the Oglalas, Brules, and Cheyennes of the Upper Platte in a state of utter demoralization for several years. In ordinary times the killing of a Sioux by a fellow tribesman was an event of rare occurrence, but with liquor entering the camps freely such murders happened every day. (Hyde, 1937.)

Even in the late 19th century, one finds liquor associated with anger and impulsive aggression. Lieutenant Casey, an envoy from General Brooke, was sent to ask Red Cloud to come out for a parley. Richard, a half-breed relative of Red Cloud, advised Casey to leave, since Red Cloud was going in to talk with General Miles. Richard told Casey that at present the young men were dangerous because they were drunk or crazy, and one might take a shot at the blue uniform. The lieutenant did not leave soon enough; he was shot by a brave named Plenty Horses. This incident took place on Jan. 7, 1891 (Utley, 1963). Liquor had facilitated a type of behavior which a Sioux would associate with the mood for battle and brave deeds.

Though the missionaries, some of the agents, and all of the important chiefs urged the soldier chiefs to rid the Indian lands of liquor traders, they nevertheless remained where they were or travelled from place to place, leaving trails of dead Sioux killed in drunken fights (Hyde, 1937). Although the majority of accounts stress the results of drinking, certainly not every Sioux who drank became involved in such exhibitions. *Drunken Comportment* by MacAndrew and Edgerton (1969) stresses the complexity of the Indians' response to liquor. There were many episodes of drinking which produced no hostility. Many Indians did not drink, or if they did, did not become drunk. Others, though they became very drunk and aggressive never touched the missionaries or whites who reported these episodes. So cultural and moral codes were still in effect. This must be stressed, since it demonstrates the falsity of the stereotyped notion that Indians are hereditary alcoholics and uncontrolled drinkers.

Yet one must not forget the reaction of the Sioux leaders themselves to the question of liquor. Spotted Tail considered it so destructive of his Brules that he moved them to Rosebud, where they might be isolated as much as possible from the Missouri River liquor traffic. Though the effects of drinking began to destroy the communal fabric of the tribe, liquor also brought a substitute for the powerlessness engendered by the deculturation process. Red Cloud spoke of both themes when he said:

Friends, it had been our misfortune to welcome the white man. We have been deceived. He brought with him shining things that pleased our eyes; he brought weapons more effective than our own. Above all he brought the spirit-water that made one forget old age, weakness and sorrow. But I wish to say to you that if you wish to possess these things for yourselves, you must begin anew and put away the wisdom of your fathers (Maynard, 1969).

In the old ways, as we have said, men sought a position of power through personal action in battle, the hunt, horse stealing, or a vision. An individual's competence in these matters led to respect in terms of tribal values. When the white advance brought the complete destruction of many of these tribal ways, liquor became a substitute for action. It led to feelings of euphoria and strength reminiscent of the successful theft, hunt, or battle. Perhaps such temporary states of euphoric assertiveness served a positive function in preventing total despair and self-destruction. But the widespread use of liquor also led to the disintegration of social controls on interpersonal behavior among tribal members. Drinking made brawls and other out-of-character behavior more likely. For instance, among the Teton there are cases of feigning drunkenness as an excuse for some act, such as assault or stealing, which formerly would have been boasted about. With assertive behavior now not for the nation but against it, they were ashamed and had to excuse their behavior by claiming to be drunk and therefore not accountable for their acts, in a manner common in many groups (see MacAndrew & Edgerton, 1969).

TWENTIETH CENTURY DEVELOPMENTS

After the turn of the century, the Sioux were settled on the reservations of South Dakota. The Brule reservation was very distant from any city or even from any small off-reservation town. Such isolation had in the days of horses and poor roads led to the solidification of a reservation life. The inhabitants lived by subsistence farming and practiced many of the old tribal festivities. The opening of ranges to white leasers in 1918, however, led to the sale of large herds of Indian cattle and an economy whereby, rather than farming or ranching, the Sioux began to live on cash from leases. When a more complex reservation economy failed to materialize, the cash economy became stable and in many ways remains so at present. The availability of liquor is a difficult matter to ascertain. Though many old-timers talk about bootleggers and home-made liquor, they agree that liquor certainly was not as common in the past as today. They also say that there was not as much violence or destruction of family life associated with liquor. The introduction of the car brought easier access to liquor. The reservation

CCC projects, cash income, and the availability of autos in the 1930's led to evenings spent in off-reservation towns where booze from bootleggers was available and "heavy drinking was always part of the evening" (White, 1964).

World War II brought job opportunities off the reservation for many, and military service for others. The off-reservation work led to the pattern which one still sees today:

> These Sioux had more money in their pockets than ever before, but they found that it was easiest to move in circles where a rough, fast life was the norm. Heavy drinking and carousing during after-work hours became the rhythm of their life, and for the Indian man who had had little job experience before, saving money and job stability were less important. (White, 1964.)

When the end of the war brought a decline in the number of jobs, many of the Sioux returned to the reservation with no jobs and only lease money on which to live. Their early lives in the isolated communities had given them certain tribal values, and most had drunk and seen drinking in these communities. Now, however, they had had new experiences in the city or military service, where liquor was readily available and where a lower-class culture of excitement looked upon heavy drinking as the norm and Indians as born drinkers. At the same time their contacts with the American middle class had made them want to "get ahead" like other Americans. On their return to the reservation, the isolation of the past was broken, and many of the old values conflicted with the middle-class goals they had observed—for instance, the sharing and cooperation of the Sioux versus the saving and competition of the middle class. The outside world was moving in on the reservation—in the form of radio, TV, movies, relocation, white ranchers, and relatives from the city who continually "talked up" achievement. Yet the reservation Indians, with no means to achieve in the white middle-class sense, felt basically alienated from the wider American community. As White says:

> The Sioux are rapidly losing their distinct reservation culture and with their constant contact with the American social class system they are becoming a lower-class proletariat. Instead of being a culturally and socially distinct group with a simple rhythm of life they are the "failures" of American society. (White, 1964.)

From such a viewpoint the reservation became a dead end; yet the urban ghetto offered little more. Boredom, lack of job opportunities, inferior education, prejudice, and the language barrier began to accentuate the old motivation for drinking—to overcome feelings of powerlessness and lack of respect resulting from all these barriers. The result has been as White describes:

This (chronic drinking) is the easiest way to a quick elation and excitement, a way to relax and forget the fears and insecurities of one's life. It is also a means for the Sioux who by tradition is dignified and reserved to be loud, raucous, and cocky in his repartee. In his elation he forgets any inferiority and gains a feeling of power and assurance—ready to accept and dare. (White, 1964.)

To speak of powerlessness as a central motive in Sioux drinking does not deny the complexity of their motivation. Certainly they drink because they desire intimacy, wish to excuse and escape responsibility, and desire excitement. Yet the majority of Sioux the author has spoken with on this matter report a definite pattern in their drinking, which is also supported by statistical data (Maynard, 1969). The Sioux tends to drink most when he experiences chronic unemployment, failure or rejection, or when he is at a crisis point requiring that he decide whether or not to go forward into the future, e.g., to college, a new job, or a new area of responsibility. At these times, when he is most concerned with his personal desires to become respected and worthwhile, he simultaneously feels most powerless. To exemplify this theme of powerlessness, the following cases of three adolescents and an adult are presented.

ADOLESCENT CASES

Case I

Jim was approaching the end of his high school career. Though he had lived off and on with a brother or relatives, he had no stable family. Fortunately he was very close to one girl in the school who encouraged and respected him, and he was involved in athletics and school leadership. Recently, he had expended himself considerably in a number of activities, only to be rejected by many of his fellow students who favored another boy.

One evening after Jim had been drinking heavily, the author was called to help control him. After being carried to his bed, Jim grew incoherent and began to swing at another adult. When he realized what was happening, he broke into tears and sobbed for five or ten minutes. After we had talked briefly, he began to say how he had been rejected by the students after so much work. He said these kids meant nothing to him. If they wanted someone who had no real interest in them, who cared? Yet he admitted he did care, was depressed about it, and wanted to get drunk. Secondly, certain administrators, he felt, had not respected him, but rather favored other students who, he felt, were not as capable as he. Though Jim reiterated that he did not care about them and hated them, he also insisted that they should respect him. He had given his best and had been degraded and to hell with them. The way he felt, he just wanted to get drunk.

One must realize that Jim did have close friends, and the affection of many. He felt, however, that he did not have their respect. He had wanted to find prestige by exercising his competence for the school's improvement. After his rejection, though the affection of the students and administrators was still his, he felt his personal competence had been denied. So he drank to show that, at least, others had to notice and deal with him.

After this episode the boy went back to working hard in school and even accepted extra work. Yet basketball brought more frustration, and losses and suspensions led to more depression. He wanted to get married (another student and friend of his had done so two months previously), but at the same time he wanted to finish school and do something with his life. The advent of a basketball game with a close rival broke his abstinence; drunk, he assaulted some teachers and students, destroyed property, and was jailed. His expulsion from school followed. Jim was a person who tried but consistently failed. He feared general failure from a basketball loss; he feared the future, which he wanted so much to be worth while. No one seemed to give him enough support to let him feel secure of his own worth. The only way he knew to break this powerlessness was to drink heavily, to "show them."

In this case we have a boy concerned with his capacity to achieve success in athletics and school activities, but at the same time convinced that few respected him, especially those for whom he had expended so much energy. Such rejection meant to him that he was worthless. His response when these developments "got him down" was to show those who rejected him how tough he really was. By violent actions he seemed to place himself outside of their control; his whole thrust while drinking was to assert his fearlessness and physical prowess. Though he had wanted to be considered competent and important through student leadership and athletics, he had not succeeded, and his desire for personal power had been blocked. Hence he turned to alcohol for the strength to become bold and daring, for the fear and respect he would gain from those he attacked while drunk, and from the stories he would tell after the whole episode was over. The warrior of old who died counting coup could not tell his stories, but others could, and while he lived he would be able to see fear in the eyes of those he attacked so bravely. Jim saw such fear in the eyes of those he attacked, and he was able to live to tell and hear stories of his exploits. As Red Cloud said, liquor does remove weakness.

Case II

Joe had drunk previously, but had abstained for at least four months during which time he worked to save money for school. Suddenly, however, two of his close relatives were killed, and members of his family began to drink heavily almost continually. After the second relative had died, Joe began to drink excessively on the weekends. He would talk openly of his reasons for drinking, saying, "No one at home likes me. They are all drunk." He would say: "I am going to get killed this weekend. I will get killed on the road. Get drunk and get killed."

When the author talked with Joe about doing something to prevent death, his fatalism became more pronounced. He was preoccupied with thoughts of dying. A strange mixture of voluntary and involuntary themes came out during his irritation at any exhortation. He would say: "It's my life, I'll lead it. Let me alone." Yet a moment later he would say; "I will die. There isn't anything I can do." Like Jim, he mentioned rejection by his family. "What can I do? No one cares. No one does any different." Joe wanted to overcome the fate that had conquered his closest relatives, but his own family seemed to be headed for the same fate. He was unsure of his own power to master the forces leading inevitably to death. At these times he drank heavily.

As Joe's pattern developed, the theme of death came more and more to the surface. No longer did he speak of getting help but he talked of death as inevitable. He had fantasies of a spirit-life of great power in which one could do much for the living. He seemed overcome with the feeling that he had no way to escape death and had better get ready for it. He said he felt more inclined to die when drunk, so why not face it?

In Joe's life one sees not only rejection, but the effects of familial drinking and an inability to escape fate in the form of death by auto accidents. This all led to a strong sense of hopelessness and fatalism. Feeling himself unable to do anything to affect his future, he seemed to sense that he had to try to face death on the highways.

This case presents striking contrasts. Here was a young man who seemed to drink in order to have the courage to carry out his death. He honestly believed that he had no way to avoid it. So by drinking he could bring it closer, face it, and see what it was all about. At the same time when he drank he very often sought out teachers, or counselors, to whom he would talk pessimistically about his feeling of being doomed. The more he talked, however, the more aggressive he became. If the author tried to persuade him to go home or to stay out of cars, he would become angry and say, "Go to hell. I'll do what I want to do. Stay out of my life"—and would walk away. The next day, however, I would discover that shortly after he had walked away from me, he had gone home.

Like a warrior risking death in battle, Joe put his life in jeopardy in a car while drunk. He defied death and proved his control over it; such a risk was an ultimate test of his power. In defying me he also said to me in a sense, "I don't need you. I am strong enough myself to control death and to stop drinking." His defiance proved his strength. Liquor provided the strength to defy both death and authority.

Case III

Mark, who was approaching his final year of high school, wanted to go to college and eventually to professional school. Although his previous school record had been poor, he wanted to make something of his last year. He was drinking heavily when I talked to him, and admitted that that was pretty much all he was doing. As we talked, he focused on his inability to get an education which would prepare him for a good college. "I'm an Indian," he said. "You know what that means. Bad education, people calling you dog-eaters. I can't stay in South Dakota. They don't give an Indian a chance." At the same time he considered his record too poor to allow him to transfer to a good high school in another state for his last year. His reasons for drinking became clearer when he said, "Why not drink? They [his friends] don't want any help. They don't deserve it. They hurt me. Why help them? They're Indians. We can't do anything anyway." In other conversations during drinking, Mark retraced the same steps: "I'm an Indian. Why not drink? What else is there?" Again the striking sense of personal powerlessness in the context of intense desires to be somebody comes through.

This boy drank not only because he felt helpless, but because he could also harm the reputation of those he thought had hurt him. By getting them to drink excessively and so become future drinkers and bums, he would repay them for their lack of respect for him. By drinking he could even reject the teachers who exhorted him to try harder; his interaction with me indicated his knowledge of all of these factors. In a sense he was telling me, "You may think I am a drunken Indian, but look: I can tell you as much about myself with no education as you can with all of yours." In defying my advice, he validated his own intellectual competence.

The adolescent cases described here are not atypical, though many drink for fun or to be with friends. Friends can exert great pressure on each other to drink because of the strong value placed on friendship and sharing; refusal indicates selfishness and identification with whites. Not drinking separates one from his peer group; the adolescent would be blamed for trying to be better than anyone else. Drinking maintains the friendship circle, which in turn provides money, transportation to exciting places, and the feeling of being needed and important. One young married man told me, "While I was drinking, I had all the friends I wanted; I had plenty of money in my pockets, and gas in my car. Now I have got no friends. My car has no gas. And I don't have any money. I work and work and just don't seem to get going." Friendship-drinking has then a strong connection with the Sioux's need for power and respect.

From the author's close friendships with many Sioux adolescents, he feels that those who drink heavily as adolescents express the same concern about lack of respect. They feel powerless to prevent themselves from recapitulating their parents' or families' lives. Everyone at their home has drunk continually. As one girl commented in a depressed tone, "Here it is Wednesday and my parents are drunk already." The weekend previously she had had to wade through a house of drunken, violent people. She had had to bandage hurt people, cook food, and defend herself. As she often said, "What can I do except the same?"

The adolescents who drink heavily go over and over in their minds the problem of their worthlessness and that of their adult models. In general, the image one boy used when he talked of why he drank seems typical. He said, "I drink when I feel trapped, like the walls were closing in or the trap door was locked, and I escape by drinking." Again we see the historical theme of Red Cloud—drink removes weakness and sorrow. Consequently the adolescent does not drink heavily when he experiences success in school or in a job or when family members are sober and concerned for him. Unfortunately such security is unstable and cannot be trusted. Too often that trust has been broken by troubles arising from heavy drinking. These are the adolescents who when asked what they want to do, say, "I just want to live out another month or year."

Dr. Carl Mindell summarizes much of this motivation for drinking when he says:

> I see many young people, adolescents, who have reached that point in their lives when they and others may feel they should make a decision. . . . They feel weak, inadequate, powerless, afraid to try anything, feeling certain they will fail. They seem to be drawn to the image of the bum, the loafer. When you ask them what they want to be, they answer first "Not a bum" and yet they seem drawn to this role, this identity as a temporary or permanent solution to "What will I be when I grow up?" Many people unfortunately see being a drunkard and being an Indian as synonymous. (Maynard, 1969.)

In the cases above, we have seen how a young person will fight at times against his feelings of helplessness and at other times give in to them. Liquor provides him with the strength to do one or the other. In the following case history one can see how these concerns about power-motivated drinking have persisted throughout the life of a man who is now an adult.

Case IV

John was raised on the reservation on a simple subsistence farm, far from excitement or fast living. Horses and the freedom to roam were his early interests. He did not enjoy school work, but some activities led him to a sense of leadership and accomplishment. Like many Indian boys John remembered taking his first drink at around 14 years of age. The way he acted after this first drink shows the influence on him of those he had seen drink:

> I had my first bottle of beer when I was 14 years old. I drank and drank. When I was going home I threw my hat away, because I had seen drunks do this and others talk about this. So I went home without a hat. A lot of people have this idea, to act drunk.

Two elements are clear. First, John drank many beers rather than a few, and as a result became drunk. Second, the only way he knew how to act was the way he had seen others act.

Throughout the rest of high school John said he did not drink heavily, but when World War II began, he dropped out of school and entered the service. The military was a great contrast to the reservation with respect to liquor. On the reservation liquor was illegal and one had either to get it from bootleggers or make his own. Being in uniform made liquor easy to get. John drank heavily at times in the service, though drink was not a constant problem to him and did not lead to personal harm or injury to others. The main reason he drank then, he said, was that he "could get it easily." In a sense he saw himself able to exercise a right that he did not have on the reservation. After the war when he returned to the reservation, the "problems" began. As he said:

> I tried to get into jobs, good paying jobs, and for some reason I was always turned down. And I think this is why I started drinking when I came out of the service. When I came back on the reservation, that empty feeling took over me and I started drinking again and thereafter I seemed to get into a rut that I can't get out of.

As John explained further, the limited education of the full bloods—only five or six years of school—did not qualify them for jobs. And as he said: "Naturally we turned to drink." The high incidence of drinking, then, was related closely to their sense of futility in attempts to get ahead. Unable to get a job, John became tired, lonely, bored, and began to drink. A cycle was established: no work led to drinking; but when he did have a job, he became unreliable at work—hence more drinking. Soon he was unable to get jobs because of drinking. Finally, he began to drink continually. The feeling of emptiness became almost pervasive: "It's like a merry-go-round. We jump off someplace. We try to get something and we don't get it. The only place we can go is back to the merry-go-round and drinking again."

The way in which the majority of Sioux drank had taught John that to drink meant that he must get drunk. To understand the continued effect of such beliefs one must realize that the Sioux seldom drink alone; solitary drinking is unheard of except perhaps among some mixed bloods. John's remark becomes even more important when this is understood:

> I believe that if a person don't want to get drunk, they don't have to. But this is something that is with us as Indians. We believe that—alcohol: beer, wine, whiskey—when you drink the stuff that you have to get drunk. This is the way I believed.

He had watched other Indians to discover what to do about his problems, and had learned that the only way to overcome them was to drink. This solution became a set of behaviors, a pattern to which he and his friends conformed while drinking. In the first stage they drank a great deal, felt happy, and sometimes would sing or dance and tell stories. Often these stories shaded over into bragging about unreal exploits—for instance beating up two or three men. These tales, John said, made him "feel good—like somebody—I was really like somebody. It made me feel good—like a big man." Though what he said was unreal, the whole fabrication led to feelings of power and greatness.

The next stage brought the group into a "laughing spell." They would tell funny stories, and laugh and laugh. Their laughing boosted their spirits as it became progressively uncontrolled. After this came a final stage in which they would become aggressive and hostile. John nevertheless called this stage part of "the good times." One time he tried to find out about these good times, and what he discovered was, "I was a bad actor. I wanted to fight. Go tear something or break down a door or something." At this stage he felt that "he could whip the whole town." He would look for people on the street to fight. Yet soon he felt that he had become an animal. "You become like a bull charging everything that moves. Man, I would do that." His body felt powerful and able to do impossible things; he was somebody.

John's drunken behavior seems highly related to his concerns while sober. He wanted to be somebody; he tried to get jobs, but failed. The same concern gave rise to his behavior when drunk. Though his bragging was unreal and his aggressiveness unsocialized, these were expressions of his desire to be someone prestigious and powerful. The similarity to the way the Sioux drank in the old days is apparent. Blocked in their attempts to feel effective, they found themselves progressively more empty and weak. Like the early Sioux who had seen whites act big and strong when drunk, they too had learned to imitate those around them.

Thus when John felt empty, tired, and weak, he turned to the bottle. The sacred water imbued him with strength and happiness, even with powers beyond the mortal, which he described in such terms as fever, a spell, greatness, bigness. In a strange, almost self-destructive way, he transcended his circumstances, but then found himself under the control of a force that led him to misery. When he realized what he was doing and what he was going to lose, he decided to quit drinking. Why he did not on the contrary turn completely to alcohol, he did not know. He said he was alone and miserable and did not want to lose his family and home; this gave him the strength to take the first step toward complete abstinence. The program he devised was simple but strenuous. Even if he got no salary, he found a job and worked from sunup to sundown; then he would spend his time with his family or working on the homes of relatives. When he felt like drinking he would think of what he had done and how he had felt during his worst spells. At the same time he became involved in civic and church activities, and gradually such activities replaced the merry-go-round of liquor.

Thus the concerns that motivated him to drink also helped him to stop. He saw distinctly that he was becoming a bum, and was heading for death and possible injury to others. Yet he loved his family and wanted to keep them and his home; he wanted to be respected not only personally but in terms of others—his family, his relatives, and the Indian community. Gradually he began to see himself as changed: "Then after a while I got strong enough. Of course I went to church on Sundays and even at other times. I gained more strength and will power to fight off the urge."

Gradually he removed his weakness by action: a job, time with his family, civic and church involvement. Though still he felt the need for liquor, that need was balanced now by a sense of competence and a trust in his own strength, together with a concern for what others thought of him. Perhaps such values are the rebirth of tribal concerns that motivate him further toward social power.

Chapter 13

Examining the Research Basis for Alternative Explanations of Alcoholism

by David C. McClelland

The studies reported in this volume gradually led to the formulation of the hypotheses that drinking serves to increase power fantasies and that heavy liquor drinking characterizes those whose personal power needs are strong and whose level of inhibition is low. In formulating and testing these hypotheses we have only occasionally referred to other theories of drinking or the research findings obtained in other investigations. How well does the new theory fit all the known facts about alcoholism and heavy drinking? Does it fit the facts better than alternative theories?

For all practical purposes theorists of the psychodynamics of alcoholism can be divided into two groups—those who believe that no general theory is possible and those who accept some form of the hypothesis that heavy drinking is due to oral dependency needs. The former argue that there is no "pre-alcoholic personality type," that alcohol solves different problems for different people or different societies. Blum (1966) in reviewing psychoanalytic contributions to the theory of alcoholism concluded: "It would be an error to attribute to them a unitary theory of alcoholism, or of its etiology, or of the alcoholic personality type, as has been done" (p. 264). She asserts that if one assumes "multiple determination instead of a unitary etiology of alcoholism" much confusion is avoided. Similarly MacAndrew and Edgerton (1969) have argued from a cross-cultural standpoint that drinking does not even universally "disinhibit" but simply leads a man to behave in whatever way his society has taught him a drunken man should behave. Such a relativistic view may be correct, but it essentially abandons the attempt to find some scientific generalization across people or across societies as to why people drink. We are left instead with the task of describing how alcohol functions in a number of unique individual cases, or societies.

The dominant theoretical view, however, is that the person who is most likely to become an alcoholic has some kind of dependency conflict, and that the society which fosters dependency conflicts will promote heavy drinking. R. W. White expresses this position very simply and very well. "There is a *repressed* but still active craving for loving maternal care. There is also a very strong aggressive need, *suppressed* by circumstances to the extent that it comes to expression only in verbal form. Alcohol does a lot for these two needs. It permits the young man to act as aggressively as he really feels, without forcing him to assume full responsibility for his actions. It permits him to gratify his dependent cravings without forcing his consciousness to become aware of them" (quoted in McCord & McCord, 1960, p. 35).

This is a simpler restatement of the psychoanalytic view carefully formulated by Knight in 1937 which is summarized by Maccoby in Chapter 11, as follows. "The alcoholic's childhood experiences with a characteristically over-protective mother has produced excessive demands for indulgence. Disappointment and frustration of these oral needs trigger rage, but the individual feels guilty about his hostile impulses and punishes himself masochistically. He needs excessive indulgence to pacify his guilt, thus stimulating a vicious cycle. Alcohol smothers the rage and disappointment and it is a symbolic substitute for affection. But it serves also to spite those who withhold affection and results in masochistic debasement." Sanford (1968) agrees that "in at least some male problem drinkers an underlying dependence with overcompensatory strivings for 'maleness' is an important predisposing factor" (1968, p. 15).

The McCords conclude, after their extensive analysis of the personalities of boys who later became alcoholic, that "underneath his façade of self-reliant manhood, the typical alcoholic, we have proposed, continues to feel anxious, to suffer conflict, and to be desirous of dependent relationships. If one assumes that his traumatic early experiences produce a permanently heightened desire for dependency, then it follows that his conscious attempt at suppressing these desires is doomed to failure" (McCord & McCord, 1960, p. 154). "Alcohol would be a major outlet available to such a person. When intoxicated, he could achieve feelings of warmth, comfort, and omnipotence. His strong desires to be dependent would be satisfied. At the same time, he could maintain his image of independence and self-reliance. The hard drinker in American society is pictured as tough, extroverted, and manly— exactly the masculine virtues the alcoholic strives to incorporate into his own self-image" (p. 155).

As we have pointed out earlier, Bacon, Barry and Child (1965) adopted a similar view: "We have found strong evidence that frequency of drunkenness and general consumption of alcohol are related to deprivation of dependency needs in infancy, childhood and adulthood and to strong demands for self-reliance, achievement and responsibility" (1965, p. 45). They postulate that "dependence is a basic need, common to all people" (p. 30) which would be heightened by low indulgence in infancy. They find a significant correlation between drinking and low indulgence in infancy, which is assumed to imply frustrated dependency needs. Reasoning in terms of their general theory, they propose that "as a reaction to dependency conflict, alcohol has a triple function: it reduces anxiety and tension; it permits the satisfaction of desire for dependence; it permits uncritical indulgence of unrealistic fantasies of achievement. By this view, alcohol would be peculiarly rewarding to individuals with exaggerated dependency conflict" (1965, p. 31).

Tähkä (1966) agrees on the basis of his extensive clinical studies of Finnish alcoholics. "The effects of alcohol seem to be able to restore an emotional state comparable to that of a newly fed infant. These effects seem to be capable of giving the predisposed persons a strong and significant experience of passive gratification, characterized by pleasurable sensations of being filled with something that makes them feel warm, comfortable, secure and accepted" (1966, p. 214). "Owing to the infantalizing attitudes of their mothers and their insufficient identification with a paternal person" alcoholics seem to be struggling "for independence that is doomed to failure, because it is not possible for the alcoholic to abandon the infantile form of passive gratification, which often has probably been the only significant and meaningful instinctual satisfaction in his life. He tends to get rid of his humiliating dependence on his mother by trying to regain an early experience of illusory omnipotency and self-sufficiency where he simultaneously plays the roles of the giver and the receiver" (1966, p. 222).

In short, while the phrasing differs somewhat from theorist to theorist, the consensus is great. And it should be remembered that these conclusions are based on very different types of data—the McCords worked from longitudinal data; Bacon, Barry and Child from cross-cultural data; Tähkä from detailed clinical analyses of 50 cases. Why and in what ways do our data force us to disagree with such a widely accepted viewpoint?

At the outset we did not disagree with it. We had no reason to. On the contrary, because we had read the literature on alcoholism, we expected to find signs of dependency in our subjects' fantasies. We began to have doubts about the theory only when we found that there were no more fantasies of aroused or satisfied oral dependency needs during drinking periods than during non-drinking periods. All of the theories above make assumptions about the state of mind of the drinker while he is drinking. Though we were coding as carefully as we could the thoughts that went through the drinker's mind while he was drinking, yet we could find no clues that pointed toward "satisfaction of desires for dependency" or feeling "warm, comfortable, secure and accepted." We searched long and hard for an increase in such *sentient*, dependent feelings during drinking, but as the results of Chapter 2 show, the data did not permit us to draw the conclusion that there was an increase in these feelings. On the contrary, the thoughts and feelings which did increase nearly all centered around power, either in a socialized or in a personalized form. At this point we had a choice: we could stick to the dependency theory by arguing that the dependency urges were so deeply *repressed* that they would not show up even in fantasy, or we could accept our findings at face value and try to work out what their implications might be for a revision of the prevailing view of the dynamics of alcoholism. We chose the latter course, partly because we believe that resort to unmeasurable, inferred variables leads to sloppy and untestable theorizing and partly because we wanted to see if a revised theory would account for the known facts about alcoholism as well as or better than the dependency theory. As we reviewed other studies of the psychological and physiological effects of alcohol, it became apparent that our results were by no means unique. No one else had found increased feelings or thoughts of warmth and dependency during drinking, and nearly all had noted an increase in aggressiveness or feelings of strength.

Both Takala *et al.* (1957) and Ekman *et al.* (1962) found increases in mood variables like exuberance, talkativeness and happiness about an hour after drinking. Takala (1957) also reports increased aggressiveness in the themes of TATs written during intoxication. Trentini *et al.* (1963) obtained somewhat similar results on Italian subjects, although the measures used are a little harder to interpret. They employed three experimental groups, one of which received a highly spiced placebo drink, another the same spiced drink laced with brandy, and a third, brandy mixed with mineral water. They then asked the subjects to rate a long series of adjectives as to their personal or social desirability. After drinking, the subjects rated such adjectives as the following to be more personally than socially desirable: *happy, daring, diverting, elegant.* These all suggest a mood of heightened lively social presence (see Chapter 10). On the other hand, there were no increases in the drinking as compared to the placebo condition in the personal desirability of such adjectives as *faithful, generous, nice, loyal, sincere* and *good.* If a person during drinking is in the frame of mind the dependency theory suggests he is in, why should he not feel such interpersonal qualities are more important?

Pollack (1965) carried out a study of experimental intoxication of alcoholics and normals. While many of the tests he administered during drinking yielded scores that are not easily interpretable in terms of our theory, the changes in self-descriptions during drinking reveal similar trends. Using a Q-sort technique, he found that normals described themselves during drinking as more *warm* and *affectionate, optimistic, self-confident, good-natured, clever* and *amusing.* Most of these changes are in the interpersonal area. His alcoholics on the other hand described themselves more often as *intelligent, optimistic, idealistic, natural leader, straightforward* and *direct, careful* and *cautious,* as well as *friendly* and *out-going.* Both groups also ascribed to themselves many more bad characteristics during drinking, but it is at least interesting to note that the alcoholics, who according to our theory have a stronger personalized power concern, tend to show more increases in self-descriptions having to do with assertiveness (leadership, intelligence, directness, and so forth) rather than with interpersonal relations.

Perhaps the results of these drinking studies may best be summarized in the words of McGuire, Stein, and Mendelson (1966) who, after a careful clinical study of alcoholic and nonalcoholic subjects undergoing prolonged experimental intoxication, concluded:

> During the pre-drinking period, the chronic alcoholic subjects expected transformations in their relationships and feelings when they became intoxicated. They believed they would become "masculine," "admired by women," more sociable, and better able to carry out tasks, and that they would have a better estimate of themselves, feel less "anxious," and become more "integrated" as individuals. No similar expectations or beliefs were noted in the non-alcoholic subjects.
>
> When drinking began, the alcoholic subjects actually felt that the anticipated changes occurred. To explain these findings we postulated that a kind of "ego integration" occurred in the early days of intoxication.... Our findings further indicate that a mystique of chronic alcoholism was cherished by these subjects; it had many of the attributes of the secret society, especially in terms of the requirements for continued membership. These subjects believed that by belonging to and participating in this society they became "men," and would therefore be accorded the prerogatives they imagined were with being a man. (1966, p. 25.)

While the positive "ego-enhancing" effects of drinking have been noted in some of the reports mentioned above, on the whole they have tended to be underplayed in reports by American scholars, perhaps because the heritage of Prohibition and studies of motor coordination may have led them to expect that all of the effects of alcohol were negative, and partly because they believed so strongly in the tension-reducing, dependency-gratifying effects of alcohol that they simply overlooked the ego-enhancing effects. For example, Cahalan *et al.* (1970) in their nation-wide survey of drinking habits in the United States, used a number of items to find out what motives people had for drinking. The items, drawn from two previous studies of the reasons for drinking, include such statements as the following:

(a) I drink because it helps me relax.
(b) I drink to be sociable.
(e) I drink when I want to forget everything.
(f) I drink to celebrate special occasions.
(g) A drink helps me to forget my worries.
(j) A drink helps cheer me up when I'm in a bad mood.
(k) I drink because I need to when I'm tense and nervous.

(Cahalan *et al.*, 1970, p. 199.)

Even a cursory glance at these items reveals that none of them gives the respondent an option of saying that he drinks because "it gives me a lift" or "it strengthens me." Instead the items nearly all suggest that the only reasons for drinking are to reduce anxiety in social situations, to cause a person to forget, to get rid of anxiety and tension, to cheer him up when he is in a bad mood, etc. The bias of course is not just in the scientist; it is in the respondents themselves who, even when given a free response question, seldom in the United States mention the "pick-up" function of drinking (see Cahalan, *et al.*, 1970, p. 160). Contrast this with results from France, for example, where over 55 percent of the respondents in a similar nation-wide survey said that wine is nourishing, gives a lift and strengthens, completes a good meal, and cheers, making one happy (Sadoun *et al.*, 1965).

Such results make it important to stress that most of our studies do not deal with the conscious reasons people think they have for drinking, which may vary widely from culture to culture, depending on expectations of what the effects of alcohol are supposed to be. Instead our subjects for the most part scarcely knew that alcohol was the object of study; and even if they did, they could not have controlled their fantasy responses in a way calculated to give the reactions they might have thought on the basis of cultural tradition would be expected.

PHYSIOLOGICAL BASES FOR POWER THOUGHTS AROUSED BY DRINKING

It is our conviction that the fantasy measures are closer to representing, directly and sensitively, the physiological effects of alcohol than are self-reports of states of mind which may be heavily influenced by what a person thinks the effects of alcohol should be, as defined in his culture.

What physiological effects might prompt thoughts of increased power and strength in men everywhere? As noted in Chapter 6, alcohol produces some changes in the body which in the initial stages at least might well make a man feel stronger. It may well stimulate the secretion of adrenalin (Keller, quoted in McCarthy, 1959) which mobilizes body resources generally and increases alertness (Patkai, 1969). Its effect on the sympathetic nervous system serves to dilate blood vessels, giving a temporary feeling of warmth. It may increase pulse rate slightly (Pihkanen in Takala *et al.*, 1957). In small amounts, it serves as a quick source of caloric intake, since it is absorbed directly into the bloodstream through the walls of the stomach. Finally it dulls pain, relieves aches, and may stimulate appetite. All of these effects are more marked and more immediate for distilled spirits than for beer, because the former increases the percentage of alcohol in the blood more quickly than the latter (Pihkanen in Takala *et al.*, 1957). So there is ample basis for assuming that alcohol produces a number of changes in the body which ought easily to give rise in men to thoughts about increased power. At a secondary level the drinker may react to such thoughts or the symptoms of motor uncoordination that also develop with heavier drinking in a variety of ways, depending on the culture and his personal attitudes toward drinking.

So our finding that alcohol increases power fantasies should not have been surprising. It is supported by many other studies, including the conscious reasons given for drinking in countries outside the United States. If it is surprising, it is only because negative attitudes towards alcohol in the United States have led s ientists and respondents to underplay this function of drinking. It remains the primary reason for doubting the hypothesis that drinking arouses or satisfies dependency feelings.

OTHER REASONS FOR DOUBTING THE DEPENDENCY HYPOTHESIS

The first reason lies in the need to explain why so many people drink in small quantities so often. The dependency conflict theory primarily explains heavy drinking or alcoholism; that is, presumably only heavy drinking produces a state of near infantile dependency. But what then is the explanation for light drinking? Should one assume that, since everyone wants dependency to some extent and is partly frustrated in this desire, many will have a cocktail or two before dinner daily in order to gratify a frustrated dependency urge? None of the theorists quoted above has gone so far as to advocate such an explanation for ordinary drinking. In fact many of them have really not concerned themselves with the problem of light drinking, except to suggest that since we are all beset by anxieties, a few drinks daily should help reduce the tensions of normal life. As the findings reported in Chapters 1 and 2 show, however, one or two drinks do not reduce anxiety. For the average person five or six are necessary. Thus, explaining why many people frequently take only one or two drinks remains a problem for the traditional dependency conflict theory. It seems best solved by our finding that even a drink or two can increase thoughts of power and strength of a socialized nature. According to our view light drinking and heavy drinking both increase power thoughts, though of a different sort. Light drinking increases thoughts of socialized power, heavier drinking thoughts of personalized power. Heavy drinking occurs addictively in those whose personalized power concerns are already notably higher than their socialized power concerns. This heightened concern with personalized vs. socialized power is confirmed in the cross-cultural study of folk-tale themes which showed personalized power tags, like Violent Physical Manipulation (*cut, chop*) and Entering Implements (*arrow, knife, spear*), to be more common in heavy drinking societies, and socialized power tags, like War and Capability, in more sober societies.

The cross-cultural study of folk tales provided another reason why we came to doubt the dependency conflict explanation for heavy drinking. All the tags we had included to get at dependency conflict failed to show any significant correlations with heavy drinking in a society. To be sure, we did not know whether the folk tales were told during drinking and therefore whether themes of dependency would be expected to be increased for this reason. Even so, we fully expected that tribes which drank heavily, if in fact they had dependency conflict problems, would certainly project these conflicts into their folk tales whether told when drunk or sober. Yet the only clue we uncovered that might point in this direction was the increased frequency of the *Oral Body Parts* tag among the heavy drinking societies. Even that had another possible interpretation to which we will return later. In any case it seemed a very weak straw on which to base a dependency conflict theory.

Furthermore, Bacon, Barry and Child (1965) present no direct measures of dependency strivings in their cross-cultural study. Their argument for the hypothesis of dependency conflict is based on indirect measures—namely, lack of infant indulgence, and pressures toward independence and achievement in adulthood. They inferred that such harshness would frustrate universal instinctual desires to be dependent and cared for. In other words, it is an interpretation of their data that supports the dependency conflict hypothesis, not the data themselves directly. Their findings are similar to those obtained here: societies which drink heavily are hard on their children and on their adults. They push them toward independence, achievement and manliness from infancy on, so that in time they become obsessed with "manly" virtues. It is not *necessary* to assume that this concern for masculinity is a defensive façade that hides a deep-lying, heightened desire for dependence, particularly if one can find no *direct* measure of that desire.

Finally we have come to doubt the dependency conflict theory of drinking because, as Davis reports in Chapter 9, we could not alter the amount a man drank by manipulating his dependency feelings, though we could by changing his feelings of power.

EVIDENCE SUPPORTING
THE DEPENDENCY CONFLICT HYPOTHESIS

But are there other facts that point more unequivocally to a heightened dependency need in heavy drinkers? On what other studies was the consensus as to the etiology of alcoholism built?

Much of it derived from extensive individual case studies, such as those published by Tähkä (1966). The case study, however, is a very blunt instrument for testing or refining a scientific hypothesis. The observer knows that he is studying an alcoholic. He also knows, if he is a well-trained psychiatrist or clinical psychologist, what the prevailing opinion is as to the etiology of alcoholism. He expects to find oral dependency, and in fact he often does. The problem is not so much that it isn't there; rather, oral dependency is undoubtedly present to some degree in every person. It just tends to stand out as figure on ground for the psychiatrist studying an alcoholic, partly because he knows drinking is an oral activity, partly because he expects oral involvement on theoretical grounds, and partly because he has no control subjects among whom he can observe comparable levels of oral dependency.

But the longitudinal studies of the McCords (1960) are not open to these objections, and they have been interpreted as giving major support to the dependency hypothesis. As these investigators point out (1960, p. 133), their studies correct for the biases of other investigations in several ways: "first, the analyses were based on direct observations of the adult alcoholics (or pre-alcoholic children) within their homes over an extensive period of time; second, the original observers did not know that any study of personality would be based on their report; third, the reports were made by a variety of observers whose possible biases would tend to cancel one another; fourth, neither the original observers nor the raters focussed on the problem of the alcoholic personality, and thus conscious theoretical biases were minimum; finally, the sample of alcoholics contains men who had never come to the attention of official agencies dealing with alcoholism." The last point is particularly worth mentioning because it can be argued that the average alcoholic seen by a psychiatrist ought to be a more dependent type than those who never go to seek help. With all these corrections for theoretical or sampling bias, the McCords clearly come to the conclusion that "dependency conflict is a key factor in producing alcoholism." For instance, they provide a table (1960, p. 89) showing that among those boys who had satisfied dependency needs (as derived from ratings made at the time) only 6 percent became alcoholics as contrasted with 18 percent of the boys with frustrated dependency needs and 34 percent of the boys with conflict over dependency needs. The difference between 6 percent and 34 percent is highly significant statistically. Is this not incontrovertable evidence for the dependency conflict theory?

It is not. As in the case of Bacon, Barry and Child, the McCords did not have a direct measure of conflict over dependency, but rather inferred it from some other observations that were made. Their two direct measures—mothers' encouragement of dependency, and oral tendencies present—did *not* relate to subsequent alcoholism. Rather, their *interpretation* that dependency conflict was involved relies heavily on the finding that mothers who alternatively loved and rejected their sons tended to have more sons who later became alcoholic. They *infer* that this pattern of maternal behavior should increase dependency conflict, although of course it is not the only problem it might create, and although Bacon, Barry and Child argue that rejection rather than alternation of love and rejection should maximize dependency needs. They also obtained many other findings. So, rather than quibble over the interpretation of one or another, let us lay them all out systematically in Table 13.1 and see whether as a whole they tend to support a dependency or a power-conflict theory.

All the characteristics listed in the table were significantly more common in the backgrounds of boys who became adult alcoholics as contrasted with comparable boys who did not become alcoholics. The two groups of boys were very much alike in the beginning in socio-economic status and other background factors. Yet they differed in personality characteristics as rated from observations made at the time. Boys who were to become alcoholics were more active, assertive, and aggressive than comparable boys who did not become alcoholics. These characteristics suggest to us that they were already more concerned with being powerful. They also had fewer fears and were less over-controlled or inhibited.

Jones (1965, 1968) found similar differences in traits displayed in junior high school by boys who later became alcoholics as compared

Table 13.1—Developmental characteristics of alcoholics contrasted with normals and criminals (*from McCord and McCord, 1960*)

Significantly more common ($p < .05$) in alcoholic than in normal group	Other notes
As pre-alcoholic boys	
(a) "Power concern":	
more self-confident,[1] assertive,[2]	No greater oral tendencies
more aggressive, sadistic,[1,2]	
more active,[1] talkative,[2] expressive[2]	
(b) "Less Inhibition":	
fewer abnormal fears,	
less overcontrolled,[2] fastidious[2]	
(c) "Other":	
disapproved of mothers more,	See mother's treatment below
more indifferent to siblings	
Mothers of pre-alcoholic boys	
(a) "Power concern" antecedents:	
alternated affection and rejection,[1]	All techniques designed to undercut
especially if low esteem of father,	sense of male authority and
rejected both son and husband,	importance
criminally or sexually deviant,	
rejected role in the family	
(b) "Less Inhibition" antecedents:	
subnormally restrictive,	
less strongly Catholic	
(c) "Other":	No greater encouragement of
escapist reaction to crises	dependency or masculinity
Fathers of pre-alcoholic boys	
Low esteem for wives	More evidence of battle of
	sexes over male authority
Escapist reaction to crises,	Also characteristic of fathers of
rejecting, or punitive and	boys who became criminals. The
non-affectionate	latter differed from fathers of
	alcoholics by being more dominating,
	aggressive, physically punitive.
Family climate	
Outsider, opposes parents	Unique to pre-alcoholic syndrome,
	source of power conflict.
Parental antagonism,	Source of power conflict,
lack of supervision of child	source of low inhibition.

[1] Confirmed at $p < .05$ for alcoholics from the control group also.
[2] Significant differences between adult problem and moderate drinkers when they were junior-high-school boys (M. C. Jones, 1965, 1968).

with boys who did not. The evidence is very good that the pre-alcoholic boy tends to be more self-confident, assertive, active, talkative, and uninhibited than comparable boys who do not become alcoholics. Whatever an alcoholic may say as an adult about his childhood to the skilled clinician, when he is a boy, to the outside observer who knows nothing of his future as an alcoholic, he does not appear dependent with strong oral needs. It is at least curious that he shows no direct evidence of a greater dependency concern in adolescence—unless one wants to make the reaction-formation assumption that whatever a person does signifies its opposite. Thus one might infer that because the boys are more assertive, they are really more dependent. But the assumption of reaction formation is not parsimonious, and it leads to great difficulties in measurement in determining when a thing is what it is and when it is just the opposite.

As to the characteristics of the parents of future alcoholics summarized in Table 13.1, first of all they were less restrictive, less religious, and generally less strict in supervising the child. These appear to be the child-rearing antecedents of the low level of inhibition found in adults who drink heavily. Next, as already noted, maternal alternation of affection and rejection goes with future alcoholism, but so do a number of other characteristics that fit less easily into the hypothesis of dependency conflict. Why should mothers who reject their husbands, and husbands who have low esteem for their wives, and parents who fight all the time tend to produce alcoholics? Could all these characteristics produce increased dependency conflict in their sons? Possibly they could, but isn't it more likely that all these and other signs of the "war between the sexes" will result in a sense of doubt about male worth and importance? If a mother alternates affection with rejection for her son, especially if she holds the father in low esteem, one likely outcome would be that the son would have doubts about his worth as a *male*. At times his mother would seem to value him, but at other times she would seem to reject him and all other males in the immediate family. She further rejects her role in the family, either directly or by being criminally or sexually deviant, so that she is obviously not fulfilling the traditional female role of a wife and mother who supports and builds up the sense of importance of the males in the family.

It may be worth trying to state as precisely as possible the difference between this interpretation and the one given by the McCords (1960). They argue that almost everyone feels a dependent desire "to give himself over to unquestioning, undemanding maternal care, to be comforted, and to be guided by someone else." It is this childhood desire, according to the McCords, which is erratically satisfied and frustrated in the case of the pre-alcoholic. Our interpretation, on the other hand, is that males in all societies are expected to be assertive and strong, instrumental in supplying the needs of the family vis-à-vis the outside world (see Parsons & Bales, 1955; Zelditch, 1955). The male sense of self-worth and self-esteem depends on his ability to fulfill this role, although it is of course stressed to a greater or lesser degree in different families and in different societies. One of the chief sources of such self-esteem is the crucial support a son or husband gets from the women in the family. The mother can undercut a sense of self-worth in the son by alternatively loving and rejecting the boy or by consistently showing that she has no respect for the male role. Another way the sense of male efficacy might be undercut is by the presence of an outsider influential in the family who consistently opposes the parents in their directives to the child. As Table 13.1 shows, such an outsider was more common in the families of boys who later became alcoholics. A person of this sort is obviously a source of power conflicts in the home and a source of contradictory expectations as to what the son should do. However the boy attempts to assert himself, someone—either his parents or the outsider—is likely to try to stop him or to undercut what he is doing. It is difficult to see how this particular variable—the presence of an outsider who opposes the parents—would increase dependency conflict, although it is not so difficult to see it as a source of damage to male self-esteem and assertiveness.

It is worth noting also that the chief difference between the fathers of those who became criminals and the fathers of those who became alcoholics is that the former were consistently more dominating, aggressive and physically punitive to their sons. In terms of the present interpretation this makes sense, because a consistently physically aggressive father provides for the boy a model for assertiveness in the male role which he can and does adopt. Though it is a deviant male role model, it is nevertheless a consistently strong one, which the boy can emulate. On the other hand, the fathers of the pre-alcoholics are both undercut or derogated by their wives and do not adopt a consistently aggressive pattern with which the boys can identify. Rather they show "escapist" reactions to crises. Thus their sons have doubts about how to be an assertive male, and no model in the family to follow. Our interpretation of all these findings is that the central concern for the pre-alcoholic boy lies in the area of male self-esteem, in the desire to demonstrate male strength—personalized power; we do not find evidence for dependency conflict, in which the chief issue is the wish for undemanding maternal care versus the desire to be free of such a weakness.

ADULT CHARACTERISTICS OF ALCOHOLICS

Let us now turn to the characteristics of adult alcoholics as discovered by many different investigators. They have been listed in Table 13.2. Again with few exceptions to be discussed in a moment, they do not seem to require an interpretation in terms of dependency conflict. On the contrary, many of them appear to point not only to the usual lack of inhibition, but also to a heightened concern over potency.

Certainly the aggressive rebelliousness found to characterize alcoholics by nearly all investigators (see Chapter 10; Jones, 1968; and the McCords, 1960) is one of the key defining attributes of a need for power at least at the impulse level (see Chapter 8). Furthermore the intense husband-wife conflicts which characterize male alcoholics suggest they are having problems with the assertive male role. The alcoholics' touch of paranoia in feeling victimized or grandiose (see Table 13.2) is also characteristic of a heightened power concern. There is some conflicting

Table 13.2—Characteristics of adult male alcoholics or heavy drinkers contrasted with moderate drinkers or normals

"Power concern"
> Assertive anti-social behavior (Chapter 10)
> Intensive husband-wife conflict (M)
> Erratically punitive and lax (M)
> Feel victimized (M, Mo)
> Feel grandiose (M)
> More unrestrainedly aggressive (M, J), rebellious (J, Je)
> Passive parental role (M)

"Lack of Inhibition"
> Lack of order (Chapter 10)
> Undercontrolled (J)
> Fluctuating moods, unpredictable, disorganized (J)
> Less fastidious, overcontrolled, conservative (J)
> Rapid tempo (J, T)
> Seek immediate enjoyment (M), sensuous (J)

"Other"
> Less formal group participation (M, Je)
> Lively sociability (Chapter 10), gregarious (J, Chapter 8)
> More dependent (M)
> More field dependent (W)

Note: All characteristics listed have been found significantly more often among alcoholics or problem drinkers than among comparable normals.
M   = McCord & McCord, 1960
J   = M. C. Jones, 1965, 1968
T   = Tähkä, 1966, p. 74
Je = Jessor *et al.*, 1968
Mo = Moore, 1962
W   = Witkin, 1965

evidence as to whether alcoholics are more or less sociable. In one group the McCords found them to participate less in formal groups, as did Jessor *et al.* (1968); but in another group the McCords found them to be more sociable. Jones reports that they are described as more gregarious, and in Chapters 8 and 10 we found a sociability factor that was associated with heavy drinking. There are two clues here which help resolve the conflicts in the evidence. According to the analysis in Chapter 8 one must distinguish between the true alcoholic or addictive liquor drinker who is concerned with establishing personalized power over an opponent, and the heavy beer drinker who spends a lot of time being sociable and attending sports events. Since it is always difficult to get a precise definition of what constitutes an alcoholic, some of the conflicts in the evidence about sociability may be due to the fact that some investigators include heavy, convivial beer drinkers in their sample of problem drinkers. In fact it appears to be rare that a beer drinker ever becomes a true "alcoholic."

Another clue is provided in Chapter 10, where it is suggested that one must distinguish between "lively acting out" so as to be the center of all attention in a party—which is a sign of a desire for personalized power—and prolonged social attachments to others—which may be a sign of an interest in socialized power or more simply of a genuine affection for others. In other words, there are two kinds of "gregariousness" which may be confused in a judge's mind, but the evidence is clear that alcoholics show the first or narcissistic type.

But what are we to make of the McCords' finding that adult alcoholics are rated significantly more often as dependent (Table 13.2)? Is this not direct evidence for the dependency hypothesis? In a sense it is, but it is also worth noting that the scale the judges used to get this rating ran from *highly masculine* through *normally masculine* to *dependent* and *effeminate*. At least to us, the *dependent* category seems a little out of place on this dimension. That is, it should be possible to be less than normally masculine without being dependent, although it was not possible for the McCords' judges to make such a rating. It is crucial to our theory, because we too are saying that these males should be less than normally masculine because they have real doubts about their efficacy as males, but this does not necessarily imply that they are dependent.

One other consistent characteristic of alcoholics suggests that they may be more dependent. Witkin and his associates (1965) have regularly found that an alcoholic is less able to adjust a rod to the upright vertical position when its frame is tilted, or to adjust his body to the upright when he is seated in a tilted chair in a tilted room, or to locate a simple figure embedded in complex designs. These are all considered to be signs of "field dependence" in the sense that the alcoholic seems to be more dependent on external cues than on his own internal frame of reference. Can this characteristic be taken as evidence of a *repressed* need for "undemanding maternal care" or for guidance by someone else? Not really. Witkin (1965) does not tie this type of cognitive style *directly* to interpersonal dependency needs. Rather he shows that field independence is associated with better articulation of the body concept (clearer body boundaries), with a better sense of separate identity, and with certain specialized defenses. He noted that alcoholics show a relatively global body concept not only in their greater field dependence but also in their figure drawings (1965, p. 325). He, along with most observers, accepts the view that alcoholics have dependency problems and that this cognitive style may indicate the presence of such problems.

But again we would give it a different interpretation. Males are consistently more field *independent* cross-culturally than females; that is, they have a concept of the body with clearer boundaries, and a better sense of separate identity as assertive individuals acting on the environment. Women, on the other hand, are consistently more contextual in their approach to perception and interpersonal relations (see McClelland, 1965). From this point of view the greater field dependence of alcoholics suggests the doubts about their masculinity which we have been arguing characterizes them in particular. They have a more confused sense of identity, a desire to express their power vigorously, to overcome their doubts about their potency. So their cognitive style is less articulated than it would be in a normally self-confident male. Thus the field dependency finding appears to confirm our theory as much as it confirms the dependency conflict theory.

Table 13.3 lists some of the rather unusual items on the Minnesota Multiphasic Inventory which, according to MacAndrew (1965), differentiate alcoholic from other psychiatric out-patients. The list of such items is more extensive than this, but three types of responses have not been included because they do not need further interpretation: (1) items expressing the greater aggressiveness of alcoholics, (2) items showing greater lack of inhibition in alcoholics ("I readily become 100 percent sold on a good idea."), and (3) items which are related to symptoms of the disease ("I have had blank spells. . . ."). This leaves a number of "odd" items which one can either regard as the result of some chance background factors in the composition of the alcoholic sample, or try to interpret as psychologically meaningful.

The two items at the bottom of Table 13.3 seem related to oral dependency and will be discussed later. Many more—11 in all—appear to be power-related responses. For example, liking to wear expensive clothes (prestige supplies), reading newspaper articles on crime (aggressive impulses), being a sports reporter, all refer to activities we have shown to be related to power needs and drinking (Chapter 8). A concern for magical (religious) transformation (MMPI item 483) we have also argued is related to an infantile power concern. See the discussion of the *Change of State* tag in Chapter 3. It is as if the alcoholic were appealing to powers outside himself (Christ changing water into wine, praying, prophets predicting what would happen, powers that take my soul outside my body) to bring about radical changes in the world because he views the world in terms of such acts of personalized power.

Table 13.3—MMPI item responses which differentiate significantly between alcoholic and other psychiatric outpatients (from MacAndrew, 1965)

MMPI item Number	Alcoholic's response	
		Power-related responses
529	True	I would like to wear expensive clothes.
6	True	I like to read newspaper articles about crime.
283	True	If I were a reporter I would like very much to report sporting news.
86	False	I am certainly lacking in self-confidence.
		* * *
59	True	My soul sometimes leaves my body.
27	True	Evil spirits possess me at times.
58	True	I know who is responsible for most of my troubles.
413	True	I deserve severe punishment for my sins.
		* * *
483	True	Christ performed miracles such as changing water into wine (see *Change of state* tag, discussed in Chapter 3).
58	True	Everything is turning out just like the prophets of the Bible said it would.
488	True	I pray several times a week.
		"Oral dependent" responses
140	True	I like to cook.
562	True	The one to whom I was most attached and whom I most admired as a child was a woman. (Mother, sister, aunt or other woman).

What is not wholly clear from the evidence is exactly *why* he is so concerned about personalized power. Our best guess is that it is not *purely* defensive in the sense that he is compensating for a felt weakness or lack of power. Thus we need not disbelieve him when he says he feels self-confident, despite the fact that he also says others are responsible for what happens to him. Rather we would argue that personalized power as a theme is just more salient for him in every way—in himself and in others. It may have become salient in part because he was undercut and has doubts about his potency, or because anyone who sees power in this way is always testing to see if he has it. Thus his concern for personalized power may have developed in part defensively—to compensate for felt inferiority—and in part offensively—to support an aggressive stance toward life which had proved satisfying in the past. Genetics may even play a part, for boys with strong mesomorphic bodies are more likely to be aggressive, and as Table 13.1 shows, more aggressive boys are more likely to grow up to be alcoholics. A successful assertive stance toward life may help create the need for personalized power which is the drinking man's key concern.

While some of these interpretations may appear strained, the reader might try accounting for these findings in terms of the dependency conflict hypothesis. To us at least it seems easier to account for more of them in terms of power concerns than in terms of dependency problems, although we fully recognize that psychological theorizing in its present stage of development is so loose that almost any theory can account for almost any set of facts.

DRINKING AMONG ANGLO-AMERICANS, SPANISH-AMERICANS, AND INDIANS

A group of researchers led by Richard Jessor (Jessor *et al.*, 1968) has conducted a major study of the interaction of social structure and personality variables in producing deviance, particularly drunkenness, in a southern Colorado town. They have developed a complex theoretical model with attendant measures of its key variables, which demonstrates that deviance is a joint function of societal factors (such as lack of opportunity and exposure to illegitimate means) and pre-disposing personality factors (such as personal disjunctions and tolerance of deviance). What is particularly important theoretically is the finding that if opportunity is held constant, personality predispositions make a difference in deviance (drinking) rates, whereas if personality predispositions are held constant, opportunity makes a difference in deviance (drinking) rates. For our limited purposes here, there is no necessity to go extensively into the theoretical model or the measures used to test it. Instead, we have singled out for comparative purposes in Table 13.4 a few of the key measures that they found predisposed to drunkenness.

As the table shows, the Spanish-American residents of the town drink a little more on the average than the Anglo-Americans, although they are not drunk quite as often. On the other hand, the Indians drink far more and are drunk much more often than either of the other two groups. Why? In terms of opportunity measures (not shown in Table 13.4), the Indians are actually somewhat better off economically than the Spanish-Americans. A large land claim settlement, and income from the production of natural gas and sale of lumber on their land has resulted in payments to an average Indian family of five of between $4000 and $6000 per year in recent times (Jessor *et al.*, 1968, p. 9). Thus it certainly cannot be argued that the Indians drink more than the Spanish-Americans because they are poorer. On the other hand, they do have somewhat greater exposure to illegitimate means (see Table 13.4) such as having a drunken or delinquent parent, not being part of a sanction network, or being a young man living in town and unemployed. To some extent of course the access to illegitimate means is circular: alcoholics are more likely to be unemployed or irregularly employed, so that one cannot argue that in any simple fashion that unemployment is a cause of drunkenness. Even so, the difference in access to illegitimate means between the Spanish-Americans and Indians hardly seems large enough to account for the big difference in rates of drunkenness—particularly when a similar difference between the Anglos and the Spanish-Americans does not produce greater drunkenness among the Spanish-Americans. Thus one has to search among the personality variables for explanations of differences in rates of drunkenness among the three groups.

The investigators asked each of the adults in a community survey study to rate how important to him were such things as "the love and affection you get in the family," "the good opinion of the family for the things you do well," and "being able to do things in the family in your own way." (See Appendix II.) Each respondent made a total of 20 *value* ratings, five under each of four headings—affection, dependency (wanting help), independence, and recognition. They were then asked to rate how much they really *expected* to get the various things of which they had just rated the importance. That is, a man might consider it

Table 13.4—Drinking rates, access to illegitimate means, personal disjunctions, and attitudes toward deviance among Anglo-Americans, Spanish-Americans, and Indians*

		Anglos (N = 93)	Spanish (N = 60)	Indians (N = 68)	Significance of diffs. A vs. S	A vs. I	S vs. I
Quantity-frequency of alcohol	Mean oz. per day	0.3	0.6	2.0	n.s.	$p < .01$	$p < .05$
Times drunk previous year	mean	2.0	1.5	14.4	n.s.	$p < .01$	$p < .001$
Access to illegitimate means[1]	mean	3.15	4.10	5.28	$p < .001$	$p < .001$	$p < .001$
Personal disjunctions[2]	mean	2.8	5.7	5.7	$p < .001$	$p < .001$	n.s.
("Power Concern") Recognition expectations	mean	10.0	10.3	9.1	n.s.	$p < .05$	$p < .05$
Deviance disapproval[3] ("Inhibition")	mean	70.7	85.9	67.9	$p < .01$	n.s.	$p < .01$

* From Jessor *et al.*, 1968, Community study.
[1] A composite measure consisting of exposure to deviant models (such as a drunken or delinquent parent), absence of sanction networks (e.g., no family, low church attendance, no telephone), and deviance opportunity (e.g., greater if male, young, living in town rather than country, unemployed).
[2] Differences between how *important* Dependency, Recognition, etc. are and how much the respondent *expects* to get Dependency, Recognition, etc.
[3] Wrongness rated on a scale of 0 to 9 of such activities as "driving over the speed limit," "a married woman fooling around with other men," "a woman being a heavy drinker," etc.

very important to be able to do things in his family in his own way, but estimate that in fact he did not really expect to be able to do things in the family in his own way. The difference between the value rating and the expectation rating yields a disjunction score. Table 13.4 shows that the gap between goals and expectations is much higher both for the Spanish-Americans and the Indians than for the Anglo-Americans. Once again it is not altogether clear why the Indians drink more than the Spanish-Americans if they both feel it unlikely they will get what they value in life. There is one area, however, in which there is a significant difference between the Spanish-Americans and the Indians: all three groups wanted Recognition to about the same degree, but in this area alone, the Indians had significantly lower expectations of achievement than the Spanish-Americans or the Anglo-Americans. In the areas of Independence, Dependency and Affection, there were no significant differences between the Spanish-Americans and the Indians.

So the data clearly suggest that a greater disjunction in the area of Recognition may have something to do with the greater drunkenness among the Indians. This conclusion agrees with what the Indians themselves give as the explanation of why they drink so much. They feel that they have been exploited so long by whites and treated so consistently as wards of the Federal government that they have lost their sense of self-respect and their ability to make self-reliant decisions on their own. Even their recent economic affluence cannot wipe out the years of discrimination which have undermined their pride. After all, they were in no sense responsible for the fact that natural gas was discovered on their land and brought important financial returns. In short, they have doubts as to whether they are really *men*. They have a power need and attempt to prove their personal power through drinking, since their sense of being unable to gain recognition prevents them from adopting more socialized means of gaining power. In short, these results seem to us to bear out our general theory as to the nature of alcoholism, and to cast some doubt on the alternative theory of the key problem as dependency, since there were no differences between the Spanish-Americans and the Indians in disjunctions in the Independence or Dependence areas. Unfortunately, as we pointed out in Chapter 8, this interpretation, while plausible, is not the only possible one. The felt lack of Recognition may be a result of drinking so much, rather than its cause. Our own preference for a causal interpretation depends not so much on the correlation itself, as on general theory and case reports from the sample of Indian men.

The last line in Table 13.4 illustrates the importance of the other factor which we have repeatedly found to have a bearing on sobriety—namely, the level of inhibition. It is clear that the Spanish-Americans disapprove much more highly of all sorts of deviance than either the

Anglo-Americans or Indians. Thus even though other pre-disposing factors in the environment or in the individual might push them towards drinking, their high level of inhibition should and did control drunkenness.

VARIATION IN RATES OF HEAVY DRINKING

Certain facts about drinking are seldom discussed when theories of the psychodynamics of alcoholism are being elaborated from clinical or personality data. These are the marked differences in rates of heavy drinking among various population sub-groups. If the dependency conflict theory is to be taken seriously, it would have to be expanded to explain why some social groups drink much more heavily than others.

It is our belief that these differences can be more easily explained in terms of the personalized power theory than the dependency conflict theory; all the facts are laid out in Table 13.5, so that the reader may try his own interpretations. Some of the variations in drinking rates are striking. For instance, on the average, men always, everywhere, in technologically complex and in primitive societies, drink more heavily than women (Child *et al.*, 1965). Why? Don't women want undemanding maternal care, comfort, and guidance by someone else as much as men do? And if so, isn't it at least probable that in some societies this need would be frustrated more in women than in men so that they would be more likely than the men to take drink? Cross-cultural evidence does not suggest that there is a universal difference between men and women in the dependency area, but it does show that men are almost universally expected to be more self-reliant, assertive and achievement-oriented than women (Zelditch, 1955). Thus it would seem more sensible to relate a universal sex difference in drinking to a universal difference in the way men and women are expected to behave. Since men are more likely to be expected to be strong and assertive, they are more likely to become excessively concerned with exercising personal power.

Why should middle-aged men drink more heavily than younger or older men? (See Table 13.5.) Again, it seems easier to find an explanation in the power than in the dependency area. Generally speaking, more strength and assertiveness is expected of middle-aged men with heavy family and work responsibilities than of either younger or older men. Yet this increase in responsibility is associated with a regular physical decline in potency both in the sexual and aggressive senses of the term. What is more likely than that men faced with high demands for assertiveness and a lessening capacity should turn more often to the artifical sense of increased potency that drinking produces?

Table 13.5—Variations in rates of heavy drinking explained in terms of power concern theory

Rate Differences	Explanation
1. Heavier drinking among men than among women in all cultures (Ch, Ca, Sa)	Men are cross-culturally expected to show more personal assertiveness.
2. Heavier drinking among middle-aged men than younger or older men (Sa, Ca, p. 32, p. 222; Ma, PG)	More power is expected from middle-aged men than younger or older men.
3. Heavy drinking among manual workers (Sa; Ca, p. 222)	Because their work exhausts physical strength, they turn more often to alcohol to regain a feeling of strength
4. Heavy alcoholism rates among Breton deep-sea fishermen (Sa; Hugues & Lavenir, 1959)	Conditions of work requiring bravery and prowess in face of constant possibility of failure maximize personal power concern (see Chapter 4)
5. Heavier drinking in northern than southern France, in north Europe than Latin Europe (Sa; Lolli *et al.*, 1958)	Absence of male solidarity rituals, presence of strong females in North
6. High drinking rates among the Irish (Bales, 1962, Ca, p. 66) Low drinking rates among Jews (Snyder, 1962; Ca, p. 72) and Chinese (LaBarre, 1946, Chafetz, 1964)	Assertiveness expected in Irish sons, undercut by long dependency; male solidarity rituals among Jews and Chinese
7. Higher drinking among men with poor marriage records (unmarried, broken or quarrelsome marriages) (Sa, p. 108; Ca, p. 46; Tähkä, 1966, p. 275; M)	Marriage relation especially difficult for man with power concern. Fears wife may undercut potency. She may do so by nagging which leads to more drinking to gain strength.
8. Lower drinking among highly religious (Ca, p. 147, p. 191; Ma; Je)	Either power is gained directly from religious supports (e.g., God) or operation of general inhibition factor.

Ch = Child, Barry and Bacon, 1965
Ca = Cahalan, Cisin and Crossley, 1970
Sa = Sadoun, Lolli and Silverman, 1965
Ma = Maccoby, Chapter 11
PG = Pittman and Gordon, 1958
M = McCord and McCord, 1960
Je = Jessor, Graves, Hanson and Jessor, 1968

A similar explanation can be given for why manual workers drink more heavily than intellectual workers or professionals (particularly if the capacity to purchase alcoholic beverages is equalized). (See Table 13.5.) Because physical work exhausts one's sense of potency and strength at a more basic level than intellectual work, men who are more exhausted should turn more often to alcohol to regain a feeling of strength and power. Also manual work involves a concern with personal force more than professional work, and the latter often involves a concern for social power which is increased by smaller amounts of drinking.

Alcoholism has been such a special problem among the Breton fishermen that it has been singled out for special study. Could it be that the mothers of Breton fishermen behave in some significant way different from the mothers of other workers in Brittany, so that the fishermen grow up with a greater dependency conflict? It does not seem likely. On the other hand, their deep-sea fishing seems very likely to require a personalized power concern in the same way as the hunting cultures described in Chapter 4; that is, the work requires bravery in the face of constant challenges (storms at sea, big fish, inability to catch fish). This is the ideal situation according to our theory for focussing concern on personal prowess, both because the occupation requires it and because results are highly variable over time and among individuals. It is not surprising that the person turns to alcohol as a means of reinforcing this concern for personalized power.

It has frequently been observed that drinking is heavier in the north of Europe than in the south; it is heavier in France than it is in Italy, and even in northern France than in southern France (see Sadoun *et al.*, 1965). What major cultural differences would account for these differences in drinking rates? Explanations have tended to be somewhat *ad hoc*. For instance, it has been argued that Italians do not get drunk as often as Frenchmen because when Italian children learn to drink, it is part of a family meal. Thus drinking is subject to all the family controls normally exercised over excesses of any kind. The same explanation has been advanced for low rates of drunkenness among Jews. Yet it scarcely goes deep enough: *why* is wine drunk only with meals more often in Italy than in France? One suspects that there may be more of a positive push for masculine drinking outside the family in France and northern Europe than exists in a country like Italy. Italian males certainly *could* drink outside the home in the north European pattern, but they don't feel the need to.

Again, it would seem better to look for an explanation in the cross-cultural findings reported in Chapter 4. There it was found that in societies with high male solidarity, drunkenness tended to be less frequent. In such societies, it was argued that men could consolidate their positions with reference to a cohesive group. They did not have to prove continually that they were "men" like the hunters. This predicament seems to be more characteristic of north than south European families. In the former the male has to prove his worth, earn by assertive behavior the right to be admired by women. Furthermore, women in northern Europe have always had more "rights" than in southern Europe; they too can vote, inherit property, become the "man" of the family if they are competent enough, and so forth. In other words, in northern Europe both men and women are judged more by achieved than by ascribed status standards. This obviously creates a climate in which a man is much more likely to become concerned about his personalized power, either because he is not in fact very competent, or because he could be out-performed or despised by women. Veroff and Feld (1969) have documented the fact that men with high n Power are less happy in democratic families in which their wives have more power. As Tähkä points out, the most usual motive reported for initial drinking by his Finnish subjects was a desire to demonstrate "one's manliness to a group of peers." (1966, p. 206). On the other hand, it is not necessary for an Italian male to demonstrate his manliness. He becomes a member of the sacred fraternity of males at the moment of his birth; he is constantly admired, rewarded and supported just because he is a male—by his mother, his sisters, and all the females in his environment (see Strodtbeck, 1958).

A somewhat similar contrast in the way men are treated may explain the well-documented difference in drinking rates among the Irish and the Jews. Irish boys are often close to their mothers, being nurtured and protected by them well beyond adolescence, but Jewish boys are just as close to their mothers. In fact, the extent to which the middle-class Jewish mother feeds, looks after, and attempts to supervise everything her son does is proverbial in contemporary U.S. culture. Such a mother fits in many particulars the description of the over-protective mothers whose behavior Tähkä found to be responsible for producing alcoholism in his Finnish subjects. He reports, for instance, that "over-protective and markedly narcissistic maternal attitudes could frequently be inferred from the information provided by the subject" (1966, p. 199). If Jewish mothers are at all like these Finnish mothers of alcoholics, as would seem to be the case, why shouldn't the rate of alcoholism among Jewish males be unusually high instead of unusually low? The key to the difference does not appear to lie in the maternal care and protectiveness area but in the ease with which one can become a "man" in the two cultures. A Finnish boy must prove he is a man; a Jewish boy knows he is one always and is constantly reminded of it by his mother and by certain ritual observances like the Bar Mitzvah.

The contrast is even more marked with the Irish. The Irish male is expected to be tough and assertive, but as Bales reports,"a son cannot marry until his father is ready to sign the farm over to him and relinquish control. Until that time the son is called a 'boy,' and has the social status of a boy, no matter how old he may be" (in Pittman & Snyder, 1962, p. 168). In other words, Irish culture creates the classic concern for personalized power for sons, which leads to heavy drinking. A male is expected to be a "man" and a "boy" at the same time. Since there is no realistic way for him to escape either horn of the dilemma, he chooses the bottle as a way of enhancing his sense of personal strength for the moment.

The Jewish boy is in quite a different situation. Once again, though his mother may attempt to feed, dominate and protect him, she makes it clear always that she is doing it because he is her *son*, a male infinitely worthy of attention and respect. In fact, in older Jewish tradition her spiritual salvation depended on her having a son. Thus the son knew that by his very existence he had performed an important part in helping his mother (an act of *social* power). The rites of circumcision and Bar Mitzvah assert the boy's incontestable maleness as an ascribed fact of his existence. Confirmation in the Catholic church does not serve the same function, because there is nothing uniquely male about it. It is probably also true that traditional Jewish culture has many of the inhibitory characteristics found in sober societies in Chapter 4, which also tend to reduce drinking rates. However, the pressure to prove one's manliness through drinking should also be less among Jews.

Low drinking rates among the Chinese and other ethnic groups can be explained on similar grounds. In the traditional Chinese family, once again the son did not have to earn his right to be considered masculine, but was ascribed a good deal of authority from the mere fact of being born a male. In other words, all these ethnic or sub-cultural variations become simply other instances in the general test of the hypothesis confirmed cross-culturally in Chapter 4.

Another characteristic of alcoholics reported in Table 13.5 is that they tend to have significantly poorer marriage records than the average male; that is, more of them remain unmarried, or if they marry, the marriages are more likely to break up or to degenerate into a continuous "war between the sexes." Tähkä found for his 50 alcoholic subjects that nine were unmarried, 18 were divorced or separated, and 18 of those still married had quarrelsome or moping wives. This leaves a total of five who were "normally" married. The usual explanation for these facts is that heavy drinking makes a man a pretty unattractive marriage partner. His wife nags because he drinks; supposedly he drinks because his wife nags. While the definitive formal study has probably not yet been made as to which came first, the nagging or the drinking, the situation described by Maccoby in Chapter 11 is thought to characterize what often happens. He reports that the Mexican alcoholics more often had nagging mothers and nagging wives; further-more, they often passed from a dominant mother to a dominant or a nagging wife. He describes one case of a man who stopped drinking "after marrying a motherly and gentle woman ten years older than he." These findings suggest that the data on marital discord in general support our hypothesis that one of the chief causes of alcoholism is a concern about male superiority and power. The marriage relationship is critical for a man who needs to demonstrate his personal potency. He may even choose a strong wife in order to prove his masculinity by winning out over her. If so, the choice is a self-defeating one, because such a wife will tend to fight back and weaken what may already be a shaky sense of male power. Or, in order to avoid the fatal test of strength, he may not marry at all. According to the theory, doubts of sexual dominance and potency should particularly plague alcoholics, and this seems to be in general true. For instance, Tähkä reports (1966) that 30 of his 50 subjects used regular drinking for asserting manliness or approaching girls. Unfortunately, since he reports no control figures, it is not certain that these motives characterized alcoholics more than normal men; but certainly his detailed individual studies suggest that this is the case. What often results is a vicious cycle. A man who has doubts about his power with women is sensitive to the least sign of rejection, drinks to strengthen himself, and thereby puts himself in a more likely position to be rejected, so that he drinks even more.[1]

Finally, in Table 13.5, we note that drinking tends to be much lower in highly religious people. The explanation probably lies in the general inhibition factor that we have repeatedly found tends to promote sobriety, either in individuals or in societies. In short, religion *socializes* personal power and redirects it to altruistic ends. However, it is also worth noting that religion may provide a substitute form of "ego enhancement" for a man with a personalized power drive. If he is truly religious, he tends to get the same strength and power from God that he might otherwise get from drinking.

The founder of Alcoholics Anonymous appears to have hit on this fact in diagnosing the alcoholic's central problem. He writes in *Alcoholics Anonymous* (1955, p. 60): "Our description of the alcoholic, the chapter on the agnostic, and our personal adventures before and after make clear three pertinent ideas:

(a) That we were alcoholic and could not manage ourselves.
(b) That probably no human power could have relieved our alcoholism.
(c) That God could and would if He were sought."

The therapeutic effectiveness of Alcoholics Anonymous derives from this correct diagnosis. To join it, an alcoholic must admit his complete weakness and inadequacy and accept wholeheartedly the belief that to

[1] Unfortunately an attempt in the two bar studies to relate marital problems to drinking and power needs yielded conflicting results. See Appendix V. It is probable that our measure of "marital problems" was not sensitive enough, for in one study marital problems did not even appear to be related to heavy drinking.

live a normal life he must be utterly dependent on a power greater than himself. In other words, he must accept the power of God as a substitute for the power of the bottle to enhance his sense of potency. God "inspirits" him, strengthening him in place of liquor.

This completes the review of known facts about alcoholism in the light of the traditional dependency conflict theory and our personalized power theory. At a minimum our goal has been to show that the facts do not *require* interpretation in terms of dependency conflicts. Even further, we feel many of the facts can be more easily interpreted in terms of a personalized power theory. To some extent, of course, the difference between the two theories has been exaggerated for the sake of exposition. Most dependency theorists also talk about inadequate masculine identification, which they tend to interpret as resulting from dependency needs. By way of summary, Table 13.6 has been prepared to contrast the two models of the psychodynamics of alcoholism. On the left is presented a somewhat simplified version of the McCords' careful

Table 13.6—Two contrasting models of the psychodynamics of alcoholism

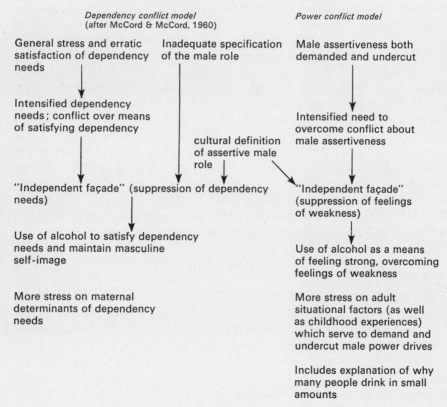

presentation of the dependency hypothesis which, as shown, also includes an element of "inadequate specification of the male role." Thus they, and other such theorists, would accept much of the presentation of our theory laid out on the righthand side of Table 13.6, but would argue that male assertiveness becomes so important largely because the male is ashamed of unconscious dependency on his mother. As explained above, we have been led to doubt the importance of this factor, both because we can find so little direct evidence for it and because for us many of the conflicts in the male role found in adult situations are more important determinants of heavy drinking than is the way a boy was treated as a child by his mother.

Our theory is necessarily somewhat unspecific as to exactly how a person develops such an exaggerated concern with personalized power. Much of the evidence points to the importance of some kind of power *conflict*—in which a man is both expected to be strong and is yet undercut, so that his concern can be seen as *compensatory* or *defensive*. Yet not all of the evidence points in this direction. As Davis reports in Chapter 9, it is men who feel *more* powerful, not less powerful (e.g., undercut) who drink more. So it is possible that any event which heightens a man's concern with his personalized power—be it a success or a failure—also heightens his tendency to drink and thereby to reinforce his feeling of power under conditions of low responsibility for his actions. Both Davis (1964) and MacAndrew and Edgerton (1969) suggest that drinking may signify a kind of "time out" in which a man cannot be held accountable for his acts, because alcohol is a known "incompetence producer." According to our theory he can feel powerful and socially irresponsible at the same time after drinking. Or to use the terminology of Chapter 8, heavy drinking encourages his fantasies of personalized, narcissistic power over fantasies of socialized power. A further advantage of our theory, we believe, is that it incorporates more easily the results we have obtained as to why normal people drink alcohol in small amounts—namely to increase socialized power thoughts. Drinking liquor is a way of feeling stronger; it is resorted to addictively by men who have exaggerated needs for personalized power.

SOURCES OF THE NEED
FOR PERSONALIZED POWER

The type of power need that leads to heavy drinking can be exaggerated in several ways:

1. Strong Demands for Male Assertiveness. As we have pointed out above, at certain times in life and in certain societies and in certain types of occupations, and with certain (mesomorphic) types of bodies, males are expected to be particularly strong, brave and assertive. This expectation increases the likelihood that some men in those situations will end up with exaggerated needs for personalized power that can be enhanced by drinking liquor. On the other hand, there are cultures and occupations in which a man is simply not expected to be personally strong and assertive or in which social power is required. Some men, for instance, make a feminine identification in American culture. They do not tend to be heavy drinkers (cf. for example, Harrington, 1970, p. 66ff.), as we would predict. They have no strong personalized power concern because they do not accept in the first place a strong, assertive male ego ideal. It remains to be seen whether the image of male assertiveness can be entirely rejected with psychological impunity, but certainly it can be rejected enough to reduce personalized power concern to a very low level, or to sublimate it in a social direction as in the ministry, social work, etc.

2. *Low Support for the Male Role.* If the occupation or the society strongly demands male personal assertiveness, then lack of support for the male role will accentuate the personalized power concern. On the other hand, it is quite possible to have a high-demand, high-support culture, such as Arab culture, in which traditionally bravery and male assertiveness are strongly demanded, but at the same time male solidarity and female support are strong enough to remove all possibilities of the average Arab having doubts about his superiority and manliness. Thus, drinking rates in Arab countries have remained low, and Islam actually prohibits drinking alcohol. Instances of cultures with high demand and low male support already have been given above—e.g., the Irish or the north Europeans.

3. *Lack of Socialized Power Outlets.* In our view power concerns may be channelled along social lines; and when they are, drinking decreases in amount, though possibly not in frequency. Even when a man's life situation produces power demands of the sort described, it is possible that he may find alternative socialized ways of feeling strong, if they are available. But they may not be available, as in the case of American Indians deprived of traditional methods of demonstrating their prowess in hunting, and reduced to a state of weakness on a reservation (see Chapter 12), or of American blacks prevented from showing normal male vocational success by racial discrimination. In such cases the lack of outlets for socialized power channels the power drive in the personal direction, encouraging such expressions of it as heavy drinking and gambling.

Power needs may arise out of cultural, structural or developmental sources. Maccoby has described in Chapter 11 one of the clearest instances of a culturally defined image of the male role which tends to produce a personalized power concern and drinking in Mexico. The

Mexican male is expected above all else to be *macho*—hypermasculine, aggressive, sexually potent, dominant over women. Yet in point of fact he finds it very difficult to live up to this ideal. To some extent the lower-class Mexican unrealistically dissipates the economic resources which would make it possible for him to be socially assertive and dominant. His money, as the Mexicans say, goes "up in smoke" (in the rockets and firecrackers he frequently sets off) or "down in drink." Both may make him feel personally strong, but weaken him for the next round. Furthermore, the lower-class Mexican family has tended to be matrifocal. The men come and go, but the mothers remain the strong, stable element holding the family together (see Lewis, 1961). Thus, the idealized patriarchal family structure is in fact undercut by the power of wives and mothers. (See Chapter 11.) Furthermore there are no institutions of male solidarity other than the drinking groups which collect in the *cantinas*. Since unfortunately this type of male solidarity requires drinking, it cannot very well cut down on the necessity for drinking, as other male solidarity rituals do.

High drinking rates among lower-class black Americans have a similar explanation. Again, there is the ideal of the strong aggressive, sexually potent male, and the fact of a matriarchal society in which the women have economic and social power, undercutting male importance at every turn. It is small wonder that many lower-class black males turn to drink as a means of asserting their manliness. Recent movements stressing more socialized forms of "black power" ought to cut down on drinking, according to our theory.

The personalized power need may also be conditioned by positions in the social structure. The three most important are sex, occupation and age. Being a male renders one more likely to be faced with a demand to show personal power. Being in certain occupations which demand bravery and daring in the face of danger has the same effect, and aging for a man often puts him in a situation where he feels steadily less able to cope with the high demands for male assertiveness and responsibility that go with middle age.

DEVELOPMENTAL SOURCES
OF A PERSONALIZED POWER CONCERN

These deserve a somewhat more expanded treatment, because it is in this area that the present theory differs chiefly from the dependency conflict theory. Clearly family influences must be important; the longitudinal studies cited above show that alcoholics differed consistently from non-alcoholics even when they were boys. One might argue that these differences are due to heredity, except for the fact that the mothers of pre-alcoholics also behave significantly differently. Clinical psychologists like Tähkä and Maccoby have particularly stressed that the mothers of future alcoholics are somehow different. They have dominated and infantilized their sons. We have protested that this evidence is suspect because it comes from biased observers, because it is not specific enough to differentiate, say, between Irish maternal dominance and Jewish maternal dominance, and because in any case it need not be interpreted as leading to heightened dependency conflict in the son. But can it be ignored altogether?

One argument for not ignoring it altogether lies in the bits and pieces of evidence for oral involvement that have been noted in the above factual review and put aside for later comment. Let us pull these facts together and see what they add up to: (1) The *Oral Body Parts* tag was significantly more frequent in the folk tales from heavy drinking societies (see Chapter 4). (2) Rorschach studies have regularly reported a higher frequency of oral responses among alcoholics than non-alcoholics (see Nezei & Erdly, 1966); Tähkä (1966, p. 88) found significantly more food responses in the Rorschachs of his alcoholics than his controls, and also significantly more passive food receivers (pigs, fetuses, etc.). (3) MacAndrew (1965) found that alcoholic out-patients agreed more often than other psychiatric out-patients with the items, "I like to cook," and "The one to whom I was most attached and whom I most admired as a child was a woman." (4) Wolowitz (1964) has developed a food preference questionnaire in which the subject is forced to choose between a sweeter, softer or more liquid food and a sour, harder, or more solid one. His assumption is that preferences for sweeter, softer and more liquid foods indicates greater oral passive gratification, and he found alcoholics showed a significantly higher preference for such foods. Alcoholics generally, more often than the controls, said they preferred such foods as apple-sauce to a raw whole apple. (5) Smoking, another "oral" indicator, is significantly related to drinking in many studies, although the evidence in Chapter 8 suggests that it belongs in the beer-drinking, sociability factor rather than in the liquor-drinking, power cluster.

None of these signs of greater orality has been shown to characterize young men *before* they become alcoholic. The one test of the hypothesis that alcoholics have a greater oral involvement made before the subjects became alcoholic failed to show a significant difference (Table 13.1). So it would be possible to argue that these signs of oral involvement simply reflect the fact that the men are alcoholics, and as alcoholics they have chosen the gastrointestinal system as the place in which to work out their conflicts. After all, they suffer much more oral, gastrointestinal stimulation than people who do not swallow such large quantities of alcohol. Many of them abuse their gastrointestinal system practically every day of their lives. They experience hangover symptoms, vomiting, stomach aches and cramps, and diarrhea, so that sensations from their "oral body parts" must absorb a lot of their waking thoughts every day. To use an analogy, if a man chose to work out some psychodynamic conflict by pounding his thumb with a hammer daily, it would scarcely be surprising if such a man included more "thumb imagery" in his Rorschach. Similarly an alcoholic may think more often about oral or gastrointestinal sensations because his drinking in fact focusses his attention on them. Or he may prefer soft foods because they seem easier on an upset digestive system.

Thus although the more frequent oral references do not point unequivocally to some special kind of dependency relation to the mother among alcoholics, the clinical evidence is still hard to explain away entirely. And what about the fact that alcoholics say more often than other patients that they were particularly attached to a woman when they were children? There is another theory which would explain a special female involvement among alcoholics in a way which is consistent with the power concern theory. It is Whiting's cross-sex identity theory (Whiting *et al.*, 1960).

He argues that in certain families (typically where the boy sleeps exclusively with his mother, and the father is outside the household) the boy forms a primary feminine identification because his mother is perceived by him to be the adult who supplies all important resources. Thus the boy envies her and wants to be like her and has no alternative adult male to emulate at this period of his life. In many such societies, as the boy grows older, initiation ceremonies serve to mark the end of his "feminine identification." Circumcision at puberty, for example, symbolizes the breaking of his ties to women, and signifies that he has become a "real" male. From then on his male status is more or less ascribed (though he may have to carry out some feat as part of the initiation to validate fully his male status) and he does not have to keep proving his masculinity.

But in other societies the transition to maleness may be less marked and definitive. Then a phenomenon called "protest masculinity" may develop, which is much like the *macho* complex among Mexican men. The boy retains a primary unconscious feminine identity, but keeps trying to prove that he is not feminine by a kind of defensive hypermasculinity. Whiting has proposed measures of the two levels of sex identity. At the level of primary sex identity, he has recommended the use of the Franck test which presents to the subject a number of half-finished designs which he is to complete in any way he likes. Franck and Rosen (1949) found that there were large sex differences in the way these designs tended to be completed and were able to develop a coding system which clearly differentiated between male and female completions. Thus, a boy with primary cross-sex identity should show a higher proportion of female to male completions on the Franck test than a boy with normal primary masculine identity. As a test of secondary sex identity, Whiting recommends the use of any of the various masculinity-femininity interest scales that have been developed by personality testers. For example, Strong on his Vocational Interest Blank noted that boys liked certain hobbies, occupations and types of reading more than girls; hence he reasoned that a boy who has more of the interests that boys in general have should be considered to be more masculine. These interests, attitudes and choices are obviously at a much more conscious level than the figure completions to the Franck test designs. The boys know when they choose these items that driving cars fast, like mechanics magazines, shooting and hunting are considered masculine. According to our theory, boys who have a primary feminine identification along with a secondary masculine identification ought to be heavier drinkers, because they should have precisely the concern about their masculine image which we have argued is a cause of alcoholism.

There is one investigation which reports that this is the case. Harrington (1970) studied a group of adolescent boys labeled deviant by their parents or the community in appearing for help at various mental health agencies in upstate New York. He was primarily interested in showing that those boys who showed "protest masculinity" (who were defiant, aggressive trouble-makers) had higher femininity scores on the Franck test, combined with much higher masculinity scores on the Strong Vocational Interest Blank. This turned out to be the case. Furthermore, in his sample there were ten adolescent boys who already had heavy drinking problems. (Harrington, 1970, p. 65.) They too, as our theory would predict, showed primary feminine identity (above average feminine score on the Franck test) and secondary masculine identity (above average masculine score on the Strong test). The sample is not large and cannot be considered a definitive test of the theory. Nevertheless it is well known that drinking is part of the *macho* or protest masculinity syndrome, and if it can be shown more generally that protest masculinity is a result of this type of cross-sex identity, then a more solid basis will have been laid for arguing that this is one of the major sources of personalized concern in males that leads to alcoholism. The further advantage of this hypothesis is that it explains the strong attachment to female adults found clinically among alcoholics and mentioned specifically by them on the MMPI. But according to our theory the connection with a strong female is interpreted not in terms of a mother creating dependency in her son, but in terms of her providing an occasion for cross-sex identity which may lead to a defensive concern with personalized power in a culture which stresses masculine prowess.

While the cross-sex identity hypothesis seems reasonable, it will be remembered that we made an attempt reported in Chapter 3 to check its validity cross-culturally using various folk tale themes. We reasoned that if cross-sex identity was promoted by a culture, then males would be more often described in ways that are in most cultures considered to be more characteristic of females. In this way we derived a Man-Feminine tag which supposedly reflected the degree of cross-sex identity in a culture. This tag, however, did not correlate with amount of drinking in a culture, suggesting that cross-sex identity is not cross-culturally associated with heavy drinking. The measure may however have been at fault. At the individual level, as we have already noted, men who accept a feminine style do not drink heavily, and that may be what the man-feminine tag was measuring as a cultural characteristic. It is the men who have primary feminine identification, but who strongly reject it consciously, who drink heavily; and we did not find a way to measure these two levels of sex identity in the folk tales. So at a minimum, cross-sex identity as a reason for doubt about masculinity remains an interesting possible source of the personalized power concern that leads to heavy drinking.

SOLUTIONS TO POWER NEEDS

If the alcoholic's central goal is to reinforce his sense of personalized power, then as we showed in Chapter 8, it is evident that drinking is only one of several methods that may be employed to reach such a goal. Gambling and accumulating prestige supplies are others. It is worth outlining some of these other strategies, partly to give a clearer picture of the "alcoholic personality," and partly to point the way to therapeutic interventions which might strengthen solutions to power problems which are less self-destructive than heavy drinking.

1. Reduce the Need for Personalized Power. As a first possibility it should be mentioned that in theory at least the need for personalized power can be reduced if a man can simply give up some of his desires to be powerful or strong. He might be converted to a more "feminine" way of life, or at least to accepting a less aggressively masculine ideal for himself. A Breton fisherman might give up going to sea and become an innkeeper, thus reducing the personalized power demands that deep-sea fishing makes on him. To some extent such "natural therapy" occurs in much older men who presumably give up heavy drinking in part because they gradually come to accept the fact that they are weaker and cannot be expected to live up to high standards of masculine assertiveness. Therapeutic programs to lower the power drive have not to our knowledge been attempted, though in theory they might prove effective in reducing one of the root causes of alcoholism.

2. Borrow Strength. Given that the power need remains high, it may be satisfied by wholehearted acceptance of a power outside oneself, like God, which guides, directs, and in a sense is responsible for one's every act. The person feels strong because at every moment he has God on his side. As already noted, religion or Alcoholics Anonymous can be sources of strength, and inspiration which can take the place of alcohol. Some of the antipathy between many religions and drinking may derive in part from the folk psychological recognition that they are competing sources of inspiration. The man who uses alcohol to get a feeling of strength presumably does not need God so much. When Marx claimed that "religion is the opiate of the people" he may have reversed the true state of affairs. It may be more accurate to say that "an opiate (alcohol) is the religion of the people." Thus if the Russian Communists, following Marx's dictum, tried to abolish God, they may only have increased alcoholism by eliminating one of the alternative outside sources of strength that men turn to when they have power problems. Alcohol may truly become the "religion" of the people, at least in the limited sense of providing men with the strength they need in time of trouble.

Strength may also be borrowed from identifying with or following any strong charismatic leader. Attendance at mass meetings may make a man feel more powerful because a leader makes him feel strong and important. Recall how Winter showed in Chapter 5 that young men watching a film of Kennedy's Inaugural Address had their power drives enhanced. Alcoholics like revival meetings, even though they may not be "cured" by them; they feel uplifted or stronger under such circumstances. Men may glory in their military past or currently participate in parades in order to revive the feeling of borrowed strength that comes from identifying with powerful groups.

One of the most curious outside sources of strength that alcoholics sometimes seek is a strong wife. As we have already noted, many clinicians report that alcoholics tend to marry strong wives, although Lemert (1962) has raised some questions as to how common this is, statistically. Obviously, it is an extremely maladaptive solution to the alcoholic's problem. Although he may blindly reach out to such a woman in the hope that she will provide him with the strength and guidance that he needs to be strong and effective, she can of course only serve to make his problem worse if we are correct in diagnosing his basic problem as a need to show his personal strength as a male. Drinking and marrying strong women are as symptoms psychodynamically similar.

They are both aimed at a feeling of temporary strength, but they both undermine whatever real sources of strength the man has and make him less able to be powerful in any socially effective way.

It is worth stopping for a moment to note that we have now outlined three distinct mechanisms which may be responsible for the close ties sometimes observed between an alcoholic and a strong woman. First, a close tie between a boy and a strong mother, in the absence of a father, may lead to cross-sex identity which produces protest masculinity and drinking. Second, a man who wants to assert his masculinity may maladaptively marry a strong wife in order to prove "that he is a man." And third, an alcoholic may marry a strong wife in the misbegotten belief that she may provide him the strength and inspiration he needs to be powerful. One might legitimately ask at this point if we have not in these ways simply reintroduced the widely accepted notion that alcoholics both want to be dependent on women and independent of them. Particularly in the third case, is it not true that the man has a dependency conflict? He wants to be dependent on a strong wife, yet at the same time he doesn't want to be.

It is necessary to be as precise as possible in defining what is meant by dependence. A person can be dependent on another for a variety of reasons—to get good and loving care, to get expert advice, or to borrow strength and guidance to meet life's crises. According to the classic theory of dependency conflict in alcoholics, what the alcoholic seeks (and is ambivalent about) is maternal care. Prototypically he wants to feel cozy and warm like an infant at the breast. His deepest, most repressed motives are regressive. He seeks the total care of infantile satisfaction—presumably because, as the McCords (1960) and Bacon, Barry and Child (1965) argue, he has at one time had these satisfactions and then been denied them. As we have repeatedly noted, we simply have found no clear evidence for such strivings in alcoholics or pre-alcoholics. Instead what they appear to be after is strength. The difficulty lies not in their security feelings but in their self-image. They may ally themselves with strong women to borrow strength, but not to seek an infantile regressive satisfaction. While these two types of dependency are phenotypically similar, they are genotypically different. Thus it is easy to see how they could be confused. Observers have noted close connections between pre-alcoholics and strong women—both as wives and mothers. In terms of classic psychoanalytic theory, such close relationships mean typically one thing—namely, the desire on the male's part for infantile oral gratification. Thus, these close relationships have tended to be universally interpreted in this way, particularly in view of the fact that alcohol is something taken through the mouth and therefore qualifies by definition as an "oral" sign. What we hope our data have introduced into these interpretations is a greater precision in defining the reason for the close relationships sometimes observed.

3. Act Out Aggressively. In Chapter 8, we demonstrated how a personalized power drive has several primary effects in action, among which drinking assumes a very special place, because it has important and mostly anti-social secondary effects, like car accidents, fights, aggressive acts, etc. Among college students (Chapter 5) drinking belongs to the "stud" cluster which also includes exploitative sexual activities. All of these behaviors are methods of acting out a personalized power drive exacerbated often by drinking. The aggressive hold-up man or murderer is demonstrating his personal power. So is the "Don Juan" who repeatedly conquers or rapes women. Most of these strategies of handling power problems are ineffective in two senses. They often leave the person in trouble with the law, which makes him feel less powerful than ever; and even if they do not, they seldom satisfy him for long because he knows that society does not recognize him as "really" strong. So over and over again he must reassure himself that he *is* strong by aggressively "acting out" in various ways.

4. Satisfy the Power Drive Vicariously. As noted in Chapters 5 and 8, a man with a high need for power tends to surround himself with *prestige supplies.* He drives the most powerful car he can afford. He collects credit cards. He tends to buy expensive clothes or jewelry or anything that in his social class indicates how big and important he is.

He can also seek other types of symbolic satisfaction. He can go to the "fights" or watch boxing, wrestling and football on television. He can read sports or "girlie" magazines. In all of these ways he can feel more powerful vicariously.

One of the less obvious strategies for feeling powerful is to redirect the drive toward one's self, deriving satisfaction from self-control or asceticism. If a man can exercise control over himself as in fasting, dieting, complete abstention from drinking, or muscle building, he is demonstrating in a direct way how powerful he is. He is not yielding to impulses the way more ordinary mortals do. No one has made a particular point of the fact that alcoholics very often "swear off" drinking. Whenever this occurs, it is normally attributed to the alcoholic's feeling of guilt or disgust at his own behavior. But there is another likely reason for it, which derives from his central problem. Self-denial—the refusal to have even one little drink—is another strategy for showing one's strength. After all, why isn't it just as reasonable if a man feels guilty about his drinking behavior for him to reduce it *gradually* to a more normally acceptable level? Our theory explains why such an approach to improving one's condition is in fact less likely to be adopted by alcoholics than "swearing off" drinking completely. Extreme ascetic self-discipline can also cure alcoholism for the same reason. For instance, the Black Muslim movement in the United States has succeeded in converting many heavy drinkers into total abstainers who are ascetic in other areas of life as well. The appeal of such total self-discipline and control among the Black Muslims has worked because it is an *alternative* method of giving a man a sense of power, the desire for which caused drinking in the first place.

5. *Socialize the Power Drive.* The strategies just listed are more effective than the acting out strategies, in an individual as well as in a social sense. That is, they do often succeed in bolstering a person's sense of strength and importance, whereas the acting-out strategies almost by definition undermine that sense of strength at the same time they are enhancing it. More effective than either are methods of socializing the power drive, or increasing the person's ability to control and regulate behavior in order to effect cooperation with others. As the data summarized in Chapters 6–8 show, high s Power people do not drink as much as high p Power people; their power drive has been channelled along socialized rather than personalized lines.

To encourage this end, a man may *join an organization*—a church, a social movement or a political party—in which he may work with others and for others to gain power in the real world. Even though he may be only a low-level participant in organizational work, he may get a sense of social power from being part of an institution having a major social impact, or he may work his way up in the organization to positions of power and influence and gain in this way an even greater realistic sense of his social influence.

Or he may *help others*, exercising the most elementary form of socialized power. If A can give something to B—either time, attention or material resources—he is by definition more powerful than B. Though it is not often noted, the helping relationship is one of the most regular ways in which a person can validate his own sense of worth and social importance. Alcoholics Anonymous again makes use of this simple psychological fact, by insisting that one of the ways alcoholism can be cured is for the ex-alcoholic to be continuously helping other people with alcohol problems. This strategy differs from more supportive ones like driving an expensive car because in fact the person giving the help is realistically more powerful, important and worthwhile in the social sense.

6. *Succeed at One's Work.* In American society, as in north European society generally, a man's worth is often judged more by what he can do than by the mere fact of his being a male. Thus if a man can get to be good at something, he is more likely to be held in high esteem by his fellows and himself (to have socialized power). He may get to be good at sports—at golf, ping pong, bowling or fishing. Or as he grows older,

he may turn to other less physical games or skills at which he can show his prowess; he may work hard at being a skillful card player, bowler, or gardener. But of course in his occupation lies the chief source of his self-esteem, at least when he is of working age. Many men "take to drink" as a source of regaining a sense of power when they cannot achieve their occupational goals. A classic case is provided by the black American who has been prevented by racial discrimination from even the normal chances of advancement open to whites in his occupational position. He has been powerless to alter this situation as an individual in the past. How can he "be a man" in the American sense of occupational achievement, if he can't even find a decent job? So he turns to alternative ways of being a man, like drinking and crime in lower social-class areas. Clearly one significant answer to such a power problem is to make it possible for such men to succeed by training them, by giving them opportunities to succeed vocationally and by removing racial discrimination which undercuts their sense of self-worth.

This analysis of alcoholic and other solutions to power problems is not just a theoretical exercise. It has been undertaken to get a more complete picture of the ways of satisfying a man's power needs other than by heavy drinking. If our diagnosis of the alcoholic's problem is correct, it should lead to the design of more effective types of therapy. And in fact the pilot therapeutic program described in Chapter 14 was based on the analysis of the alcoholic's problem just completed. It began with the hypothesis that the typical alcoholic has a power problem: he wants especially to be strong, masculine and assertive, and he has adopted drinking as a way of feeling personally powerful. We thought he might be persuaded to use the drinking solution to his problem less often if he could learn to gain power satisfaction in other symbolic or socialized ways.

For one way to test the validity of a theory is to see whether acting in terms of it improves therapeutic success. Our theory of the etiology of alcoholism has certain clear implications as to what type of therapeutic program would be most likely to succeed, and we were determined to test these implications in part to see how valid our theory was. Similarly it is our belief that the dependency conflict theory of the origins of alcoholism also has specific therapeutic implications which should be tried out. One additional way to test the relative validity of the two theories is to see whether a therapeutic program built on one or on the other is more successful. If what an alcoholic really wants is tender loving care, and a feeling of infinite warmth and gratification, it should be possible to find ways of giving him this kind of support without undermining his sense of independence. Our expectation would be that a therapeutic program based on this assumption will be less successful than one based on the assumption that the alcoholic needs other ways of solving his power problem. But we are not so convinced we are right that we think an actual comparison of the efficacy of the two types of therapeutic programs is unnecessary. It should be carried out by "believers" in the alternative theories to equalize experimenter bias. For what the field of alcoholism needs is more careful experimental research and analysis, and less undisciplined, often prejudiced thinking. If this chapter has accomplished nothing else, it should at least have laid out all the known facts about heavy drinking which, together with the facts presented in other chapters, will have to be taken into account in any future explanations of alcoholism.

A Pilot Attempt To Help Alcoholics by Socializing Their Power Needs

by William N. Davis

Far too often, promising empirical results on alcohol are reported in scientific journals only to languish there, apparently unnoticed by professionals who are working clinically with problem drinkers. Consequently, such results remain nothing more than promising. On the other hand, when professionals, who see alcoholic patients, publish their clinical insights, their potentially valuable ideas frequently are ignored by experimental investigators. There is a need for closer cooperation between experimentalists and clinical practitioners in the field of alcoholism and problem drinking. Without it, there is the danger that treatment approaches to alcoholics will become rigid and doctrinaire, while research on alcohol and alcoholics will become academic, disregarding the realities the clinician must deal with daily.

It was with the importance of integrating research with clinical practice in mind that the project to be described was undertaken. We decided to attempt a treatment program based upon the empirical findings and the theoretical conclusions reported in this book. Our task seemed quite straightforward: what was necessary was a treatment program founded on the idea that a heavy drinker is an impulsive person whose need to think of himself as powerful is strong and unfulfilled, and whose drinking represents a way to gratify temporarily his quest for personal power. Our expectation was that such a program, properly designed and implemented, would produce some beneficial changes.

This chapter contains, first, a full description of the treatment program and an account of the way in which it was carried out. There follows a small amount of clinical data, based upon four-month follow-ups of the first six problem drinkers who participated in the program. The chapter concludes with a retrospective appraisal of what the program did and did not accomplish.[1]

THE PROGRAM

Stated in the abstract there were a number of treatment "inputs" which underlay our therapeutic attempts. Basically didactic and descriptive in orientation, we endeavored (1) to acquaint participants with the idea of psychologically examining themselves and others; (2) to make them aware that a desire to feel powerful can be an important part of a person's life, with a number of different avenues to satisfaction; (3) to demonstrate that drinking increases one's power thoughts and that therefore this kind of behavior is one way to satisfy a desire to feel powerful; (4) to explain that drinking, among other things, is typically an ineffective, inappropriate way to gratify power needs; (5) to suggest other more appropriate and more effective methods of gratifying a desire to feel powerful; and (6) to encourage support, and if necessary assist participants in planning how to achieve more effective means for gratifying their desires to feel powerful.

The treatment inputs were based in part upon some implicit assumptions, in part upon the results of previous research, and in part upon the structure of the treatment program. We assumed that since other, more depth-oriented, therapies generally have not been outstandingly successful with problem drinkers (Mindlin, 1959), it was not unreasonable to suppose that a more directive orientation might produce better results. Further, we assumed that it was important to give every participant a relatively specific frame of reference from which to view, discuss, and understand his problem drinking.

Research reported by McClelland and Winter (1969) demonstrates that teaching people how to examine their fantasies, and how to pro-

---

[1]Because the treatment program was designed and carried out *before* the final data analyses reported in Chapters 6–8 were completed, it is based on a less complete understanding of the power theory of drinking than we now have.

duce fantasies of an achievement-oriented nature, can in fact make people behave in a more achievement-oriented way. While our orientation was not exactly the same, we felt that if we could show problem drinkers how drinking increases unrealistic fantasies of power, then perhaps they could use this information to change their lives—that is, to find more effective and appropriate ways to satisfy their power needs.

The structure of the treatment program influenced our inputs because it was necessary to limit the total time spent with any one participant to one three-day weekend. In such a short span of time it would have been difficult to implement anything more than a relatively didactic program even if we had wanted to do something else. Financial considerations were responsible for the short time spent with participants. But it was hoped that if our approach had anything to offer, then there should be some demonstrable effect even after a weekend.

All of the weekend sessions were held in an outlying suburb of Boston, Massachusetts, where we used the facilities of a non-denominational religious retreat for the treatment program. These facilities included a cottage, where the participants slept and took part in the various treatment activities, and a nearby lodge, where the participants ate their meals.

The weekend sessions were always group sessions, typically composed of four to six problem drinkers, four or five non-problem drinkers and at least two trainers. Non-problem drinkers were asked to participate for two reasons. First, we felt that unless moderate drinkers were included, the problem drinkers might quickly coalesce into a group with a negativistic, self-defeating attitude toward the treatment program and themselves. Second, we wanted to demonstrate as best we could what kinds of differences—in drinking habits and in life styles— there were between problem and non-problem drinkers. The most forceful way to do this seemed to be to include non-problem drinkers in the group. The trainers, who were responsible for leading all the group activities, all belonged to a private, largely black organization known as Massachusetts Achievement Trainers (M.A.T.), hired to implement the treatment program. These men had been trained for and had had extensive experience in giving achievement motivation development courses, but none had had formal psychological training.

All of the participants, both problem and non-problem drinkers, were recruited by M.A.T. The program was introduced by asking potential participants if they would like to learn how to be more effective or successful men. This was true for non-problem and problem drinkers alike. No mention was to be made of the relationship between problem drinking and the treatment program, partly in order to encourage moderate drinkers to participate, and partly to prevent problem drinkers from thinking that the program represented "just one more attempt" to cut off their liquor supply. In practice, however, many problem drinkers immediately associated the recruitment procedure with their own major problem, and so in some cases the set was created that the program specifically was aimed at stopping their drinking.

Participants were recruited from a number of different sources. Most of the non-problem drinkers were acquaintances of the trainers. The problem drinkers were recruited from either local clinics or treatment centers for alcoholics, or from bars and taverns known locally for their high percentage of alcoholics. No rigorous criteria were used to determine whether one was a problem drinker or a non-problem drinker. It was felt that because this was a preliminary or pilot project, more than anything else it was more important to recruit willing participants than to wait patiently to find people who matched perfectly precise, predetermined criteria. Thus, whether participants came from treatment centers or were recruited in "seedy" bars, they were arbitrarily pronounced problem drinkers. Those who participated by virtue of the fact that they were acquaintances of the trainers were assumed to be non-problem drinkers unless they specifically indicated that they had a drinking problem.

Even with this less than systematic selection, it was difficult to recruit participants. Problem drinkers who were involved with some kind of clinic were especially hard to recruit, because medical authorities were dubious about the wisdom of the proposed treatment program and its auspices. The chief difficulty lay in the fact that part of the treatment program included serving alcohol to the participants to show them the effects on their thought processes. Knowing this, many clinics in the area were reluctant to have their patients participate. Another difficulty grew out of the fact that since most of the trainers were black, they found it relatively easy to recruit black participants, but more difficult to find white participants, and especially white non-problem drinkers.

At the beginning of every weekend, which usually was at dinnertime Friday, one of the trainers briefly introduced the program and described in general terms what would happen during the next three days. The trainer emphasized at this time that the program would be intensive, that the participants would be together constantly during the entire weekend, and that with the exception of time spent eating and sleeping, everyone would always be engaged in some kind of group activity.

Typically, the introduction was followed by a "Who Am I?" session, during which participants were asked to say something about their lives and their current problems, and to respond to any questions asked by other members of the group. The "Who Am I?" was intended to have a dual purpose. First, since most of the participants did not know each other beforehand, the "Who Am I?" was a good way for people to learn something about those with whom they would be spending the weekend. Second and more important, "Who Am I?" was the initial representation of the first therapeutic input mentioned above. It was hoped that through group discussion and individual histories, participants would be stimulated to begin to think about themselves and others in a psychological way. Although "Who Am I?" was the first and only activity directed specifically at this input, everything that followed was also designed to stimulate psychological awareness. Thus, in one sense, all the treatment activities were related to the first treatment input.

The course of the treatment program was not always the same after this point. Consequently, rather than outline the course of a "typical" weekend, or try to describe the changes in format that took place from weekend to weekend, we will concentrate in the discussion to follow on the treatment inputs—the activities connected with them, and where in general they were introduced during a weekend.

The second treatment input was intended to make participants aware of the psychological importance of feeling powerful or powerless, as well as describing how different people cope with their desire to feel powerful. The specific activities centered around this input included role plays, films, and trainer-led group discussions.

The role plays, of which there were two or three, were always acted out by members of the group. The general purpose of these was to demonstrate that sometimes people feel very helpless and very powerless, and that when feeling like this, different people react in different ways. For example, one role play depicted a scene between a personnel manager and an employee. The employee, who had worked effectively for the company for 20 years, had come to the personnel manager to convince him that he was the right man for a new, higher paying job that was opening up. The personnel manager, however, was under strict orders to refuse this job to the employee because of a new company directive requiring for the new job a certain amount of education which the employee did not have. The new job actually did not require any more training and in fact before the directive was issued the employee would have been the best man for the new job. With this information members of the group were asked to act out the parts of personnel manager and employee. The role play was usually performed several times. Observing members of the group were asked to watch the actors closely and try to emphasize with what the employee in particular was feeling. After five minutes or so of acting out the parts, the role play was stopped and a general discussion ensued. The trainers emphasized the frustration and powerlessness that the employee almost always felt.

Then the discussion became general, and observing members were asked if they ever felt so helpless, and how they reacted in such situations. At the conclusion of the discussion the general point was usually made that most people experience moments of powerlessness; that some people have feelings like this a lot of the time; that there are differences in how people deal with the situation, some strategies being more effective than others. Often some time was spent on the strategies people use. It was suggested, for example, that in the case of the employee role play, it would have been more effective to talk to the personnel manager's supervisor than to punch the manager in the nose (which many of the group said they would have done).

Several films were presented during the course of the weekend, one of them directed specifically at the second treatment input. It described a man who had a poorly paying job in a penny arcade. This man was continually yelled at by his supervisor, and finally was rejected by his girl friend because he was not advancing in his job. In response to his realistic life situation, clearly portrayed as one of powerlessness, this man day-dreamed of having supernatural powers—with beautiful women at his beck and call and, eventually, absolute control over people who looked like his supervisor at the penny arcade. The discussion following this film stressed the powerlessness that this man must have felt, and how he had coped with it. Again the discussion was purposely generalized, and participants were asked to relate similar experiences and feelings. Again, the ineffectiveness of the strategy was stressed, and alternative methods of dealing with the situation were exemplified and discussed.

A trainer-led group discussion of power and psychological research relating to it usually was introduced towards the end of the weekend, so that feelings engendered by the role play and the films could be related to it. The trainer's remarks concentrated on the importance of power as a psychological need, and on research (e.g. Chapter 8) which delineated different ways in which people try to gain a sense of power.

The third treatment input was designed to demonstrate that drinking increases a sense of subjective power, and that therefore drinking is one way to satisfy a desire to feel powerful. There was a series of activities centered around this input. On Friday night, either during or just after "Who Am I?" all the group members were served at least two and sometimes as many as five or six drinks, generally of their own choice. Amount of consumption was determined mostly by individual preference, with an upper limit set by the trainers. This particular part of the procedure, as we have said, was objected to by many of the clinics contacted for potential participants. It was the primary reason why M.A.T. was forced to recruit problem drinkers from bars or taverns. This part of the treatment was considered extremely important, however, because it provided an opportunity for participants to learn something first hand about the effects of alcohol on them.

Near the end of the drinking session the trainers distributed a short version of the TAT, containing four pictures especially selected for their relevance to power imagery; this was a written TAT with standard instructions. The stories written at this time were later used to illustrate the psychological effects of alcohol.

At some time on Saturday morning another TAT was administered. The pictures used here were different from those in the first set, but they also were chosen for their relevance to power imagery. This TAT was considered a "dry" TAT in contrast to the one administered Friday night under "wet" conditions. The thought was that the thematic differences in the stories written under the two conditions would serve to demonstrate that alcohol increases fantasies of power, as demonstrated in Chapter 6.

Immediately after the dry TAT had been completed, the trainers introduced a power scoring system that was to be used to score the TAT stories for power imagery—the earlier system described in Appendix I. When the explanation was completed, participants broke up into small groups to score their own stories with the aid of a trainer. A general discussion typically followed the scoring. At this time trainers demonstrated by illustration how drinking seems to increase feelings and thoughts of power, and pointed out also that since drinking has this effect, it is one way for people to satisfy their desire to feel powerful.

The fourth treatment input was based on the fact that heavy drinking is an inappropriate, ineffective way to gain a feeling of power. And the fifth involved suggesting other more effective ways of gratifying a desire to feel powerful. These inputs were frequently introduced alongside one another towards the end of a weekend by means of a trainer-led discussion. It was pointed out that while alcohol may temporarily increase a sense of power, it cannot serve as a permanent solution because heavy drinking actually decreases the ability to cope with real problems. In order to avoid the realization of this unpleasant fact it is necessary to drink more and more heavily and more and more frequently—all the while decreasing realistic power. Thus begins a vicious cycle which ends with the drinker in a continual stupor bereft completely of any realistic basis for feeling powerful. The ineffectiveness of drinking as a means of achieving a sense of power was associated during this discussion with anti-social methods of gaining power, such as criminal activity, and with the ineffective methods the group had observed in the role plays and in the films.

The discussion then shifted to more realistic and effective means. First, supportive and vicarious sources for a feeling of power were mentioned, including such things as driving a fancy car and wearing flashy clothes, or attending lots of sports events and mass meetings. Activities like these can, in an indirect way, help one to feel bigger and more powerful, and they do not in themselves represent anti-social behavior, or behavior that necessarily interferes with more direct ways of gaining a sense of power.

Supportive and vicarious ways of gaining power shade over into direct, effective, and realistic methods of attaining a sense of power. It was explained to the participants that activities like joining an organization and becoming active in it, or trying to help others were excellent ways to gain realistically a sense of power. Most of the emphasis here, however, was placed on the importance and value of work as a source of power. Members of the group discussed the idea that there is no activity more important to a man's sense of power, and therefore to his self-respect, than consistently working and consistently earning money.

The sixth treatment input usually followed the group discussion of ineffective and effective means of gaining power. Participants were first encouraged to think of ways in which they could increase their own sense of power, and then were required to make some sort of concrete plan to this end. To help with this stage of the treatment program, a "Future Planning Manual" was given to every participant. Completing the manual forced each person to specify both the immediate and the long-term goals he would try to realize. The manual itself places emphasis on immediate goals, requiring an outline of the specific steps necessary to gain them.

After the "Future Planning Manual" had been discussed and filled out, each treatment program usually came to an end. Typically, however, there was a short rehash session before the weekend was officially terminated. Participants were asked to reflect on their weekend experience and make any suggestions they cared to about how to improve the program.

SOME DATA

Altogether, the treatment program was conducted four times during April and May of 1967, and then temporarily discontinued for lack of funds. Thirty-five men took part in the four programs, 20 of whom were problem drinkers and 15 non-problem drinkers.

The data to be presented pertain to the first six problem drinkers who participated in the program. Follow-up information was gathered four months after their participation, and in four cases a personal interview was conducted. Each man was asked about his drinking history, his experience while in the program, and his current situation. Since the other two who were followed could not be reached directly, reliance was placed upon material supplied by a third party, who knew them well and had recently seen them. When contacted for an interview, all four men readily agreed to participate. Although there was little information available when the four were recruited for the treatment program, the interview established that each had a serious alcohol problem.

John B., 62, white, married, a barber, had been drinking steadily for about 40 years. When recruited he was an in-patient at a small private hospital for alcoholics. Over the years he had lost numerous jobs and had been hospitalized several times because of his drinking.

Norman B., 23, was white, unmarried, an unemployed beautician. He was an in-patient at the same hospital as John when he agreed to participate in the treatment program. Norman had had a short but stormy drinking history. He had begun to drink heavily in high school. Since that time he had been arrested three times for being drunk and disorderly; he had been hospitalized once for drinking; he had experienced numerous blackouts and some hallucinations as a result of drinking; he had lost at least one job and alienated most of his family by his drinking.

Carl P., 40, married, a black employed in the poverty program. He had been drinking heavily for a great many years. Recently he had nearly lost his job because of drinking, and his problem had come very close to ruining his marriage.

Dennis C., 43, was white, widowed, a cook. He also was recruited while hospitalized for drinking. Dennis had been drinking since he was 17, but it had become a problem for him shortly after he was discharged from the Army. Since then he had had innumerable contacts with alcohol treatment agencies, had lost at least three jobs, and had been arrested twice because of his drinking. With the exception of Carl, each of these men had at one time or another been associated with Alcoholics Anonymous.

The other men who participated in the first treatment program could not be reached for an interview. It was learned, however, that Julius G., 49, an unemployed black, had been drinking wine heavily for a great many years. He was recruited at a local mission for homeless unemployed men. His drinking had for years prevented him from holding a steady job. For quite a while he had been a member of a "wino" subculture among Boston's alcoholics.

The sixth participant, Frank D., 45, was an unemployed black, recruited from the same mission in which Julius was contacted. Frank's drinking had not only cost him many jobs, but had caused his wife to leave him. Frank had also been a member of a wino subculture.

It seems clear that each of the men who participated in the first treatment program had an alcohol problem severe enough to have seriously disrupted his life in one way or another. Given this history, what kind of gains, if any, did they realize from their treatment?

When asked if anything had changed for the better since his participation John B. replied, "Yes, I no longer get into one irritation or another, one stress or another. Where you used to say, the hell with this, send out for a fifth and get loaded, I accept what comes along, change it if it should be changed, accept it if it should be accepted, and I am more objective in everything." At another point John called the program "very valuable," and a "benefit" to him. More specifically, John had not had anything to drink since he participated in the program. He reported that he was getting along very well with his wife, something that seemed to amaze him after the years of difficulty and turmoil. When he left the treatment program John returned to his job after a three-month lay-off due to drinking and hospitalization. He said that he had been able to accomplish this fairly well and that things were going quite smoothly at work.

A short phone contact was made with John eight months after his participation. At that time, he felt he was still doing pretty well, although he was drinking a little and was not sure he would be able to control it. His job and family situation were still fairly good, but he did complain about having had some differences with people at work. John also mentioned, however, that he was learning to talk with people better, and to be cooperative rather than obstinate.

From one point of view John's situation began to deteriorate at some time between four and eight months after he was in the program. He had begun to drink again and apparently was becoming somewhat depressed. Nevertheless, there is little doubt that he had realized some benefits as a result of his treatment.

At four months after his participation in the treatment program Norman B. reported he was working steadily, drinking less, and getting along better with his family. His first four months, however, were not as smooth as John's. Norman had remained sober for seven and one-half weeks, something of a record for him during recent years. Then he went on a binge to "lift a depression," and as a result lost his job. Since then he had been drunk at least once a week, but only on the nights preceding the days when he did not work. He liked his current job and wanted to stay. Although he attended A.A. meetings faithfully during his periods of sobriety, his attendance had begun to fall off.

There was also a brief phone contact made with Norman eight months after he had been a member of the treatment program. At that time he had still another job which he liked better than the previous one because it paid better. His drinking had increased somewhat over the past four months, although he claimed he had not gone on any binges. Norman had made a few friends but was depressed about his inability to find a really close friend.

As with John, Norman was obviously not "cured" by his treatment experience. The phone contact made in the eighth month gave the impression that he was headed in the direction of heavy drinking again. Still, some changes had occurred. He had remained sober for some time, worked steadily for a while, and had made some effort to improve relations with his family. These were improvements, even if temporary, and they seemed to be a direct result of Norman's participation in the treatment program.

Carl P. was perhaps the most successful "graduate" of the treatment program. Following his weekend experience, he returned to the job he had almost lost because of drinking and in a short time achieved a substantial promotion. He reported that his relationship with his wife had improved a great deal, as had his relationships with the friends whom he had begun to alienate. Carl said that he was still drinking lightly but claimed he was in good control of it. Carl was extremely enthusiastic about the program and the benefits he had derived from it— so much so that he was hoping to join M.A.T. and to become an active advocate of this organization's ability to help people in general and problem drinkers in particular.

Dennis C. was the fourth man in the treatment program who was contacted for a personal interview. When asked if the treatment program had affected his life in any way he replied, "Yes it did. It had quite a bit of effect because when I left there, I had set three primary goals: one of them was to go to night school; another was to take a summer job in as remote an area as I could where I would be able to save enough money to pay for the night school; and the third was I was going to join the YMCA." In the four months following his participation Dennis accomplished two of his three goals. He joined the YMCA, and saved enough money working at a remote resort area to pay for the beginning of his night school. Furthermore, he looked into the question of what school might accept him, and investigated where he might receive the kind of training he wanted—restaurant management. For most of the four months Dennis stayed completely sober and frequently attended A.A. meetings.

Just before he was contacted, however, Dennis went on a binge and was eventually arrested for breaking and entering; thus he had a "slip" after a period of fairly good adjustment. As with the other cases, this history suggests that the treatment program was not a cure but that it did prove of some value for the men involved.

Julius G. and Frank D. were in the most deteriorated condition of the six who were recruited for the first treatment weekend. It was reported through a third person that Frank had obtained a steady job shortly after his treatment experience, and that at four months he was still working steadily, earning $70 a week. This was in sharp contrast both to his period of unemployment before the treatment program, and to his previously erratic job history. Frank has been saving his money to try and bring his wife to Boston and effect a family reconciliation. Apparently, he has had very few drinks since his participation, and has not gone on any binges.

Julius was less affected than anyone else by the treatment program. At four months he was still drinking wine extremely heavily. Even so, some minimum changes had been effected. Unemployed before the treatment weekend, Julius sought and obtained employment shortly after it was over, only to lose his job again because of drinking. He made some overtures, furthermore, toward entering a treatment center for more help with his alcohol problem. Interestingly, while he still drank, he was apparently ashamed to do so in front of anyone whom he knew to have been connected with the treatment program.

All in all, the follow-up data seem encouraging, even if they do not suggest that the treatment program was totally successful. Of course, six men represent an extremely small sample, and there was no control group which would have allowed a more explicit check on the program's effectiveness. Still, it seems likely that at least some of the changes reported above were due to the treatment program.

It is not really possible to draw any firm conclusions from these sketchy follow-up findings as to the comparative effectiveness of this type of treatment. Among alcoholics who visit clinics to get help, as many as 42 percent may show considerable improvement for at least a year afterwards (Gerard and Saenger, 1959). On the other hand, the alcoholics treated here had a considerable history of unsuccessful treatments and belonged to a group for whom the improvement rate is much lower. For instance, Mindlin (1959) reports that among a group of 50 Workhouse inmates committed for alcoholism, "only one . . . could be motivated by the clinic staff ever to attend the outpatient clinic" and none improved. Furthermore, the men inveigled into this treatment program for the most part exhibited characteristics like poor economic resources, low occupational skills, a record of many arrests, and poor motivation—all of which Mindlin found predicted failure in outpatient treatments. So the present form of treatment might be regarded as promising, at least for those not readily reached by other methods.

The question arises, however, concerning why the program was able to produce the changes that it did. Theoretically, the men who participated should have developed the ability to satisfy in a more adaptive way their desire to feel powerful. At the same time, their need to use alcohol as an impulsive way to gratify their need for power should have decreased. To some extent, and for varying periods of time, this is what occurred in almost all the participants. But it had been expected that changes would occur because the various inputs designed for the program would have their intended impact; that is, that participants would become aware of their need to feel powerful and of their maladaptive way of temporarily achieving a sense of power. Then they would learn and act upon more socialized or effective strategies for gaining a sense of power.

Judging from the participants' comments about the program, nothing of the kind actually occurred. None of the men who were interviewed understood why the concept of power was important, or what the TATs were intended to demonstrate. All had incorrect or extremely vague ideas about the major purpose of the treatment program. A few representative remarks will illustrate the lack of perception more clearly. Dennis said that the "pictures (TAT) were contorted like you couldn't tell what they were, but that was probably the object of the whole thing anyway." He remembered nothing about the power scoring system, and when asked what he remembered about power he said, "I have to stop and think a minute. Well, mostly that in most every-everything we do today or attempt to do in our line of work or whether we're active in sports or active in recreation of any kind, it's the actual physical act of what we do that shows power signs at all."

Norman saw no major purpose to the weekend. He had "no recollection of anything having to do with power," but saw the various role plays, movies, and tasks presented as preparation for the "tests." John was most impressed "by the complete lack of organization and planning." He had thought the weekend would be a "crash program course" but came to believe that its major purpose was "some sort of research deal." As for the TATs, John thought he was "to properly analyze what was in the picture and to get a coherent story out of it." He apparently had no idea how the theme of power came in, and admitted "that power, that kind of puzzled me."

In view of these observations it seems reasonable to assume that even though the program had some effect, it was not achieved in the way that was expected. How, then, did the program prove beneficial? Again, brief remarks by some of the participants are significant. Norman reported that he got a lot out of the program because he learned about "blocks," a subcategory in the power scoring system (see Appendix I). This helped him, he said, to analyze situations and to act in a more appropriate way. Carl also mentioned learning about blocks and their relevance to effective action. Of most importance to John was the realization that you should have short-term goals. "I always thought of goals as the ultimate end or something," he said, "but there can be nearby goals, goals in small matters. And to properly analyze this goal, set up the obstacles in front of this goal and how you can achieve this goal is something I never particularly thought about." Dennis was also impressed with learning about goals. Referring to the "Future Planning Manual" he said, "That impressed me the most because it at least gave you a brief outline so you could follow to some extent or to a great extent what you were interested in doing." It was impossible to find out anything about how Frank and Julius felt they were benefited by the program.

Those parts of the program which had the most impact on the participants may have something important in common. In each case participants mentioned what might be called a structural support; that is, each man learned a new way to structure his world, and to act upon the structure that he had imposed in a more active and analytic fashion, Superficially, at least, the theme of power seems far removed from this kind of change, which more than anything else resembles an alteration in cognitive style.

But, recognizing that this is a *post hoc* point of view, one can argue that such an alteration is strongly related to a sense of power, and that it was inadvertently fostered by the treatment program. To be able to structure one's way of looking at the world implies that one has conscious control over his behavior. It means that one has a particular frame of reference from which to make decisions and then to act accordingly. Thus, John talked of selecting a goal, recognizing the obstacles in front of his goal, and then, with these obstacles in mind, figuring out how to achieve that goal. Norman and Carl, and to a lesser extent Dennis, mentioned a similar process. This style of thinking is in marked contrast to an impulsive, non-analytical orientation, in which one tends to experience events as simply happening. There is little understanding of means-ends relationships, and there is virtually no consistent frame of reference available from which to view the world. Shapiro (1965) has written an important article on the phenomenological experience which accompanies an impulsive style. Among other things he points out that impulsive people feel that they have little control over what is happening to them, that they are passive observers both to internal and to external events that involve them. It would seem extremely difficult, if not impossible, for an impulsive man to gain a sense of power or to feel that he was having an impact on the world.

There is an abundance of literature which attributes an impulsive orientation to problem drinkers (see Chapter 10). The present theory is in agreement with this literature insofar as it hypothesizes that problem drinkers are impulsive men who have a strong unfulfilled need for power. Judging by the data from interviews, there is reason to believe that the six men who participated in the first treatment program were also impulsive.

All the participants spoke of doing things frequently on a whim. Norman declared several times that things often just "hit him." During the interview John seemed to be surprised by some of the things he said and "wondered where that came from." The erratic job history of most of the participants, as well as the frequent moves that some of them had made, also indicate an impulsive orientation. Yet as a result of the treatment weekend the participants seemed to adopt a different way of thinking. The cognitive orientation they began to use may have stimulated the feeling that they could have more active control over their thoughts, their behavior, and the events occurring around them. This, in turn, strongly implies that most of the participants experienced an increased sense of personal power and an increased awareness that they could have an impact on the world.

Although the treatment inputs were not specifically planned to achieve this result, they contributed to it. All the inputs involved an emphasis upon analysis—upon observing a movie, a role play or another man talking, then thinking about that event, and finally coming to some relevant conclusion regarding it. The TAT scoring system was, of course, the most explicit in this regard. In short, everything about the program encouraged an analytic, active style of thinking. It seems likely that it was this feature of the program to which the participants responded, and which proved most beneficial to them.

The trainers tried, furthermore, always to treat the men as "origins" capable of controlling their lives, rather than as pawns (deCharms, 1968). This aspect was underlined by the fact that the men were not in a hospital; there were no doctors or other experts to tell them what to do. In fact, John was impressed by the "complete lack of organization and planning" which resulted from the trainers' attempt to give the participants some power over what happened. If the participants in the program improved because they adopted a style of thinking that increased their sense of power, then it seems to follow that increasing a problem drinker's sense of power is, in fact, therapeutically beneficial.

In retrospect, then, the treatment program may have failed to teach the men what it set out to teach. It did not make them aware of their unfulfilled wishes for power; of their use of drinking as a maladaptive way to gain a feeling of power; of more effective ways to achieve a sense of power. Furthermore, the treatment program did not represent a really adequate application in practice of what had been learned from the research findings.

It is difficult to say why the program was unable to achieve its teaching objectives. Perhaps, as John suggested, the content was presented in a poorly organized way. Or it may have been that the participants were simply unable to grasp what was being presented.

Further follow-up studies of other participants should help to clarify this issue.

In spite of failing to teach directly what it set out to teach, the program was clearly of some benefit. The treatment and the setting may have helped the men to look on the world in a different way, resulting in an increase in their sense of power to control what they did and what happened to them. This hypothesis implies that such a cognitively oriented treatment might be extremely valuable to alcoholics. As the follow-up data suggest, however, simply modifying cognitive style may not be enough to maintain positive changes. One wonders how much more successful the program might have been if its emphasis on power had been as well understood as the style of thinking it encouraged. Perhaps the temporary gains made by the participants would have been sustained if the importance of power had been fully realized by them. If the participants had learned about their power needs and about adaptive ways to satisfy them at the same time they acquired a more analytic, proactive, self-confident style of thinking, then they might have been able, first, to recognize what they needed to do to gain a sense of power and second, with the aid of new cognitive strategies to achieve a more realistic sense of power. As it was, the participants learned how to be less impulsive, and they received some need satisfaction from this achievement alone. But they never learned how to use their new style of thinking so as to increase their sense of power maximally because they never understood its psychological relevance.

In future programs the concept of style of thinking will be made an integral part of the treatment. Also—depending on the results of other follow-up data—the power inputs will be redesigned so as to provide for a better understanding of the importance of power. We look forward to finding out whether such adjustments will produce a more effective means of treatment. For a useful therapy would be both the best test of the theory we have advanced and its ultimate application.

Chapter **15**

Summary

by David C. McClelland

What does it all add up to? What have
we found out in 10 years of studying drinking? The careful reader of the
preceding chapters will of course have realized that we have found out
many things, reported dozens of significant, often replicated, empirical
relationships. He will have accepted some of our interpretations of these
relationships and wondered if others were really supported by the data.
But even he, to say nothing of the general reader, would probably like
a straightforward summary of what we think we know now based on the
accumulated evidence.

For the sake of simplicity and readability we have decided to make
the summary non-technical, to strip it of all the usual hedges and
citations from the literature which characterize good scientific writing
and which have characterized our own summary statements in previous
chapters. Our purpose in presenting such a summary is to communicate
as directly and easily as possible the generalizations about drinking
which we feel are supported by the empirical evidence gathered by us
and by others.

It should be clearly understood of course that, like all generalizations, those that follow have their limitations. They may not apply to women, since women have seldom been a direct subject of study. They do not cover certain specialized types of drinking patterns such as religious or ceremonial drinking, very occasional outbursts of extreme drunkenness, or total abstention. And of course it should always be remembered that any of the generalizations accounts for at most 20–25 percent of the variance—which means either that the measures are providing faulty estimates of the true size of the relationship or that other factors not covered by the generalization influence drinking. In short there are undoubtedly individuals or even groups of individuals who drink for very different reasons from those about to be given. Starting then with a healthy respect for what we do not know, let us summarize what we do. As the careful reader will recall, all the statements below are backed by suitable empirical findings reported in previous chapters.

Why do men drink, and some to excess? To dispose first of one common answer to this question, men do not drink primarily to reduce their anxiety. Cross-culturally, peoples whose folk tales express more anxiety, drink less, not more. At the individual level alcohol, in the small amounts normally consumed, has little or no effect on anxious thoughts, although it does tend in fairly small amounts to reduce reality ties, particularly in the form of concern about time. At quite high levels of consumption, anxious thoughts decrease although other measures of inhibitory thoughts show no particular trend.

Nor do men drink primarily to attain feelings of being cared for or orally gratified. We found little evidence for increased concern along these lines either in the cross-cultural study of folk tales or in individual fantasies. Since we found no direct evidence of increased dependency concerns in heavy drinkers, we reasoned that the indirect evidence commonly cited to support the dependency theory could be interpreted in other ways. The fact that heavy drinkers are commonly counter-dependent and aggressive need not be interpreted as meaning that they have a repressed need for dependence, as many have argued. It may be taken at its face value as evidence for a personalized power drive. The more frequent references to oral body parts among heavy drinkers, found by us as well as by others, need not be taken to mean an interest in oral gratification. They may simply mean that since alcoholics have used the gastro-intestinal system to work out their motivational problems, their thoughts simply reflect the fact that it is more often stressed by the ingestion of large amounts of alcohol. Nor can the fact that alcoholics often seem to seek relationships with strong individuals be unequivocally interpreted to mean that they want to feel cared for, dependent and orally gratified. They may more simply want to feel strong and try to borrow strength from such people.

Nor do men drink primarily to become incompetent, to enjoy a "time out" period in which they will be free to act without being held accountable by society for their actions (see MacAndrew & Edgerton, 1969). There are elements of truth in this explanation, since after drinking men report themselves as feeling less responsible and are less concerned about time; but it is better combined with an explanation of the positive feelings they get from drinking.

Men drink primarily to feel stronger. Those for whom personalized power is a particular concern drink more heavily. Alcohol in small amounts, in restrained social settings, and in restrained people tends to increase thoughts of social power—of having an impact on others for their own good. In larger amounts, in supportive settings and in impulsive people, it leads to an increase in thoughts of personalized power—of winning personal victories over threatening adversaries. Among younger men, particularly in appropriate settings, thoughts of personal power are often expressed in terms of sexual and aggressive conquests.

Ingestion of alcohol cues off thoughts of strength and power in men everywhere, apparently for physiological reasons. Taken in distilled form, it creates burning sensations in the throat, stimulates the secretion of adrenalin which has broad mobilizing effects throughout the body, and is absorbed through the stomach wall into the blood stream, supplying a quick source of energy. These diffuse sensations of increased strength, particularly those induced by distilled liquor, are readily elaborated into fantasies of increased power—by some men more readily than others, and in some situations more than in others. The effect is much less marked for beer at the individual level in our culture. Wine drinking in our culture also appears not to be a central part of this syndrome but to be related to a more socialized form of power expression.

Who drinks excessively? The man who has an accentuated need for personalized power and who for a variety of reasons has chosen drinking as the outlet for it rather than some other alternative. In our study of working-class men, it appeared that drinking was only one outlet for a heightened personalized power drive, the other three being the accumulation of prestige supplies, gambling and more frequent aggressive impulses. The outlets for the personalized power drive appeared to be alternatives, in the sense that the man who chooses one is no more likely to engage in another. Furthermore, the personalized power drive is itself an alternative to a more socialized form of the power drive which expresses itself in thoughts about exerting influence *for others* coupled with doubts about the worth of power, and in actions such as seeking and achieving office in social organizations. Engaging in any of the alternative modes of expressing personalized, as opposed to socialized, power in the extreme leads to certain secondary "acting out" consequences like speeding, car accidents, fighting, and acting aggressively in many ways. This is particularly true of those who choose the heavy drinking alternative, because heavy drinking accentuates the sense of personalized power, which in turn leads to more drinking, drunkenness, accidents, fighting, marital discord, and sexual exploitation. In college men the pattern is similar but less marked.

Why some men choose drinking rather than accumulating prestige supplies or gambling as modes of expression for their personalized power drive is not explained by our findings. However, drinking probably costs less money than the other two alternatives and should therefore be chosen more often by men from the poorer strata of society, which in general is the case. Furthermore continued heavy drinking tends to decrease still further the economic resources necessary to pursue alternative ways of expressing the personalized power drive.

What accentuates the need for personalized power? A whole range of factors contributes. The culture may stress *machismo*, or male strength and daring. Genetic inheritance may play a part: boys with mesomorphic body builds are more likely to be aggressive, and aggressive boys are more likely to become alcoholics. Certain cultural conditions, such as those observed in hunting societies and among the Breton fishermen, demand more personalized power and prowess. Aging in men often brings increased demands for strength and decreased physical resources to meet them, which accentuates the need for personalized power. Many social situations challenge the sense of personalized power and focus attention on it—e.g. the "war between the sexes," in which women may both demand male prowess and yet find ways of repeatedly undermining the male sense of self-worth; lack of male solidarity in societies which insist that a man must prove his claim to being a male rather than get it at birth from the mere fact of being male; certain childhood socialization experiences or traumas such as achievement-obedience conflicts or a cross-sex identity which makes a man wonder if he is a man because at an unconscious level he has identified with women. In short, whatever makes power important or salient—in the family, in the culture, in the society, or in the current life situation—may lead to an accentuated power concern in some men which leads them to drink to increase their sense of personalized power.

In two studies we succeeded in increasing experimentally the amount that men would drink on the average. In one we manipulated the sense of power directly; the more powerful the men felt, the more they subsequently drank. In this instance drinking appeared to maintain their increased sense of power but without the sense of responsibility they had felt during the experience prior to drinking. Thus once more a finding reinforced the conclusion that alcohol, certainly beyond the first two drinks, tends to increase the sense of personalized power at the expense of feelings of responsibility, reality orientation, time concern, or social influence. In this sense the "time out" theory of drinking is supported, but with the important qualification that it is the feeling of increased *personalized power* that is enjoyed without the necessity for rendering full social account for its expression. In the other study, introducing an attractive female folksinger into a social drinking party for young men increased the amount of alcohol they consumed over that taken at similar parties where she was not present. Her presence apparently proved a direct challenge to their sense of personalized power as males, since their thoughts of physical sexual conquest shot up markedly. As in the first study, making thoughts of personalized power prominent led to an increase in drinking which in turn reinforced the thoughts of personalized power.

How can people be cured of excessive drinking? The simplest way seems to be to socialize their power drives. Cross-culturally, societies which are hierarchical and insist that power and authority be carefully channelled and institutionalized tend to be relatively sober. At the individual level, a person might be encouraged to express his personalized power drive through an alternative mode, like accumulating prestige supplies—a mode which is less damaging than drinking. Or more effectively, he may be helped to join organizations that will socialize his power drive by getting him *to do things for other people*— which is by definition expressing a socialized rather than a personalized power drive. Alcoholics Anonymous does precisely that by insisting that everyone who joins must spend his time trying to cure other alcoholics. Or the person may be given insight into why he drinks and trained directly to choose his own methods of socializing his power drive in a form of therapeutic psychological education which has been tried out on a pilot basis, and shown some promise of success. It would be further evidence for the personalized power theory of drinking if a careful study showed that therapy based on it is more effective than therapy based on other theories.

Our main conclusion is that the alcoholic experience has a common core for men everywhere and that they drink to get it. While individuals in different cultures embroider and interpret the experience in different ways, and while it is more marked for distilled liquors than for wine or beer, the experience centers everywhere in men on increased thoughts of power which, as drinking progresses, become more personal and less socialized and responsible. And societies and individuals with accentuated needs for personalized power are most likely to drink more heavily in order to get the feeling of strength they need so much more than others.

APPENDICES

I. Description of Power Scoring Categories Used
in Chapter 6   338

II. Activities Questions Asked in Bar Study II, with
Variants Noted for Bar Study I, If Any   342

III. Are Sex and Aggression Power Concerns in Fantasy
Alternative Manifestations of the Same Drive?   348

IV. Scoring Manual for Personal and Social Power
Concerns   351

V. Correlations of Marital Problems with Power
Concerns and Drinking in Two Bar Studies   357

VI. Correlations with Drinking of Self-Descriptive
Statements Not Grouped in Three Factors   358

VII. Picture Reproductions   360

VIII. Detailed Codes for Social Variables Related to
Drinking   368

IX. Motives for Drug Taking Among College Men   370

Description of Power Scoring Categories Used in Chapter 6

For the sake of convenience the system of scoring categories used in Chapter 6 will be referred to as the n Power[a] (for alcohol) system to differentiate it from earlier and later systems used. The n Power[a] total gives a score which correlates around .67 with other n Power total scores, but it was abandoned as a measure of n Power in favor of a later more generally applicable coding system derived by Winter. See Appendix II.

Appendix Table I.1 explains how the categories were derived from Winter's coding system in the lefthand column and how each category was classified as indicating Strong or Weak Power, depending on its loading on Factors II or VI. Factor II scores correlated highest ($r = .16$) with Office Holding for the college students in Chapter 5. So the categories loading at least $+.13$ on it were considered symptomatic of an organized or "Strong" Power orientation. Factor VI scores correlated highest with drinking ($r = .34$) and the "stud" cluster of activities (sex, vicarious power experience). So categories loading at least $+.13$ on it were considered symptomatic of an impulsive or Weak Power orientation.

Table I.2 shows how various summary scores were obtained for each individual, using this system. Note particularly that once it was decided the power theme of a story centered primarily on aggression, all of its sub-categories went into that column —so that even if a phrase in it might be scored for Exploitative Sex, it was not scored. Thus overlap was prevented as much as possible by omitting categories, referring to alternative power systems when they occurred as minor elements in a plot clearly oriented toward Sex, Aggression, or some other type of power. Similarly the sub-category of arousing positive or negative feelings in others was scored only when the emotional response was not part of an Exploitative Sex or Physical Aggression episode. There were two reasons for this decision. First, stories involving Exploitative Sex and Physical Aggression almost without exception included references to emotional responses of the victim (generally fear or anger). So scoring them also for the emotional response was in effect double scoring that would add nothing new to the over-all score. Secondly, it was felt that the emotions commonly reported did not reflect the power of the actor so much as the desire of the respondent to preserve himself. That is, the key idea behind this category is that the respondent should demonstrate the power of the actor by being happy in his presence or sorrowful in his absence. If an actor hits someone in the face, his power is already evident, and the emotional reaction of the victim is more a sign of the latter's desire to survive than a sign of the actor's power.

The *coding definitions* were the same as those reported in Chapter 5 by Winter with the following modifications or additions.

Appendix Table I.1—Source and classification of n Power[a] coding categories

n Power categories (Chapter 5)	Rotated Factor Loadings Factor II Strong Power	Factor VI Weak Power	n Power[a] categories	Sign of Strong or Weak Power
1. Imagery = Impact			all used, then story classed as: Exploita-	
a. strong action	.13	.11	tive Sex, Physical	W
b. reputation	.10	.24	Aggression including	W
c. emotions in others	.25	−.21	verbal insult, Other Power	S
2. High Prestige	.06	−.15	combined as one category, scored	
3. Self-confidence	.11	−.09	once per story	S
4. Low prestige	.19	.28	included	W
5. Low self-confidence	−.09	.59	included as "Actor Failure"	W
6. Emotions in others +	.47	−.42	combined as one category, scored	
7. Emotions in others −	.02	.08	once per story	S
8. Instrumental Act	.31	.49	included[1]	S
9. Blocks in world (Veroff)	.06	−.04	included[2]	S
10. Dramatic setting	.04	−.06	omitted	
11. Thema	.15	.15	omitted[3]	
12. Power Contrast			new category from Meaning Contrast analysis	W

Note: Categories from Winter scoring system were included under Strong or Weak Power if they loaded at least +.13 on Factors II or VI respectively.

[1] Loadings are for Veroff definition used in *n* Power[a]; included under Strong Power because it loaded .62 on Factor I which had nearly as high a correlation with Office Holding as Factor II.

[2] Included to strengthen Strong Power sub-total because it loaded .65 on Factor I.

[3] Omitted because it involved double scoring and because it loaded −.23 on Factor I.

As just noted, *positive or negative feelings in another* are scored in *n* Power[a] only when an Other Power episode was involved. Since Winter did not partition his Power Imagery, he did not make this distinction.

Negative self-perceptions or low self-confidence includes in *n* Power[a] instances in which the actor failed badly, although no negative self-perception is mentioned, e.g., "He wants to blow up the world but is exploded in his own bomb." In the Winter system actor failure was not scored as such, unless negative self-perception was mentioned.

Power Blocks include explicit mention of barriers or obstacles to attainment of a power-related goal. Almost all power-related stories contain blocks, in the sense that people are to be convinced, controlled, influenced, etc. This kind of imagery is not scored because it is too intimately connected with describing the power concern. What *is* scored is an instance of further disruption to the power-seeking behavior in a story already established as power-related. Example: "The troops are planning to attack the enemy positions at dawn. During the night they are hit by a small attack which they have to fight off first."

Appendix Table I.2—Organization of scoring system
n *Power*[a] for each individual

Type of Power Imagery:		Sex	Aggression	Other
High Prestige	S[1]			
Low Prestige	W[2]			
Instrumental Act				
Instrumental Act	S			
Block, world	S			
Power contrast	W			
Phys. Aggr.	W	omit		omit
Exploitative Sex	W		omit	omit
Feelings in				
Others	S	omit	omit	
Actor failure	W			

[1] S = category belonging to Strong Power sub-total.
[2] W = category belonging to Weak Power sub-total.

Summary scores:
1. Sum of all weak (W) categories, regardless of type of Power story.
2. Sum of all strong (S) categories, regardless of type of Power story.
3. Sum of all categories in Sex-related Power stories.
4. Sum of all categories in Aggression Power stories.
5. Sum of all categories in Sex and Aggression Power stories.
6. Sum of all categories for Other Power stories.

Power contrasts in n Power[a] covered:

1. Instances in which exaggerated prowess collapses:

" '*Wow, what a great build I have!' thinks the champ. 'How can that peon even step into the ring with* me?' *Floyd drops him in the first round with a cream puff to the nose.*"

"*He wants to be great and rule the world but gets blown up in his own bombs.*"

Note: The second portion of such contrasts was also scored for Actor Failure.

2. Instances in which some weak or ordinary person has a sudden rise to fame and fortune or dreams of it.

"*This man was a poor farm hand who fell into a wheat thresher and was mangled. He becomes a great movie star and marries Elke Sommer.*"

"*He's thinking how sweet revenge is going to be, because he's going to become great and show them all up.*"

The key to scoring this theme is that the power contrasts have a magical or dramatic quality that does not in any way involve work, effort or planning on the part of the actor. Sometimes blocks are magically removed from the actor's path to power through no action of his own.

3. Instances in which the omnipotence of the actor is so exaggerated as to suggest it contrasts with reality: "He's the great lover of the Yale campus, quite a Casanova. He has a perfect record with women."

Physical Aggression in n Power[a] included insulting, name-calling as well as explicit, intentional hostile thoughts or acts directed by an animate being toward another person or object. Excluded are (1) violent accidents, natural disasters and suicide; (2) *general* references to aggressive acts—e.g., "there was a riot"; (3) violence in defense of one's family, property or nation; (4) violence involving only inanimate objects—e.g., "the tree was demolished by lightning."

Scored:

"*He wants to blow up the whole world.*"

"*He hates the Yalie and slices him up with a switchblade.*"

"*The wolves attacked and devoured the travellers.*"

"He kicked the vase to bits."

"He slowly pulled the wings off the fly and laughed as it rolled around helplessly."

Exploitative Sex in *n* Power[a] involves sexual desires and sexual activities not involving love or affection. Statements must suggest physical aspects of sex (seduction, rape, sleeping or going to bed with someone, references to bodily parts in a sexual context, or bodily states of the actor—e.g., "he's tingling with anticipation for her.") *General* sexual references (e.g., "they are having an affair.") are not scored unless the sexual activity is further elaborated.

Activities Questions Asked in Bar Study II, with Variants Noted for Bar Study I, If Any

Activities, Interests, and Attitudes Questionnaire

Name: Address:

Occupation:

Education (highest grade finished):

Marital status:

1. What organizations do you now belong to? (Include Rotary club, church club, Masons, etc.) Have you ever been an officer in any of these organizations?

Organization	*Years a member*	*Offices held* (No. years)
_____	_____	_____
_____	_____	_____

Note: In Bar I, the question was asked so that a person could list offices held in organizations of which he was no longer a member (e.g., High School clubs).

2. Do you now participate, or have you ever participated, in any organized sports?

Sport	*Years participated*	*Type of team* (H.S. varsity, college intramural, club, etc.)
_____	_____	_____

Notes: 1. Coded for contact vs. non-contact sports.
   2. In Bar I, they were asked for *current* participation in informal sports as well (once or more a week, 1–3 times a month, a few times a year, or never). These were also coded for contact vs. non-contact sports.

3. Do you now participate, or have you ever participated, in outdoor activities such as camping, hunting, golfing, and so forth? Please list the activity and the number of years participated.

Activity	*Number of years*
_____	_____

Note: Not asked in Bar I.

4. On the average, over a year, how many college sports events do you attend in person?

Bar I

_____More than thirty   _____Once a week or more
_____Between ten and thirty   _____1–3 a month
_____Between five and ten   _____5–11 a year
_____Less than five   _____1–4 a year
_____None   _____None

5. On the average, over a year, how many professional sports events do you attend in person?

Bar I, as in item 4.

_____More than thirty
_____Between ten and thirty
_____Between five and ten
_____Less than five
_____None

6. On the average, how often do you watch sports on television?

Bar I, as in item 4.

_____One or more a week   If you watch sports on TV what kinds
_____One to three a month   of events do you mainly watch (e.g.
_____Five to eleven a year   football, baseball, golf, etc.)?
_____One to four a year   _____
_____None   _____

7. Suppose you were drinking beer at a party, a bar, or some other place where you normally drink. On the average, how many cans of beer would you finish?

_____9 or more   _____1–2
_____6–8   _____less than 1
_____3–5   _____don't drink beer

8. How often during the past year have you been at a party, or a bar, or some other similar place where you were drinking beer?

_____4 or more times a week   _____6–12 times a year
_____2–3 times a week   _____1–5 times a year
_____2–4 times a month   _____never

Note: In Bar I, they were asked how often they had four or more drinks using the same frequency code.

9. Now, suppose you were drinking hard liquor at a party, or a bar, or some other place where you normally drink. On the average, how many drinks would you have?

_____9 or more   _____1–2
_____6–8   _____less than 1
_____3–5   _____don't drink liquor

10. How often during the past year have you been at a party, or a bar, or some other similar place where you were drinking liquor?

_____4 or more times a week   _____6–12 times a year
_____2–3 times a week   _____1–5 times a year
_____2–4 times a month   _____never

Notes: 1. See note to item 8.
  2. In Bar I, they were also asked if they ever get drunk; ____never, ____once or twice before, ____a few times a year, ____1–3 times a month, ____one or more times a week, and also; if they had ever been in trouble because of drinking on the same frequency scale.

11. If you were going to buy any car costing $7000 or less, what kind of car would you buy (new car only)

Make _____ Model _____

Body type _____ Approx. horsepower _____

Note: In Bar I, they were asked the cost of their ideal car and its maximum speed.

12. What is the fastest speed you have ever driven a car? _____MPH

Note: In Bar I, they were also asked how fast they had ever ridden.

13. How many times have you driven a car over 90 MPH? _____times

14. What magazines do you read or look at regularly?

_____ _____

_____ _____

Note: Coded for *Playboy*, other sex magazines, *Sports Illustrated*, *Hot Rod*, etc. vs. other types.

15. What television shows do you like to watch?

_____ _____

_____ _____

Note: Coded for shows noted for violence, drama, intrigue, etc. (Examples: I Spy, Man from U.N.C.L.E., Mission Impossible, etc., or sports shows or other types.)

16. Do you own any of the following? How many of the following would you like to own? How many do you expect to own some day?

	Own	Like to own	Expect to own
a. color television			
b. tailor made suit			
c. Playboy club key			
d. second home (cabin, etc.)			
c. country club membership			
f. rifle or pistol			
g. fully equipped bar			
h. convertible car			

Note: Summed to get number of prestige supplies. In Bar I the measure was the number of prestige supplies listed in response to the question: "If someone gave you $10,000, what would you do with it? List three alternatives."

17. How many credit cards are in your wallet right now? _____

18. Have you ever been involved in an automobile accident, as the driver?

_____yes _____no If yes, how many times? _____

19. Have you ever received a ticket for a moving traffic violation?

_____yes _____no If yes, how many times? _____

Note: Answers not coded in Bar II.

20. Within the last three years, have you been in a physical fight (not a verbal fight)?

_____yes _____no If yes, how many times? _____

Note: Not asked in Bar I.

21. Below is a list of various behaviors or actions. For each one, please check the appropriate column.

	have done often	have done once or twice	haven't but would like to	never considered doing
a. yelled at someone in traffic				
b. threw things around the room (books or magazines, etc.)				

c. destroyed furniture or
glassware   _____ _____ _____ _____
d. tore up books, telephone
directories, etc.   _____ _____ _____ _____
e. stayed up all night for
no reason   _____ _____ _____ _____
f. got into a car and drove
a long distance, on the
spur of the moment   _____ _____ _____ _____
g. made insulting remarks
to storekeepers, clerks, etc. _____ _____ _____ _____
h. didn't show up for
work because you just
didn't feel like it.   _____ _____ _____ _____
i. played out a role that
you didn't really have   _____ _____ _____ _____
j. walked off, leaving your
wife or girl to fend for
herself the rest of the
evening   _____ _____ _____ _____
k. took towels from a
hotel or motel   _____ _____ _____ _____
Note: Not asked in Bar I.

Gambling (Not asked in Bar I)

1. On the average, how often do you make bets of $1 or more?
   _____Twice a week or more
   _____Once a week
   _____Once or twice a month
   _____Once a year
   _____Never

2. On what form of gambling do you bet the most money?
   _____Racing (dogs or horses)
   _____Other sports events (football games, etc.)
   _____Numbers
   _____Card games
   _____Casino games (dice, roulette, keno, bingo, etc.)
   _____Other: Specify_____

3. After winning at gambling, do you have a strong urge to return and win more?
   _____No
   _____Yes

4. After losing, do you often want to return as soon as possible to win back your losses?
   _____No
   _____Yes

5. Have you ever borrowed money in order to gamble?
   _____No
   _____Yes

6. Have you ever felt sad or angry after losing heavily?
   _____No
   _____Yes   Write your name_____

Additional questions asked in Bar Study I only.

1. If someone gave you $10,000, what would you do with it. List three alternatives. Answers coded for spending on Travel, Savings, Gifts, or Prestige Supplies (fancy cars, equipment, etc.).

2. How many cigarettes do you smoke a day? Check one.
   _____Don't smoke
   _____a few
   _____about half a pack
   _____about a pack
   _____about a pack and a half
   _____two or more packs

3. During the year, how often do you go dancing?
   _____more than once a week.
   _____about once a week
   _____2–3 times a month
   _____about once a month
   _____a few times a year
   _____I never dance

4. Below is a list of different activities. Indicate for each activity how many hours a week you usually spend doing that.

   Number of hours per week

	Number of hours per week
Hanging around a coffee shop, bar, etc.	_____
Read	_____
Watch TV	_____
Work	_____
Go out with your wife or a girl friend	_____
Play cards with friends	_____

In Bar Study II, the questionnaire devised and fully described by Jessor *et al.* (1968) was also administered. The scores used in Chapter 8 were obtained from questions having the following format:

Ratings: Now I'm interested in just how important you would say *each* of these is to you. Starting with the first one above, "the love and affection you get in the family" would you say that is,

(circle one)	very important	pretty important	not too important	not important at all

   Part of Affection score

Now, rate "having somebody in the family you can count on to help you."

(circle one)	very important	pretty important	not too important	not important at all

   Part of Dependence score

"the good opinion of the family for the things you do well."

(circle one)	very important	pretty important	not too important	not important at all

   Part of Recognition score

"being able to do things in the family in your own way."

(circle one)	very important	pretty important	not too important	not important at all

   Part of Independence score

The same items were repeated for importance in *work*, e.g., for "help in getting job done" (Dependence) etc. and for importance in *friendships*—e.g., for "having someone you can turn to for help when you have a problem" and twice more in general terms—e.g., "How important is it to you to get advice when you have a hard decision to make or a problem to work out?" and "How important is it to you to know you can count on some people to help you if you need it?" Thus the Dependence-Importance score is the sum of the answers to five very similar questions.

Then they were asked to think "about what you *expect* and *not* any more about what you want." For example:

This time I would like you to indicate how *strongly* you *expect* each of these to happen:

"*To be able to count on the family for help when you need it.*" (*Dependence*)

"*To get affection from others in the family*", etc.

The items parallel the importance items closely, and each person gets a summary score based on answers to five *expectation* questions in each of the four areas of Dependence, Independence, Recognition and Affiliation.

Disjunctions between values (importance) and expectations were also computed in various ways and included in the correlation matrix, but none of them showed a significant pattern of relationships with the variables in this study.

Are Sex and Aggression Power Concerns in Fantasy Alternative Manifestations of the Same Drive?

As noted in Chapter 8 (Table 8.2), Sex, Aggression and Other Power themes do not correlate significantly with each other, even though the scoring definition for each requires some type of power concern. Sex Power themes are even *negatively* correlated with Aggressive Power themes ($r = -.18$) and with Other Power themes ($r = -.14$). What right then do we have to consider them measures of the same concern or need?

As Wittenborn (1955) has cogently pointed out, and as Winter has noted in Chapter 5, the difficulty in situations like this often arises because a motive may manifest itself in alternative ways. A hungry man on a given occasion will eat chicken *or* steak, seldom both. Thus a correlation between amount of steak eaten and amount of chicken eaten on a given occasion would certainly be negative, although each is a perfectly good measure of how hungry a person is. Analogously, a man with a power need may express it in a sex-related story *or* an aggression-related story, but if he starts on one theme he will score less high on the other because he has satisfied his need in one way and doesn't need to do it in two or more. Also there are space, time and thematic limitations in writing stories. A man who starts writing about a robbery simply is less likely to be able to drag sex into the story.

But how then can we test the hypothesis that Sex and Aggression imagery are alternative manifestations of the same type of power concern? As Wittenborn suggests, one good method is to see whether they relate to a set of other variables in the same way. Consider the following set of correlations of Sex and Aggression Power scores with various activities:

	Sex Power	Score rank	Aggression Power	Score rank
Office holding	−.02	2	.22	1
Fastest speed ridden	.16	1	.12	2
Violent TV shows watched	−.12	4	.01	3
Cigarettes smoked	−.08	3	−.05	4

Here, despite the negative correlation between the Sex and Aggression Power scores, the hierarchies of their relationships to outside variables are similar: the correlation between the rank orders of the correlations with outside variables is .40.

Both are more related to office holding and speeds ridden than to watching violent TV shows and smoking lots of cigarettes.

A major difficulty with testing the alternative manifestation hypothesis this way is that the result is easily influenced by the sample of outside variables included in the analysis. For example, if only assertive activities are included, the correlation between the rank orders would almost certainly be reduced because there would be no opportunity for the alternative manifestations of the power drive to show that they were both very negatively related to passive activities (e.g., as in the cigarette smoking instance above). A particular difficulty in the present study derives from the fact that many of the measures tapped the same variable, e.g., there were five measures of rapid or reckless driving. If two power sub-scores happened to relate very differently to rapid driving, it would be possible to reduce the correlation between the hierarchies of their relationships with outside variables, simply by including many measures from this one area.

With such considerations in mind the sample of outside variables was chosen as follows. The first goal was to get a maximum range on the assertive-passive dimension represented by Factor I in Table 8.4. All variables loading $\pm .32$ or more were first selected out for examination. Then from among these only one variable from a given domain was included. It was decided that two variables came from the same domain (1) if they dealt with the same behavior area (e.g., driving speed) and (2) if they correlated significantly positively with each other at $p < .05$. Note in the final list presented in Appendix Table III.1 that average wine and liquor consumed came from the same behavior domain but they do not correlate significantly with each other

Appendix Table III.1

Variable	FACTOR LOADINGS		CORRELATIONS WITH N POWER SUB-SCORES					
	I	*II*	Sex Power	Rank	Agg. Power	Rank	Other Power	Rank
Sports participation	769	+081	040	4	245	4	274	3
Fastest speed driven	749	−016	−051	11	354*	1	304*	2
Officerships	682	+103	−008	6	209	5	054	11
Years education	631	+165	−014	7	142	8	101	8
Time with women	614	+249	033	5	157	7	160	5
Reading vicarious mags.	513	+280	076	3	258	3	341	1
Cost desired car	429	−019	113	2	181	6	−056	14
Ave. liquor consumed	425	−586	−046	10	134	9	251	4
Vicarious TV watching	416	−139	−130	16	075	12	102	7
Ave. wine consumed	410	+215	241	1	068	14	091	9
Cigarettes smoked	−295	−392	−083	13	−050	17	−104	18
Age	−443	−516	−063	12	−189	19	−204	19
Time watching TV	−399	−272	−034	8.5	−153	18	−086	16
Time working	053	+454	−113	14	281	2	−062	15
Physical health	157	+302	−116	15	078	10	053	12
Liking travel	343	−336	−034	8.5	076	11	069	10
Ave. beer consumed	076	−344	−288*	19	074	13	131	6
Freq. 4+ drinks	−029	−449	−190	17	000	15	−091	17
Marital problems	004	−638	−205	18	−030	16	019	13

* $p < .05$.

($r = .17$). On the other hand, Fastest Speed Ridden and Fastest Speed Driven came from the same behavior area but since they correlated highly with each other ($r = .64, p < .01$), only one was included.

In general when one of two or more qualified variables had to be picked in this way, the one with the highest loading on the Factor was included. In a couple of instances this rule was not followed when it put constraints on including variables from other domains. For example, Speed of Desired Car loaded most highly of the car speed variables on Factor I but it correlated significantly with Cost of Desired Car which also qualified for inclusion and which seemed to represent a domain which could be distinguished from the speed domain. So it was decided to move down to the speed variable with the next highest loading on Factor I (Fastest Speed Driven), which did not relate to Cost of Desired Car so that the latter variable could be included.

The first 13 variables listed in Appendix Table III.1 were picked in this way. Next an effort was made to add to the sample variables with the maximum positive or negative loadings on Factor II—the Inhibition-release dimension. The purpose of this procedure was to make it optimally possible to find out which Power sub-scores were more correlated with impulsive power activities, and which with more restrained power activities. As Appendix Table III.1 shows, activities loading high on restraint were relatively scarce, as were activities representing low assertiveness. It is also interesting to note that two more drinking variables qualify for inclusion because they represent lack of restraint, rather than a power orientation.

All variables loading $\pm .32$ or more on Factor II were originally inspected but some were discarded because they came from the same behavior domain already represented by another variable with which they correlated significantly. For example, Drinking Trouble qualified initially for inclusion, but was discarded because it correlated significantly with Average Liquor Consumed ($r = .44, p < .05$) which was already in the matrix. In all, six additional variables qualified for inclusion in the sample because of their loadings on Factor II, making a total of 19 variables.

Appendix Table III.1 presents the loadings of each of these variables on each of the two factors and also shows the extent to which each type of fantasy n Power score correlated with each of the outside variables. As one can observe by inspecting the rank orders of these columns of correlations, the three fantasy Power scores are all more related to the activities at the top of the table (representing assertiveness) than they are to those at the bottom, representing low assertiveness. The correlations among the rank orders are reported in Table 8.3. There is some evidence for the alternative manifestations hypothesis. The various types of power scores do relate to other variables in similar fashion, even though they are unrelated to each other. The most striking illustration is provided by the Sex and Aggression Power sub-totals which intercorrelate negatively ($r = -.18$). Yet each relates to a representative sample of outside variables in similar fashion ($\rho = .40, p < .10$). The Sex Power score also relates negatively to the Other Power score; the rank orders of their correlations with the sample of outside activities also correlate positively ($\rho = .32$), though not significantly. Aggression Power and Other Power themes relate to other variables in a highly similar way ($\rho = .63, p < .01$).

Apparently a power concern which has the same significance in a person's life can express itself either in sexual, or aggressive, or other ways in TAT stories. The lack of correlation among these alternative types of imagery in a given record does not signify that they are unrelated types of power concerns and is probably due to the simple fact that if a person starts telling one type of story he is less able to bring in other types of imagery due to time, space, and thematic limitations.

Scoring Manual for Personal and Social Power Concerns

Mary Thomas, Dan Goleman, and Ross Goldstein

Power Imagery as defined in the Winter *n* Power code is a *prerequisite* to scoring p or s Power. There must be explicit power imagery in the story which clearly meets Winter's coding criteria. The scorer should be able to point to a specific sentence or phrase in the story and name the particular power image coding criterion which applies.

If a power image is found then the p or s categories can be scored; if there is no power image then there can be no p or s scores.

Each p or s category can be scored only once in any given story.

If any one character displays power imagery, p or s categories can be scored for any and all characters in the story.

Power categories can be scored if they are wanted, fantasied, recollected, planned, or actually carried out in the story.

Step one in scoring a story for p or s Power is deciding whether there is any power imagery in it at all. The story is read through with the Winter Power Imagery criteria in mind. If there is clear power imagery in the story, then it is scored for p or s Power; if there is no power imagery, there can be no p or s score. There is no actual score given for power imagery, but it must be in the story for there to be any p or s Power.

Be conservative in scoring. Do not score on the basis of inference. Score only on the basis of what is explicitly stated in the story. As you look for power imagery and score each of the p or s coding categories, remember the rule-of-thumb: When in doubt, leave it out.

Criteria for Power Imagery (Abbreviated from Winter, 1970). See Examples at End.

1. Someone shows his power concern through actions which in themselves express his power.

a. Strong, forceful actions which affect others, such as assaults, attacks, chasing; verbal insults, threats, or reprimands; and sexual exploitation where it is clear the action does not express mutuality or love. Exclude accidents.

b. Giving help, assistance, advice, or support if it has not been solicited by the other person.

Solicited advice counts where there is evidence for power concern beyond the mere answering of questions.

    c. Trying to control another person through regulating his behavior or the conditions of his life, or through seeking important information which would affect another's life or action. Exclude routine requests for information.

    d. Trying to influence, persuade, convince, make a point, or argue with another person, so long as the concern is not to reach agreement or to avoid misunderstanding or disagreement. Do not count mere mention of an argument.

    e. Trying to impress some other person or the world at large. Such actions as creative writing, making news or publicity, trying to win an election to office, and any action that will attract widespread attention, including trying to create a public effect, or gaining fame or notoriety.

    2. Someone does something that arouses strong positive or negative emotions in others. Others show an emotional reaction to him because of something he has done.

    The action which arouses the feelings must be intentional, or under the conscious control of the actor, but the effect need not be intended by the actor.

    Do not count someone's response to natural disasters, accidents, economic depressions, and the like.

    3. Someone is described as having a concern for his reputation or position. The person is concerned about his reputation or others' judgment of his power, though no powerful actions need be mentioned.

    Or a character experiences positive or negative affect in regard to a position of high or low status or prestige.

    Distinguish affect about position or prestige from affect about achievement strivings, which does not count as power imagery.

Note: Be sure to distinguish between achievement and power in every power image category.

    "He's determined to become a world-recognized champ" would be scored as a power image (Specific criterion: concern for reputation—world-recognized—or other's judgment of his power).

    But, "He's determined to become champion" would *not* be scored for power (the concern is for achievement).

    If power imagery is clear in the story, the following p and s categories can be scored:

Personal Goal. Someone in the story is concerned about his personal or selfish power in relation to a specific other, or about his reputation or glory. His power goal is without reference to the good it may do others. He is explicitly mentioned as the beneficiary of the power goal.

    Examples of personal goal:

> *The fellow hopes to persuade his boss to give him a promotion.*
> *He's fighting the champ—a chance to win a big purse, retire to a beach in Tahiti.*
> *He wants to be President so he will go down in history.*
> *The boy is scared but will fight anyway to uphold his honor in front of the girl.*

Social Goal. Someone is concerned about using his power for the good of specified others, or for the good of some cause (e.g., mankind, people's revolution, Justice, Peace). The concern for the good of others must be unsolicited or in excess of what was solicited.

    Examples of other goal:

> *He's fighting the champ—a chance to win a big purse. His kid is in the hospital and needs a big operation.*
> *He wants to be President so he can lead the country out of chaos.*
> *He is experimenting on this patient to find a cure that will save mankind.*

Note: Don't score for personal goal or social goal unless the self interest or the other concern is explicitly mentioned. For example, do *not* score:

He's fighting the champ—a chance to win a big purse. (It could be for himself or for others.)
The fellow hopes to persuade his boss. (The beneficiary of his persuasion is ambiguous.)

Note: Not all power goals in stories can be scored as personal or social. Do *not* score for these categories when:

1. There is ambiguity about whether the power goal is for self or for others. Ambiguous cases are relatively frequent, especially in the case of a power-oriented career. In an ambiguous case score nothing.

Do score:

The captain is planning an attack on an enemy supply route. He's thinking how the general will be impressed, maybe promote him. (Personal goal)
The boy is wondering how he can get her home before the hood attacks her. (Social goal)

Do *not* score:

The captain is planning an attack on an enemy supply route. (Power goal, but not clearly personal or social).
The boy is wondering how he can get her home. (Power goal, but not clearly personal or social).
2. Do not score when the goal reflects achievement rather than power. In stories with both power and achievement imagery, personal or social goal is scored only for the power theme.
3. Do not score when the power gain accruing to self or to others was inadvertant or accidental.

Note: If *both* personal and social goal are present, clearly stated, and with no ambiguity, then score for *social*.

Example: He wants to find a cure which will save mankind and make him famous. (Score social goal only.)

Note: There may be power imagery without a power goal.
For example:

John is working late at the office and his wife is furious at him. (Power imagery: making an emotional impact on others; but no score for power goal: it was not John's goal to make his wife mad).
Power goal, both personal and social, requires a statement of intent to perform a power act.

Instrumental Activity. (s Power category.) There is an actual statement of activity by a character in the story which indicates that he is doing something about attaining a power goal. The action is independent of both the original description of the situation and the final outcome of the story. Instrumental activity in the Winter *n* Power system can also be coded when it has the effect of attaining a power goal even though the protagonist's intent is not clear. Here the actor must intend that the act is directed towards a power goal:
Example:

The scientist is working in his lab. He puts together a new bunch of chemicals and discovers a cure for cancer. He becomes famous.
Discovering the cancer cure is scored "instrumental act" in the Winter system, but not here because it is not clear he did it for the power goal of becoming famous.

Do not score statements which are simply descriptions of setting or of the outcome of actions.

Examples of instrumental activity:

Bob is wondering what to do not to lose face (setting). Bob will start the fight (instrumental activity) and drop the punk cold (outcome).

Lee and Pete are coming round the bend, each wanting to knock the other out of the race (setting). They are risking their lives by driving too fast around turns (instrumental activity). They are going to crack up and be killed (outcome).

The hood accosted the couple and asked the girl if she wanted to get laid (setting). The hood knocks out the guy (instrumental activity) and rapes the girl (outcome).

Do *not* score:

Bob is wondering what to do not to lose face (setting). Bob will start the fight (outcome).

Lee and Pete are coming round the bend, each wanting to knock the other out of the race (setting). They are going to crack up and be killed (outcome).

The hood knocks out the guy and rapes the girl (no instrumental activity distinct from setting and outcome).

Self block (s Power category). Someone is in a struggle with himself about his ability to influence, control, attract, or impress others, or about his potential for prestige and reputation.

Or, someone is involved in an interpersonal conflict that raises questions as to his competence or that spawns internal emotional confusions or conflict within him.

Insanity is routinely scored as self doubt.

Examples:

He's worried about winning the fight, he doesn't know if he can take the guy.
He lost the fight and wonders if this means he's unable to be a match for anybody anymore.
He wants recognition but is wondering if this is the best and safest way to get it.
Bob is wondering what to do not to lose face.
She wonders if she's pretty enough to get a man without going to bed with him.
This mad scientist is working on a hare-brained scheme to destroy the world.

Note: Do not score concern for reputation or status as self conflict unless there is clearly an inner struggle about ability to be powerful.

Do *not* score:

He's trying to hide his embarrassment over losing the fight. (Feeling badly about a poor performance is not the same as doubting one's ability to perform.)

Opponent block. (p Power category). Someone is engaged in a struggle with an identified specific opponent. The conflict may be sexual, physical, intellectual, economic, or moral. Both parties in the conflict must be mentioned.

Often there is a zero sum game: someone would win in his power action only at the expense of another.

Examples of opponent block:

He's thinking about stealing the car but the owner sees him.
He wants to sleep with her, she's playing it cool.
Tony the Town Hood made a derogatory comment to Eric, who retorted cuttingly.
Bill and Bob are battling 'til one of them drops.

Note: Do not score for opponent block unless the other involved in the struggle is explicitly mentioned.

Do *not* score:

He's thinking about stealing the car.
Bill is in a fight to the end.

Note: If both self block and opponent block are present in the same person, score for *self* block.

Both self block and opponent block can be scored in the same story if each is present in a different person.

Zero Sum Game. (Originally p Power category, discarded because not cross-validated). Winning for one person clearly means losing for another.

Examples:

> *The boy turns and hits the heckler, and walks off leaving him on the ground.*
> *The District Attorney wins his case and the power of the Mafia is broken in Newark.*

Power Contrast. (s Power category). The power, influence, reputation, or prestige of a person is deceptive; he has a flaw. The tone should be one of exaggeration or irony.

Or, the story has a simultaneous mixed outcome. Someone attains an outcome which is both good and bad at the same time. In defeat there is victory, or in victory there is defeat. The outcome must be related to a power act, not to achievement.

Examples of power contrast:

> *He fights the guy and demolishes him, but he feels bad because he lowered himself to the other guy's level.*
> *Chet the Jet, the world's greatest swimmer, has lost to a ten-year-old.*
> *When he finally got the girl, he was chagrined to learn she was his sister.*
> *He becomes a successful armbreaker for the Mafia and develops a bad ulcer.*

Note: Do not score sequential mixed outcomes for power contrast.

Examples for Winter's Power Imagery criteria

Category

1a. They plan to attack an enemy supply area.
    The agents will catch the suspected people.
    The company representative has bawled out the captain.
    He is trying to seduce his secretary.
    The guy will go out to do some panhandling.

1b. The older man protected the younger against others.
    The father is interested in teaching his son basketball.
    Her father went with her to help her, because she was stricken with grief.
    She is giving the kid advice.

1c. The welfare worker arranged to transfer the kid to the country, to get him under
        a new influence.
    The executive is visiting the branch office to determine whether the agency
        should handle a new account.
    They are being sent to get information on the enemy troop build-up.
    The newspaperman is trying to get the lowdown on the politician.
    Complaints kept coming into the main office, so the businessman was sent to get
        a first-hand report.

1d. His father tries to interest him in ranching.
    She tries to convince him to return home.
    The junior executive is trying to get his point across.

1e. The reporter is interviewing the farmer about a feature story that he is going to
        write.
    An author is trying to gather thoughts for his novel.

The guy is trying to impress his date.

The man is urbane and sophisticated; he knows the right places in town to be seen in, and how to be seen in these spots.

She is fed up with him and is putting on a scene.

He was seen tearing hell through town in the family automobile.

2. The professional player is giving a demonstration, and the boy is thrilled.

He has taken her to a small cafe. She is enchanted by the atmosphere, and shows her delight.

He told his mother what he had been doing. She broke down and cried.

3. The girl is thinking about the attention which is focused on her.

He has taken her out because he likes her, but also because he wanted to find out how his boss rated him on his last rating.

He wants some money, so that he can move out of the small room to a luxurious resort, where he would have a rug on the floor and a maid at the door to clean up after him.

The captain thinks he is not to blame, and wants to be vindicated.

The mate knows that his job depends on the executive, but doesn't want to let the crew think he let a white collar man tell him what to do.

They are both slightly worried about the impressions they are making on each other.

Recommended procedure for scoring a story for *n* Power
and its p Power and s Power components

	p	s	*n* Power
1. Score for Power imagery			_____
decide whether it is for			
personal goal	_____		
or social goal		_____	
2. Score for positive or			_____
negative prestige of actor			_____
3. Score for Need for Power			_____
4. Score for instrumental act			
over-all			_____
by intent		_____	
5. Score for blocks in world			_____
if in actor	_____		
if opponent		_____	
6. Positive and			_____
Negative goal anticipations			_____
7. Positive and			_____
Negative emotions			_____
8. Effect			
Power contrast	_____		
Sums	p *Power*	s *Power*	n *Power*

Categories 1–8 are fully described with examples by Winter, 1970.
See Table 7.2 for sample means and standard deviations to sets of four pictures used in bar studies.

APPENDIX V

Correlations of Marital Problems[1] with Power Concerns and Drinking in Two Bar Studies

Bar I, $N = 50$; Bar II, $N = 108$

	Bar I	Bar II
Quantity, frequency index liquor[2]	.33*	.03
Drunkenness[3]	.33*	.10
Drinking as highest alternative manifestation[4]		.22*
Before drinking		
n Power	−.04	.22*
p Power	.00	.18
s Power	−.22	.25**
p–s Power[5]	.21	−.05
After drinking		
n Power	−.06	
p Power	.09	
s Power	−.15	
p–s Power[5]	.19	

* $p < .05$, ** $p < .01$.
[1] Men reporting they were divorced or separated from their wives.
[2] At least 3–5 drinks of hard liquor 2–3 times a week or more often vs. all others.
[3] Frequency of drunkenness, Bar I; sum of beer, frequency times quantity plus liquor, frequency times quantity for Bar II.
[4] For explanation, see Chapter 8.
[5] Difference between standard scores for p and s Power.

Correlations with Drinking of Self-Descriptive Statements Not Grouped in Three Factors

Source of Statements[a]	Statement	Factor with highest loading	N = 190 r with drinking
1. CPI-302 OPI-342	I have often gone against my parents' wishes	1	.36**
2. OPI-D-64	I enjoy playing cards for money.	1	.33**
3. Yea-Nay-22	Here today, gone tomorrow—that's my motto!	1	.29**
4. CPI-250	I must admit that I find it very hard to work under strict rules and regulations	1	.26**
5. CPI-300	Police cars should be especially marked so that you can always see them coming.	1	.24**
6. OPI-D-3 CPI-170	I often act on the spur of the moment without stopping to think.	1	.22**
7. OPI-D-33	I find that a well-ordered mode of life with regular hours is not congenial to my temperament.	1	.22**
8. MMPI-56 CPI-288	As a youngster I was suspended from school one or more times for cutting up.(A)	1	.22**
9. Gough Fem-6 CPI-39	I must admit that I enjoy playing practical jokes on people.	1	.21*
10. CPI-427 CPI-34	There are a few people who just cannot be trusted.	1	.20*
11. MMPI-224 CPI-164	My parents have often objected to the kind of people I went around with.(A)	1	.20*
12. CPI-270	I often lose my temper.	1	.19*
13. OPI-D-330	I generally prefer being with people who are not religious.	1	.19*
14. OPI-D-315 T-M-I-2	I would like to hunt lions in Africa.	1	.17*
15. MMPI-446	I enjoy gambling for small stakes.(A)	1	.16
16. CPI-339	I have been in trouble one or more times because of my sex behavior.	1	.16*
17. CPI-395	It is very important to me to have enough friends and social life.	1	.15

Source of Statements[a]	Statement	Factor with highest loading	N = 190 r with drinking
18. Gough Fem-17 CPI-114 OPI-D-88	At times I feel like picking a fist fight with someone.	1	.14
19. CPI-205	I enjoy a race or game better when I bet on it.	1	.10
20. MMPI-378	I do not like to see women smoke.(A)	1	−.36 **
21. OPI-D-418	It is difficult for me to take people seriously.	2	.09
22. CPI-278 Gough Fem-38	If I get too much change in a store, I always give it back.	2	−.27 **
23. CPI-179	When I work on a committee I like to take charge of things.	2	−.20 *
24. MMPI-278	I have often felt that strangers were looking at me critically.(A)	2	−.18 *
25. CPI-27	It makes me feel like a failure when I hear of the success of someone I know well.	2	−.13 *
26. OPI-D-207	I dislike following a set schedule.	3	.38 **
27. T-M-I-8	I like people who spend freely.	3	.28 **
28. OPI-D-34	The unfinished and the imperfect often have greater appeal for me than the completed and the polished.	3	.17 *
29. OPI-D-120	In religious matters I believe I would have to be called a skeptic or an agnostic.	3	.10
30. OPI-D-375	I would consider it more important for my child to secure training in athletics than in religion.	3	.08
31. MMPI-294 CPI-212	I have never been in trouble with the the law.(A)	3	−.45 **
32. CPI-394	Even when I have gotten into trouble I was usually trying to do the right thing.	3	−.30 **
33. T-M-I-6	I like stories of home life.	3	−.30 **
34. OPI-D-335 CPI-69	I would disapprove of anyone's drinking to the point of intoxication at a party.	3	−.23 **
35. Yea-Nay-3	One should not give free rein to the passions, but rather control and weigh them up before expressing them.	3	−.23 **
36. OPI-D-354	I am more religious than most people.	3	−.22 **
37. EYS-E-I-N-8	I am inclined to be overconscientious.	3	−.19 *
38. OPI-D-133	Every wage-earner should be required to save a certain part of his income each month so that he will be able to support himself and his family in later years.	3	−.17 *
39. OPI-D-40	In the final analysis, parents generally turn out to be right about things.	3	−.17 *
40. OPI-D-161	Young people sometimes get rebellious ideas, but as they grow up they ought to get over them and settle down.	3	−.11

* $p < .05$, ** $p < .01$.
[a] See footnotes to Table 10.1.

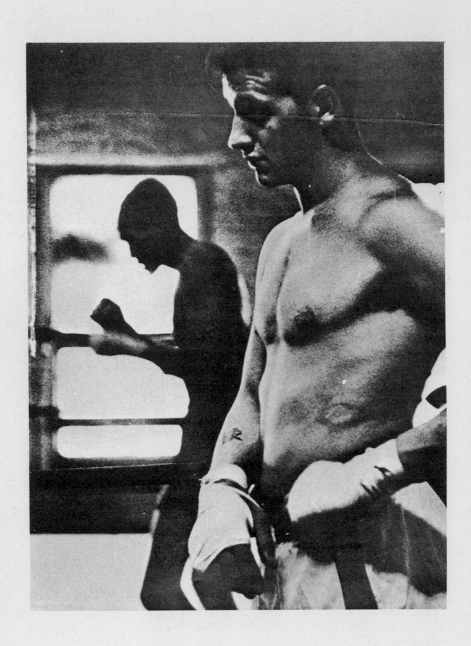

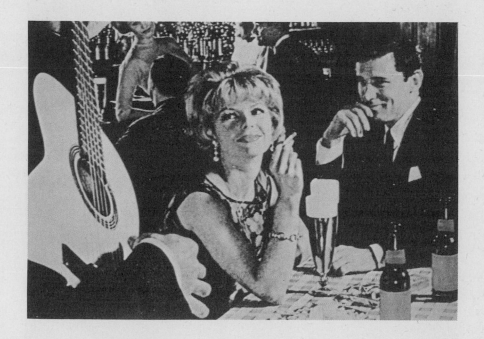

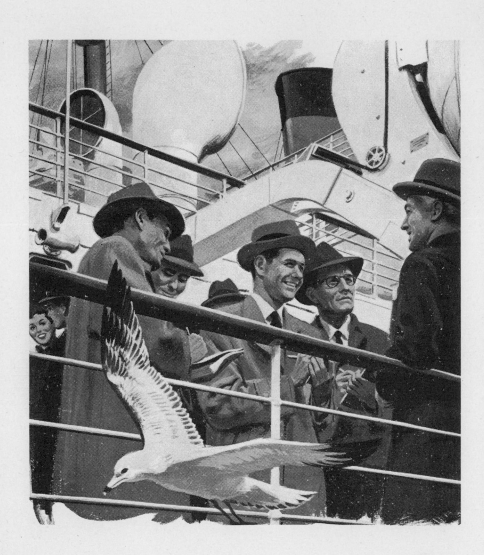

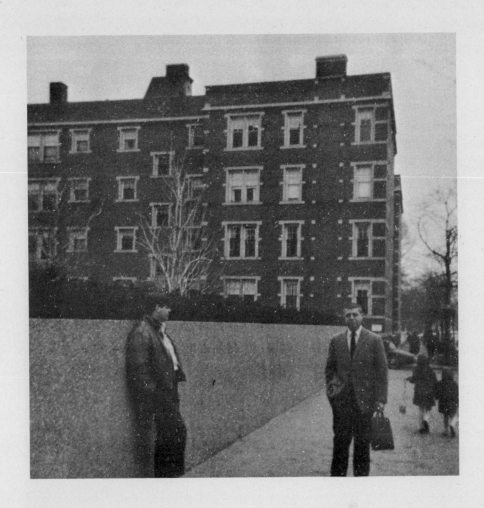

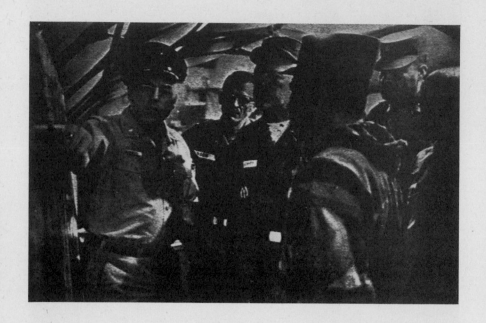

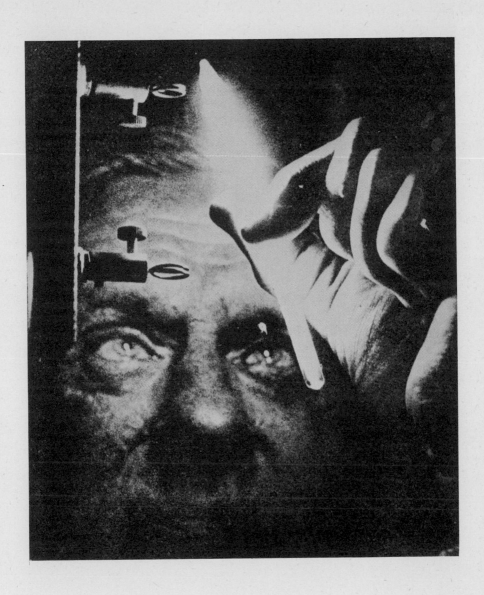

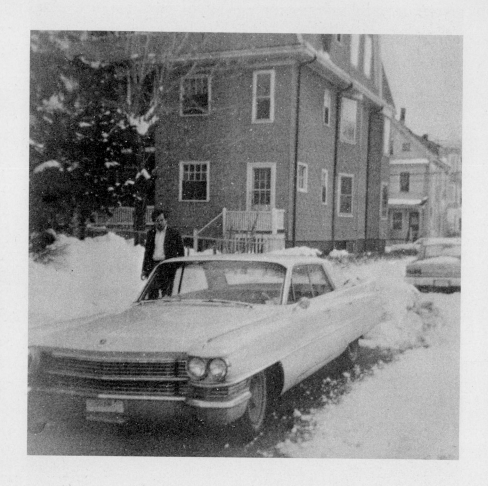

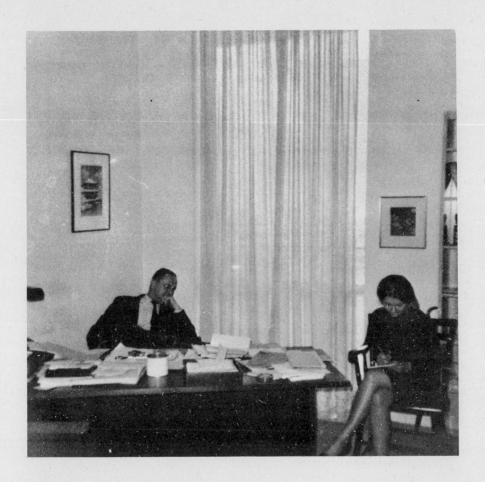

Detailed Codes for Social Variables
Related to Drinking

Variable Name	Source[a]	Description[b]

1. Variables comprising Socio-economic Complexity Scale

Hunting	Murdock—column 8	[d]scale from 0 to 9 increasing with percent of economic dependence on hunting.
Open Class System	Murdock—column 67	1 = hereditary aristocracy (D) 2 = wealth distinctions (W) 3 = no class distinctions (O)
Agriculture	Murdock—column 11	[d]scale from 0 to 9 increasing with percent of eonomic dependence on agriculture.
Degree of Jurisdictional Hierarchy	Murdock—columns 32, 33	scale from 2 to 8 representing the sum of Murdock's local and extra-local levels of hierarchy.
Permanency of Settlement Pattern	Murdock—column 30	1 = fully migratory (B) 2 = semi-permanent (S, T, W) 3 = permanent (H, N, V, X)
Size of Local Community	Murdock—column 31	[d]scale from 1 to 8 running from fewer than 50 inhabitants to more than 50,000.

2. Variables comprising the Male Institutions Scale

Presence of Male Initiation	Anthony—initiation rites Young—male sex role dramatization scale	1 = absent (Anthóny), or if Anthony lacks rating, Young's 1, 2, 3, 4.
[c]Initiation Impact	Murdock—columns 37, 38	0 = male genital mutilations before 5 years of age (0–3); adolescent segregation absent or with relatives (ARS) 1 = male genital mutilations after 5 years of age (4–8); adolescent segregation absent or with relatives (ARS)

Variable Name	*Source*[a]	*Description*[b]
		2 = male genital mutilations after 5 years of age (4–8); adolescents sleep apart from family (P)
		3 = male genital mutilations after 5 years of age (4–8); adolescents reside with peers (T)
Male Solidarity	Young—Male Solidarity Scale Whiting (1)—Men's Housing	1 = Absent: Young's 0 *or* if Young lacks rating, Whiting's 4
		2 = Present: Young's 1, 2, 3, 4 *or* if Young lacks rating, Whiting's 1, 2, 3.
Duration of Post-Partum Sex Taboos	Murdock—column 36	[d]scale from 0 to 5 running from less than a month to more than two years.
Exclusive Mother-baby Sleeping Arrangements	Whiting (2)	1 = Absent (2, 3, 4) 2 = Present (1)
Sleeping distance of Mother and Father (monogamous position)	Whiting (2)	[d]scale from 1 to 6 running from body contact to sleeping in separate villages.
Winter Temperature	Whiting (2)	[d]scale from 1 to 4 running from below 32° to over 68°
Type of Climate	Whiting (2)	1 = tropical rain forest (1) 2 = tropical savannah (2) 3 = humid climates (4) 4 = dry climates (3)

[a] References for sources are as follows:

Anthony, A., "A cross-cultural study of factors relating to male initiation rites and genital operations, Unpublished paper, Department of Social Relations, Harvard University.

Murdock, G. P., "Ethnographic Atlas," *Ethnology*, 1–4, 1960–1964.

Whiting, J. W. M. (1), Unpublished ratings assembled in J. W. M. Whiting's laboratory, Department of Social Relations, Harvard University, Cambridge, Mass.

Whiting, J. W. M. (2), "Effects of climate on certain cultural practices," in W. Goodenough, Ed., *Cultural Anthropology*. New York: McGraw-Hill, 1964, pp. 511–544.

Young, F. W., *Initiation Ceremonies*. Indianapolis: Bobbs-Merrill, 1965.

[b] Where codes have been changed from the original, the new categories are specified by name and by the original categories included in parentheses. Where codes are unchanged descriptions are marked with a "d" and are given in general form. Details are to be found in the sources cited.

[c] This recode was recommended by J. W. M. Whiting.

Motives for Drug Taking Among College Men

David C. McClelland and Robert Steele

When the research reported in this volume was started about ten years ago, alcohol was the only major "drug" or mind altering substance used regularly by a substantial proportion of the American population. In the intervening years other drugs such as marijuana and LSD have become much more popular, particularly among college students and the young. In the course of studying drinking in college students with some of the techniques described in this book, we also asked how often they had used pot (marijuana), speed (amphetamines), and acid (LSD). Thus we were in a position to find what the correlates of drug taking were in a student population—particularly the motivational correlates. Would, for example, the students who smoked pot frequently show the same motivational pattern as those who drank a lot? Or would it be a different type of student who was attracted to drug taking? In view of the intense interest today in reasons for drug taking among young people, it seemed worth working up the data for a preliminary report here, even though the information has some serious limitations. It is obtained from a small sample of college men attending a psychology course. It is garnered from what in effect was a fishing expedition in which interesting or significant correlations were selected for presentation from a mass of some hundreds of such correlations. Such a procedure necessarily capitalizes on error—some correlations would be expected to be significant by chance. And above all, the findings come from only one study—one small sample, the peculiar composition of which may have accounted for the results. The results obviously need to be checked in a number of other population groups using the same variety of research approaches employed in the study of drinking.

What follows therefore must be considered an exercise in hypothesis formation rather than hypothesis testing. Our goal was to get some preliminary idea as to what the young men who took drugs were like. The statistics employed are simply the means by which we attempted to eliminate a lot of possibilities and zero in on those which seem most worthy of further investigation. The findings gain in interest and credibility because they happen to fit pretty well with our previous work on alcohol and with certain widely held beliefs as to the characteristics of young people who take drugs.

PROCEDURE

The testing was done in a large undergraduate motivation class at Harvard University ($N = 95$, approximately ⅓ women). It was explained early in the term that a large amount of data would be collected at various times on members of the class which could be used by anyone to write research term papers focusing on correlates of particular motives. To get the motive measures, a version of the Thematic Apperception Test was administered in class early in the term, consisting of the following six pictures: ship's captain, couple on a bench by the Charles river, older man speaking to a younger man in an office, couple in a bar drinking beer, an engineer in shirtsleeves at a drawing board, a couple on a flying trapeze.

The stories written to these pictures were coded for n Achievement, n Affiliation, n Power, s and p Power, and Activity Inhibition in the standard way described earlier in this volume. Class members were also asked to fill out and hand in a long questionnaire covering many activities, as described and factor analyzed in Chapter 8, and some additional matters such as their career plans, their typical mood level, and a self-descriptive adjective check list. One item in this questionnaire asked: have you taken, or do you take frequently, any of the following? Please check:

	never	have taken once or twice	a number of times	take frequently
Pot	_____	_____	_____	_____
Speed	_____	_____	_____	_____
Acid	_____	_____	_____	_____

The answers were given completely anonymously, the connection with the TAT scores being made through a code number chosen by each student. Data obtained from the women in the class are not included in the analysis to be reported here, because the pattern of relationships for women was different, and because the focus of attention throughout this volume has been on men only. The motivational and other correlates of drug taking and drinking in women will be the subject of other reports.

This left a sample of 44 men who wrote out TAT stories and also handed in a completed questionnaire. None were freshmen, 64 percent were sophomores or juniors, the rest seniors or graduate students. Their average age was 21; approximately 77 percent of them came from middle- to upper-class families (fathers, occupation: professional or executive). They were also unusually bright, even for college students. On the SAT verbal, 76 percent scored 650 or better, and on the SAT math, 66 percent scored 700 or better. Obviously it cannot be claimed that the sample is representative even of Harvard students, let alone college students in general or young men in general. Nevertheless it probably is representative of the group which is beginning to sample extensively new types of mind altering substances.

The mode of analysis was simply to intercorrelate the motive scores and the drug taking variables with each other and with some 200 other variables derived from the questionnaire. Correlations of statistical and/or theoretical significance have been selected out for presentation below in an attempt to describe at least for this sample what the correlates of drug taking are.

RESULTS

All the students reported that they drank alcohol at least occasionally. Seventy-five percent said they had smoked pot at least once or twice; 32 percent were frequent users. Ten or approximately 23 percent had tried acid, six of whom had used it a number of times. Speed was least frequently used—only eight reporting that they had ever tried it and only three having tried it more than once or twice. In obtaining these results we used the terms the students themselves are apt to employ rather than such technical terms as marijuana, LSD or amphetamines because we were interested in the number of times they were consciously taking a "drug," as identified by such drug culture terms, rather than the technical frequency with which they had ingested a given chemical. For instance, there would have been some ambiguity in using the term amphetamines in the questionnaire, since they are taken in small amounts, especially by women, as a means of weight reduction. Only four of the sample reported themselves to be multiple drug users to the extent of having tried all of them and taken at least two of them a number of times or frequently.

The focus of this report will be on the correlates of pot smoking, because it is the only other substance besides alcohol which is commonly enough used to provide much of a basis for finding significant relationships to other variables. In a sense this may not be a serious limitation, since no one in this sample had tried either speed or acid who had not smoked pot at least a number of times. Thus using marijuana is not only the most prevalent form of participating in the "drug culture"; it also appears to be the first step that people take before experimenting with other drugs. Correlates of acid taking will also be presented for comparative purposes, but those for speed will be omitted since they yielded nothing of any significance for such a small sample of users.

Table IX.1 lays out the motivational correlates of smoking pot as obtained from the standard codes for stories written to the Thematic Apperception Test pictures.

Appendix Table IX.1—Motivational correlates of smoking pot

		Reported pot use			
Motivational variable		Frequently (H)	A number of times (M)	Once or twice or never (L)	x^2
	r	N = 14	N = 14	N = 16	
p — s Power score	.33* % p >s Power	79	43	31	7.1*
p Power score	.24 % 3 or more	50	29	19	n.s.
s Power score	−.13 % 2 or more	43	29	44	n.s.
n Power score	−.01 % 6 or more	57	36	44	n.s.
n Achievement score	−.30* % 3 or more	36	43	63	n.s.
n Affiliation score	.27⁺ % 3 or more	57	57	25 H M vs. L	4.3*
Activity Inhibition	−.07 % 3 or more	50	7	50	7.6*

$^+ p < .10$, $^* p < .05$.

The pattern of results is clearcut. The students who smoked more frequently had power motivation scores which were oriented more often in the personal than in the socialized power direction. The finding is the same as that reported for older men who are heavy drinkers in Chapter 8. Thus, using marijuana seems to be associated with the same rebellious concern for personal dominance that characterizes older men who drink liquor heavily. The next two lines in Table XI.1 show that the relationship with the p–s Power score is a product both of a positive correlation of pot smoking with the p Power score and a negative correlation with the s Power score. And there is no particular correlation with the overall *n* Power score not broken down as to its personal or socialized orientation. Furthermore a double classification by *n* Power and Activity Inhibition does not show, as it does for drinking (Chapter 7), that drug takers tend to be high in *n* Power and low in inhibition. The p–s Power score is apparently a more sensitive indicator of who is most apt to smoke pot more often. Men with high *n* Achievement smoke less and those with high *n* Affiliation smoke more. The relationship to the Activity Inhibition code is curvilinear. Those who smoke either very little or frequently score higher in Activity Inhibition than those who smoke moderately.

Apparently, inhibited people with high *n* Achievement and a socialized power drive who are "loners" (not interested in affiliation) are least apt to get involved in the new drug culture. On the other hand, those who are impulsive, gregarious (concerned about friendship), low in achievement motivation and high in a rebellious concern for personal dominance are most apt to use pot frequently. These findings fit quite well with widely held views in the university community about differences between drug users and non-users, both by officials and students. The non-users are "straight arrow"—achievement oriented, self-controlled, not particularly concerned about maintaining friendly relations with their peers, and committed to exercising power through normal socialized channels. The users, on the other hand, are impulsive, affiliative and rebellious. The only anomaly is the relatively high Activity Inhibition score for the frequent pot smokers. Two possible explanations come to mind. Either heavy users are naturally inhibited people who require pot smoking for release, or they are so involved in what is clearly an illegal activity that they are more afraid of getting caught, and hence tell more stories in which activities are blocked or stopped.

If the motivational pattern of the pot smokers is reasonably clear, what other activities are they more likely to engage in? Since they seem more concerned with personal than socialized power, it seems logical to begin by assembling the correlations of marijuana use with various types of assertive activities. In Table IX.2 the activities have been roughly grouped under what might be called normative assertion versus rebellious assertion and their relationship to acid and liquor use is also given for comparative purposes. Correlates with beer consumption were also inspected, but they add little new to the over-all picture. Unfortunately a question on wine consumption was not included.

Most striking among those who smoke pot is a predilection for a certain type of physical violence. They are more apt to participate in collision sports (football, hockey, wrestling, boxing), to have organized demonstrations of protest and to accept violence as part of them, and to have engaged in a physical fight at some time in the last three years. On the other hand, they have engaged in significantly fewer hostile acts like taking a sign from a public place, walking out on a date, throwing things around the room, yelling at someone in traffic or in a store, etc. It is not altogether clear what is going on here. Two hypotheses suggest themselves. On the one hand, it may be that pot smokers are more prone to physical violence and less prone to interpersonally aggressive acts. Such an explanation would fit with two rather commonly held beliefs about pot smokers—one, held mostly by adults, that they are more prone to violence, "trashing" and the like and the other, held more often by the students themselves, that they are more peaceable and willing to let things be. On the other hand, it is worth noting that both collision sports and violent demonstrations have a measure of social sanction by the group of which the student is a member. He is being violent on behalf of a "team." The other types of violence like walking out on a date or taking a sign from a public place are clearly selfish acts of hostility. The weakness of this interpretation is that it does not fit particularly well with the fact that they also tend to drive cars faster and get into physical fights, which are not particularly socialized acts of assertion. And furthermore their p–s Power score would also not lead one to expect them to focus their violence in socialized channels. What seems more to characterize their violence is its "impersonal" or alienated quality. They seem able to be violent against impersonal others or the system as in a collision sport or a violent protest, but not against particular individuals. Their alienation is further suggested by their more frequent statement that they would like to have not shown up for a test just because they "didn't feel like it." This is the one aggressive impulse that they significantly more often admit to having had in sharp contrast to most aggressive impulsives which they report as having had *less* often. It alone among the aggressive acts can most easily be interpreted as a kind of alienation from the system.

Appendix Table IX.2—Correlations of normative and rebellious assertive activities with use of mind-altering substances among college men (N = 44)

Normative assertion	Pot use[1] (N = 33)	Acid use[1] (N = 10)	Liquor use[2] (N = 44)	Measures
Participation in				
Collision sports[3]	.31 *	.13	.19	13 in at least one
Non-contact sports[4]	.03	−.22	.01	Median = 1.5
Attending varsity sports events	−.08	−.32 *	.17	Median = between 5 and 10 a year.
TV sports events watched	.10	−.35 *	.46 *	Median = 1–3 a month.
Rebellious assertion				
Fastest speed driven a car	.29 +	.23	.14	Median = 97.5 miles per hour.
Car accidents	.09	−.09	.25 +	20 reported at least one or more
Demonstrations, protests				
Level of participation in	.42 **	.20	.08	23 participated from 1, peripherally, to 5 as organizers.
Accept violence in	.39 **	−.01	.38	15 "yes," to: "would you participate in?"
Aggressive impulses				
To take sign in public place	−.37 *	−.29 +	.16	12 "haven't but would like to".
To walk out on a date	.05	.02	.35 *	13 "haven't but would like to".
To skip test	.38 *	.18	−.08	23 "haven't but would like to".
Hostile acts committed[5]	−.38 *	−.12	.09	No. at least once, median = 7 out of 13.
Physical fight	.28 +	−.12	.31 *	Number of fights = 12.

[+]p <.10, * p <.05, ** p <.01.
[1] Never = 0, once or twice = 1, a number of times = 2, frequently = 3.
[2] At least 3–5 drinks during at least 2–4 parties a month or 6–8 drinks 6–12 times a year (N = 22) vs. all lesser amounts (N = 32).
[3] From "don't play" through "intramural" to "varsity participation" for football, hockey, wrestling, boxing, soccer, lacrosse, fencing, rugby, judo.
[4] Same scale for crew, sailing, swimming, golf, track, cross country, bowling, shooting, skating, surfing, billiards, gymnastics, horse sports.
[5] Number of 13 activities done at least once such as those in table and "yelled at someone in traffic," "threw things around the room," "made hostile remarks to storekeepers," etc.

The contrasting pattern of relationships with assertive activities for liquor drinkers is interesting. They too are prone to physical violence, a fact which gains added significance when it is noted that pot smoking and liquor drinking in this sample are uncorrelated (see Table IX.3). Those who drink more liquor than usual—which incidentally is not a high level of drinking as contrasted with the older men studied in previous chapters—are more apt to have been in a physical fight and to accept violence in a demonstration. But there the similarity ends. The liquor drinker's hostility seems to be of a more generalized type in the sense that he is more prone to want to walk out on a date or to have had an accident while driving. He is also more likely to get vicarious satisfaction for assertive impulses by watching sports events, particularly on TV.

Acid users, on the other hand, are quite different from those who use either pot or liquor frequently. They are not particularly prone to violence or assertiveness of any kind. The low positive correlations with fast driving and level of participation in demonstrations are reduced to near zero when the correlation with pot smoking is partialed out. That is, as Table IX.3 shows, acid users are also much more likely to smoke pot and if the influence of this variable is eliminated, it is clear that violence or assertiveness is not a dimension which is associated either positively or negatively with using acid. On the other hand, acid users do tend to be significantly less interested in attending sports events or watching them on TV. They apparently have other things on their mind.

The remaining variables covered in Table IX.3 are of a more miscellaneous character but they do fill out the picture in important respects. To begin with, pot smoking is more apt to be engaged in by younger students (in this sample, aged 18–20). Probably this is not so much an age effect as a generation effect. That is, the younger students have been more exposed to pot smoking in high school whereas when the older students were in high school the use of marijuana was undoubtedly less. The fact that older students are also higher in n Achievement is not surprising since some selective factor is probably at work eliminating from school—particularly

Appendix Table IX.3—Correlations of use of mind-altering substances with characteristics of college men (N = 44)

	Pot use[1] (N = 33)	Acid use[1] (N = 10)	Liquor use[2] (N = 44)	p Power	n Achievement
Age (Mean = 21)	−.36 *	.08	−.16	−.02	.40 *
Pot use	—	.47 **	.04	.24	−.30 *
Acid use	—	—	−.24	.19	−.09
Liquor use	—	—	—	−.31 *	.01
Level of participation[3] in organized societies	−.04	.06	.27 +	.04	.21
Art works owned (N = 15)[4]	−.33 *	−.23	−.02	−.14	.35 *
Skis owned (N = 11)	.32 *	.08	.23	−.01	−.04
Postgraduation plans[5]	−.49 **	−.12	−.01	−.49	.22
Artistic career[6]	.31 *	.22	.02	−.09	−.21
Business career[6]	.01	−.14	.44 **	−.24	.06
Supervise others[7]	−.10	−.19	.45 **	−.26 +	.33
Gain reputation[7]	−.27 +	−.37 *	.38 *	−.19	.14
Released life style[8]	.38 *	−.03	.11	.18	−.29 *
Lively social presence[9]	.10	−.18	.32 *	.17	.14

+ $p<.10$, * $p<.05$, ** $p<.01$.
[1] Never = 0, once or twice = 1, a number of times = 2, frequently = 3.
[2] See footnote 2, Table IX.2.
[3] Scale of 1 (inactive) to 5 (very active).
[4] Including quality reproductions of paintings.
[5] 0 = None, 1 = escape, 2 = continue education, 3 = into labor pool.
[6] Number of mentions of a possible career in these areas.
[7] Importance on scale of 0–4 of such aspects in future career.
[8] Sum of disagree-agree scale of 1–6 for the following items:
  I enjoy playing cards for money.
  I like people who spend freely.
  I dislike following a set schedule.
  (Disagree) I always like to keep my things neat and tidy and in good order.
[9] Sum of disagree-agree on scale of 1–6 for:
  I would rate myself as a lively individual.
  (Disagree) I am inclined to stay in the background on social occasions.

graduate school—those with less of an interest in a career. As already noted, smoking pot is highly correlated with using acid and also with speed ($r = .37, p < .05$). What is new is a nearly significant negative correlation between the use of acid and liquor. In other words, people who use acid may drink less. Could it be that the newer drugs are substituting for the old one—liquor? The question is raised most sharply by the most startling finding in the top portion of Table IX.3—namely, the significant *negative* correlation between the p Power score and heavier liquor drinking. This relationship is the direct opposite of all other such relationships reported elsewhere in this book. Our major conclusion up until now has been that liquor drinking is motivated by a personal power concern, yet here we find that a personal power concern is associated with lower drinking levels. Matters are really not helped greatly by noting that the s Power score also correlates $-.27$ with liquor use which reduces the p–s Power correlation with liquor use essentially to zero. The total n Power score is also negatively associated with liquor drinking ($r = -.26, p < -.10$). No matter how you look at it, contrary to all previous findings, power concerns in this sample are *negatively* associated with heavier drinking.

Aside from cursing his luck or the instability of psychological findings, what can the investigator do to explain this paradoxical fact? The substitutability of acid for liquor may provide him with the clue he needs. As already noted, in this sample p Power or the p–s Power score are associated with use of the newer drugs. Could it be that rebellious or power-oriented young men no longer turn to liquor but to the newer drugs that are widely used? This might explain a lack of correlation of p Power with liquor consumption, but why a negative correlation? Why should the people *low* in power concerns drink *more*? Some additional facts help clear up the picture. To begin with, the upper half of the distribution of liquor consumption in this sample represents moderate, not really heavy drinking. It is considerably lower than what was defined as heavy drinking for the older men in Chapter 8. In fact the negative relationship of liquor consumption to personal power concerns becomes even more marked if the cutting point for what is considered "heavy" drinking is lowered to 3 to 5 drinks once a month or every other month. Fifty-four percent of the men who have lower p than s Power scores reached this level of consumption as compared with only 23 percent of those who had higher p than s Power scores ($\chi^2 = 4.1, p < .05$). In other words what we are comparing here is light with moderate drinking, not light with heavy drinking, and we are concluding that college men with lower p than s Power scores are more apt to indulge in *moderate* liquor drinking. Other correlates of moderate drinking in Tables IX.2 and IX.3 suggest that these Harvard undergraduates are not particularly assertive or rebellious but are fairly conventional in the sense of participating more in organized clubs and societies, wanting business careers in which they can gain a reputation and supervise others and believing that they have a lively social presence. They may not be as conventional or "straight arrow" as the men with the n Achievement, as shown in the last column of Table IX.3, but their interest in sports and more "normative" forms of violence show that they are well within the establishment mold. In other words, moderate drinking is just part of being more conventional for these college men who are not power-oriented enough to want to break the normal mold.

On the other hand, those young men who are rebellious (high in p Power) seem to turn to the newer drugs as an outlet for an anti-establishment life style. Those who smoke pot tend not to have post-graduation plans, tend not to follow a set schedule or keep things in good order, and want a career in which an artistic component is prominent. On the other hand, they are not interested in a career which would gain them a reputation or in acquiring prestigious works of art. This pattern of correlations is very similar to what it is for those with high p Power scores. The correlation between the rank orders of the correlations in the pot use column and the p Power column is .74, $N = 11, p < .05$. (See Appendix III for a discussion of the method used here.) It is worth noting that the p Power score correlates .31, $p < .05$ with mentioning a future career which involves working for the community—the poor, the discriminated against, the disadvantaged. While the same correlation is only .10 with pot smoking, nevertheless the suggestion is clearly there that p Power leads to an identification with the powerless who should react against the powerful establishment, through which s Power people normally work. This may be partly the reason for participation in even violent demonstrations against the establishment.

In contrast, the rank order of the correlations in column 1 for pot users is almost the direct opposite of the rank order of the correlations in the last column in Table IX.3 for n Achievement. The rho representing the intercorrelation of the two columns is $-.99, N = 11, p < .01$. Men with high n Achievement behave in ways opposite to those men who smoke marijuana frequently. Those with high n Achievement are likely to own art reproductions, to want to have a career in which they supervise others and to run an orderly planned life. It is small wonder that the "hippies" and the "straight arrows" have such contempt for each other. They want very different things in life and behave in very different ways.

The picture for the acid users is not so clear, particularly when one partials out the effect of pot use. They say they are not interested in a career that gains a reputation—which they shouldn't be if they continue to take LSD—and they are less often apt to describe themselves as realistic. Otherwise they behave like the pot users but to a lesser degree.

What emerges from all this is a picture of pot smoking as the mode for expressing personal power drives or rebellion among younger students which formerly was expressed through heavier drinking and which among older men is still expressed through really heavy liquor drinking. (See Chapter 8). We can understand better the by now almost classic confrontation between the pot-smoking student and the liquor-drinking older policeman, both of whom may be finding satisfaction for personal power drives in violence. Another consideration is the cross-sex identity conflict which, we have argued in Chapter 13, may be the reason for a heightened p Power concern among heavy liquor drinkers. If the students are ranked in terms of total drug use, by adding frequency of use of pot, speed and acid, the first nine all show signs of a below normal masculine orientation. As Carlsmith has pointed out (1963), college men normally score higher on the math section of the SAT than they do on the verbal section, and vice versa for college women. Men with higher verbal relative to math scores show signs of cross-sex identity. In this sample, 76 percent had higher math than verbal scores, the median advantage on the math test being 30 points. If drug use is summed across pot, speed, and acid, the first nine of the heaviest multiple drug users, scored at or below this median, as contrasted with 20 percent of the next 10 (mostly heavy pot smokers), and 50 percent of the remaining 22 who used drugs occasionally or not at all ($\chi^2 = 9.61, df = 2, p < .01$). As expected, 62 percent of those below the median in masculine orientation had higher p than s Power scores as contrasted with 45 percent of those above the median (difference not significant). What all this suggests is that both p Power and multiple drug use may represent a kind of rebellious assertiveness in men who are not strongly masculine identified. On the other hand heavy pot smoking (as opposed to multiple drug use) *is* associated in this sample with above average masculine identification. The findings are far from definitive, but they do point to the heaviest drug use among those men in whom masculine and feminine orientations are more evenly balanced—an interpretation which would not be widely disputed in the drug culture itself.

One might speculate as to whether the effects of marijuana on fantasy are similar to the effects of alcohol on fantasy as reported in earlier chapters. Unfortunately the arousal studies have not as yet been done, but one might expect them to show some similarities and some differences. That is, by analogy, if alcohol arouses p Power thoughts and is consumed by those with a high level of p Power thinking to start with, then one would predict that the same might be true for pot. However, one would also expect some differences, because the life styles of the pot users and liquor drinkers have turned out to be different in some important respects. The marijuana smokers are less conventional, more interested in "hanging loose" in a relaxed, artistic life style in which there is a significantly lower level of interpersonal hostility. On the other hand, they seem more willing and able to become physically violent in groups—in collision sports and political demonstrations, for example. Their violence is somehow more impersonal or against the system than that of the heavy drinkers, which suggests that the effects of marijuana on internal thought processes may be different from the effects of alcohol as reported earlier in this book. The matter is certainly worth investigation. What little data we have does not really permit us to disentangle cause and effect. We do not know whether the correlations obtained result from the fact that rebellious people choose to smoke pot or from the fact that pot smokers tend to have their thinking and acting altered in significant ways from the effects of the drug. To judge from our work with alcohol, we would expect that causation would run both ways in a mutually reinforcing cycle. And even with the scanty data we do have, it seems clear that the reason for taking acid and its effects are part of another mutually reinforcing cycle which only partly overlaps with the cycle for pot which in turn only partly overlaps with the cycle for liquor.

So in presenting even these tentative findings, we have succeeded only in complicating the picture and raising more questions than we can answer. To add to the investigator's problem, the scene is changing rapidly. The reasons why students try out newer mind altering substances may change as the phenomenon gets more widespread. In any case even today there is considerable experimentation with multiple drug use. A typical college party today may begin with two or three drinks and continue with a number of joints (marijuana cigarettes), and some sweet wine. All we can say with any certainty is that for at least one type of sophisticated highly intelligent male undergraduate, pot smoking appears to be replacing heavier drinking as an outlet for rebellious personal power concerns, which have somehow become associated with championing the cause of the underdog against authority.

Bibliography

Adler, N. and Goleman, D. Gambling and alcoholism: symptom substitution and functional equivalents. *Quarterly Journal of Studies on Alcohol*, 1969, 30, 733–737.

Alcoholics Anonymous. New York: A. A. World Service, Inc., 1955, pp. 60–61.

Arimoni, A. *Psicoanalisis de la Dinamica de un Pueblo.* Mexico: Universidad Nacional Autonoma de Mexico, 1961.

Atkinson, J. W. Motivational determinants of risk-taking behavior, *Psychological Review*, 1957, 64, 359–372.

Atkinson, J. W. (Ed.) *Motives in fantasy, action, and society.* Princeton, N.J.: Van Nostrand, 1958.

Bacon, M. K., Barry, H. and Child, I. L. A cross-cultural study of drinking: II. Relation to other features of culture. *Quarterly Journal on Studies of Alcohol*, 1965, 3, 29–48.

Bacon, M. K., Barry, H., Child, I. L. and Snyder, C. R. A cross-cultural study of drinking: V. Detailed definitions and data. *Quarterly Journal of Studies on Alcohol*, 1965, Supplement No. 3, 78–111.

Bales, R. F. Cultural differences in rates of alcoholism. *Quarterly Journal of Studies on Alcohol*, 1946, 6, 480–499.

Banfield, E. C. *The moral basis of a backward society.* Glencoe, Ill.: The Free Press, 1958.

Barry, H., Bacon, M. K. and Child, I. L. A cross-cultural survey of some sex differences in socialization. *Journal of Abnormal and Social Psychology*, 1957, 55, 327–332.

Barry, H., Buchwald, C., Child, I. L. and Bacon, M. K. A cross-cultural study of drinking: IV. Comparisons with Horton ratings. *Quarterly Journal of Studies on Alcohol*, Supplement No. 3 (April, 1965), 62–77.

Blane, H. T. The personality of the alcoholic. *The role of the nurse in the care of the alcoholic patient in a general hospital.* Conference at Chatham, Mass., 1960.

Blum, E. M. Psychoanalytic views of alcoholism: a review. *Quarterly Journal of Studies on Alcohol*, 1966, 27, 259–299.

Bowman, K. The treatment of alcoholism. *Quarterly Journal of Studies on Alcohol*, 1956, 17, 318–324.

Brown, J. E. *The sacred pipe. Black Elk's account of the seven rites of the Oglala Sioux.* Norman: University of Oklahoma Press, 1953.

Buchwald, C., Child, I. L. and Bacon, M. K. A cross-cultural study of drinking: IV. Comparisons with Horton's ratings. *Quarterly Journal of Studies on Alcohol*, 1965, Supplement No. 3, 50–62.

Buhler, C. and Lefever, D. W. A Rorschach study on the psychological characteristics of alcoholics. *Quarterly Journal of Studies on Alcohol*, 1947, 8, 197–260.

Bunzel, R. The role of alcoholism in two central American cultures. *Psychiatry*, 1940, 3, 361–387.

Burton, R. V. and Whiting, J. W. M. The absent father and cross-sex identity. *Merrill-Palmer Quarterly*, 1961, 7, 85–95.

Cahalan, D., Cisin, I. H. and Crossley, H. M. *American drinking practices.* A national study of drinking behavior and attitudes. Monograph No. 6, Rutgers Center of Alcohol Studies, New Brunswick, N.J.: Rutgers University, 1970.

Child, I. L., Bacon, M. K. and Barry, H. A cross-cultural study of drinking: I. Descriptive measurements of drinking customs. *Quarterly Journal of Studies on Alcohol*, Supplement No. 3, 1965, 1–28.

Child, I. L., Barry, H. and Bacon, M. K. A cross-cultural study of drinking: III. Sex differences. *Quarterly Journal of Studies on Alcohol*, Supplement No. 3, 1965.

Clark, R. A. The projective measurement of experimentally induced levels of sexual motivation. *Journal of Experimental Psychology*, 1952, 11, 391–399.

Clark, R. A., Teevan, R. and Ricciuti, H. N. Hope of success and fear of failure as aspects of need for achievement. *Journal of Abnormal and Social Psychology*, 1956, 53, 182–186.

Couch, A. S. *The DATA-TEXT system.* A computer language for social science research. Preliminary manual. Harvard University, Department of Social Relations, March, 1967.

Couch, A. and Keniston, K. Yeasayers and naysayers: agreeing response set as a personality variable. *Journal of Abnormal and Social Psychology*, 1960, 60, 151–174.

D'Andrade, R. G. Anthropological studies of dreams. In Hsu (Ed.), *Psychological anthropology*. Homewood, Ill.: Dorsey Press, 1961, pp. 296–332.

D'Andrade, R. G. Father absence and cross-sex identification. Ph.D. Dissertation, Harvard University, 1962.

Davis, W. N. A cross-cultural study of drunkenness. Unpublished A.B. Thesis, Harvard University, 1964.

Davis, W. N. Drinking: a search for power or for nurturance? Unpublished Ph.D. Thesis, Harvard University, 1969.

deCharms, R. *Personal causation.* New York: Academic Press, 1968.

Deloria, V., Jr. *Custer died for your sins.* London: The Macmillan Company, 1969.

Ekman, G., Frankenhaeuser, M., Goldberg, L., Bjerver, K. and Myrsten, A. Effects of alcohol intake on subjective and objective variables over a five-hour period. Stockholm, Sweden: University of Stockholm. Reports from the Psychological Laboratory, No. 129, 1962.

Erikson, E. H. Psychological reality and historical actuality. Chapter 5 in *Insight and responsibility*. New York: Norton, 1964.

Field, P. B. A new cross-cultural study of drunkenness. In D. J. Pittman and C. R. Snyder (Eds.), *Society, culture, and drinking patterns*. New York: Wiley, 1962, pp. 48–74.

Force, R. C. Development of a covert test for the detection of alcoholism by a keying of the Kuder Preference Record. *Quarterly Journal of Studies on Alcohol*, 1958, 19, 72–78.

Franck, K. and Rosen, E. A projective test of masculinity-femininity. *Journal of Consulting Psychology*, 1949, 13, 247–256.

Frankenhaeuser, M. Behavioral efficiency as related to adrenaline release. University of Stockholm: Reports from the Psychological Laboratories, No. 268, 1968.

Frankenhaeuser, M., Myrsten, A. L. and Järpe, Gundea. Effects of a moderate dose of alcohol on intellectual functions. Reports from the Psychological Laboratory of the University of Stockholm, 1962, No. 118.

Frenkel-Brunswik, E. Motivation and behavior. *Genetic Psychology Monographs*, 1942, 26, 121–165.

Fromm, E. *Man for himself*. New York: Holt, Rinehart and Winston, 1947.

Fromm, E. *The heart of man*. New York: Harper and Row, 1964.

Gerard, D. L. and Saenger, G. Interval between intake and follow-up as a factor in the evaluation of patients with a drinking problem. *Quarterly Journal of Studies on Alcohol*, 1959, 20, 620–630.

Goncalves de Lima, O. *El Maguey y El Pulque en los Codices Mexicanos*. Mexico: Fondo de Cultura Economica, 1965.

Gough, H. F. *Manual for the California Psychological Inventory*. Palo Alto, California, Consulting Psychologists Press, 1957.

Halpern, F. Studies of compulsive drinkers: Psychological test results. *Quarterly Journal of Studies on Alcohol*, 1946, 6, 468–479.

Harrington, C. *Errors in sex-role behavior in teen-age boys*. New York: Columbia Teachers College Press, 1970.

Hassrick, R. B. *The Sioux, life and customs of a warrior society*. Norman: University of Oklahoma Press, 1964.

Heckhausen, H. Achievement motive research: current problems and some contributions towards a general theory of motivation. In W. Arnold (Ed.), *Nebraska symposium on motivation 1968*. Lincoln: University of Nebraska Press, 1968.

Horton, D. The functions of alcohol in primitive societies: a cross-cultural study. *Quarterly Journal of Studies on Alcohol*, 1943, 4, 199–320.

Hyde, G. E. *Red Cloud's folk. A history of the Oglala Sioux Indians*. Norman: University of Oklahoma Press, 1937.

Hyde, G. E. *Spotted Tail's folk. A history of the Brule Sioux*. Norman: University of Oklahoma Press, 1961.

Jellinek, E. M. The problems of alcohol. In *Alcohol, science and society*. New Haven: Quarterly Journal of Studies on Alcohol, 1945. Pp. 13–29.

Jellinek, E. M. *The disease concept of alcoholism*. New Haven: Hill House Press, 1960.

Jessor, R., Graves, T. D., Hanson, R. C. and Jessor, S. L. *Society, personality and deviant behavior*. New York: Holt, Rinehart and Winston, 1968.

Jones, M. C. Correlates and antecedents of adult drinking patterns. Paper read at Western Psychological Association, Honolulu, June, 1965.

Jones, M. C. Personality correlates and antecedents of drinking patterns in adult males. *Journal of Consulting and Clinical Psychology*, 1968, 32, 2–12.

Kagan, J. and Moss, H. *Birth to maturity*. New York: Wiley, 1962.

Kalin, R. Alcohol, sentience, and inhibition: An experimental study. Unpublished doctoral dissertation, Harvard University, 1964.

Kalin, R. Effects of inhibition on thematic apperception. Paper presented at the meetings of the Eastern Psychological Association, New York, 1966.

Kalin, R., Davis, W. N. and McClelland, D. C. The relationship between use of alcohol and thematic content of folktales in primitive societies. In P. J. Stone *et al.* (Eds.) *The general inquirer: A computer approach to content analysis in the behavioral sciences*. Cambridge, Mass.: M.I.T. Press, 1966.

Kalin, R., McClelland, D. C. and Kahn, M. The effects of male social drinking on fantasy. *Journal of Personality and Social Psychology*, 1965, 1, 441–452.

Karp, S. A., Witkin, H. A. and Goodenough, D. R. Alcoholism and psychological differentiation: effect of alcohol on field dependence. *Journal of Abnormal Psychology*, 1965, 70, 262–265.

Keller, M. The definition of alcoholism and the estimation of its prevalence. In D. J. Pittman and C. R. Snyder (Eds.), *Society, culture and drinking pattern*. New York: Wiley, 1962.

Keniston, K. *Young radicals*. New York: Harcourt, Brace and World, 1968.

Klein, G. S. On inhibition, disinhibition and "primary process" in thinking. In G. S. Nielson (Ed.), *Clinical Psychology*. Proceedings of the XIV International Congress of Applied Psychology. Copenhagen: Munksgaard, 1962.

Knight, R. P. The psychodynamics of chronic alcoholism. *Journal of Nervous and Mental Diseases*, 1937, 86, 538–543.

Knupfer, G. Some methodological problems in the epideminology of alcoholic beverage usage: the definition of amount of intake. Drinking Practices Study, State of California Department of Public Health. Unpublished paper, 1964.

Kolb, D. A. and Rubin, I. M. An exercise in the dynamics of the helping relationship. Paper published by Development Research Associates, Inc., Cambridge, Mass. 1967.

Kuckenberg, L. G. Effect of early father absence on scholastic aptitude. Ph.D. Thesis, Harvard University, 1963.

Lazarus, R. S. A substitute-defensive conception of apperceptive fantasy. In J. Kagan and G. S. Lesser (Eds.), *Contemporary issues in thematic apperceptive methods*. Springfield, Illinois, Charles C. Thomas, 1961.

Lazarus, R. S. Story telling and the measurement of motivation: the direct versus substitutive controversy. *Journal of Consulting Psychology*, 1966, 30, 483–487.

Lee, R. B. What "hunters" do for a living: or, how to make out on scarce resources. Paper delivered to "Man the hunter" Symposium, Chicago, April 6–9, 1966.

Lee, R. and DeVore, I. (Eds.), *Man the hunter*. Chicago: Albine Publishing Company, 1968.

Lemert, E. M. Dependency in married alcoholics. *Quarterly Journal of Studies on Alcohol*, 1962, 23, 590–608.

Lentz, R. F. *et al.* Personality correlates of alcoholic beverage consumption. *Character and Personality*, 1943, 12, 54.

Levy, R. I. The psychodynamic functions of alcohol. *Quarterly Journal of Studies on Alcohol*, 1958, 19, 649–659.

Lewis, O. *The children of Sanchez*, New York: Random House, 1961.

Lisansky, E. S. The etiology of alcoholism: the role of psychological predisposition. *Quarterly Journal of Studies on Alcohol*, 1960, 21, 314–343.

Lolli, G., Serianni, E., Golder, G. M. and Luzzato-Fegiz, P. *Alcohol in Italian culture*. New York: The Free Press, 1958.

McCarthy, R. G. *Drinking and intoxication*. New York: The Free Press, 1959.

McClelland, D. C. *Personality*. New York: William Sloane Association, 1951.

McClelland, D. C. Methods of measuring human motivation, Chapter 1 in J. W. Atkinson (Ed.), *Motives in fantasy, action, and society*. Princeton, N.J.: Van Nostrand, 1958.

McClelland, D. C. *The achieving society*, Princeton, N.J.: Van Nostrand, 1961.

McClelland, D. C. Wanted: a new self-image for women. *Daedalus* issue: *The woman in America*. Boston: Houghton Mifflin, 1965.

McClelland, D. C. Longitudinal trends in the relation of thought to action. *Journal of Consulting Psychology*, 1966, 30, 479–483.

McClelland, D. C., Atkinson, J. W., Clark, R. A. and Lowell, E. *The achievement motive*. New York: Appleton-Century-Crofts, 1953.

McClelland, D. C. and Winter, D. G. *Motivating economic achievement*. New York: The Free Press, 1969.

McCord, W. and McCord, J. *Origins of alcoholism*. Stanford: Stanford University Press, 1960.

McGuire, M. T., Stein, S. and Mendelson, J. H. Comparative psychosocial studies of alcoholic and nonalcoholic subjects undergoing experimentally induced ethanol intoxication. *Psychosomatic Medicine*, 1966, 28, 13–25.

MacAndrew, C. The differentiation of male alcoholic outpatients from nonalcoholic psychiatric outpatients by means of the MMPI. *Quarterly Journal of Studies on Alcohol*, 1965, 26, 238–246.

MacAndrew, C. and Edgerton, R. B. *Drunken Comportment*. Chicago: Aldine, 1969.

MacAndrew, C. and Geertsma, R. H. An analysis of responses of alcoholics to scale 4 of the MMPI. *Quarterly Journal of Studies on Alcohol*, 1963, 24, 23–38.

Maccoby, M., Modiano, N. and Lander, P. Games and social character in a Mexican village. *Psychiatry*, 1964, 27, 150–162.

Machover, S. and Puzzo, F. S. Clinical and objective studies of personality variables in, alcoholism. *Quarterly Journal of Studies on Alcohol*, 1959, 20, 505–519.

Martinez, M. S. El Alcohol en la Salud Individual y Colectiva. *Higiene*, 1963, 2, 70–85.

Maynard, E. Drinking as part of an adjustment among the Oglala Sioux. *Pine Ridge Research Bulletin*, 1969, 9, 35–52.

Mindell, C. Quoted in E. Maynard. Drinking as part of an adjustment among the Oglala Sioux. *Pine Ridge Research Bulletin*, 1969, 9, 51.

Mindlin, D. F. The characteristics of alcoholics as related to prediction of therapeutic outcome. *Quarterly Journal of Studies on Alcohol*, 1959, 20, 604–619.

Moore, R. A. The manifest dream in alcoholism. *Quarterly Journal of Studies on Alcohol*, 1962, 23, 583–589.

Munroe, R. L. Couvade. Unpublished dittoed paper, Department of Social Relations, Harvard University, 1960.

Munroe, R. L. Couvade practices of the Black Carib: a psychological study. Unpublished Ph.D. Thesis, Department of Social Relations, Harvard University, 1964.

Murdock, G. P. *Ethnographic Atlas. Ethnology*, 1–4, 1960–1964.

Murray, H. A. *Explorations in personality: A clinical and experimental study of fifty men of college age*. New York: Oxford University Press, 1938.

Neihardt, J. C. *Black Elk speaks: being a life story of a holy man of the Oglala Sioux*. New York: Morrow, 1932.

Nezei, A. and Erdly, E. As alkoholista személyiségszerkezet megmutatkozása a Rorschachpróbában, (Personality structure of the alcoholic as reflected in the Rorschach test). *Pszichólogiai Tanulmányok*, Budapest, 1966, 639–658.

Osgood, C. Semantic differential technique in the comparative study of cultures, *American Anthropoligist*, 1964, 66, 3.

Parsons, T. and Bales, R. F. *Family, socialization and interaction process*, New York: The Free Press, 1955.

Pátkai, P. Interindividual differences in diurnal variations in alertness, performance, and adrenaline excretion. Stockholm, Sweden: University of Stockholm, Reports from the Psychological Laboratories, 1969.

Paz, O. *El Laberinto de la Soledad*. Mexico: Fondo de Cultura Economica, 1959.

Peterson, R. E. The student left in American higher education. *Daedalus*, 1968, 97: 1, 293–317.

Pittman, D. J. and Gordon, C. W. *Revolving door*. New Haven, Conn.: Yale Center of Alcohol Studies, 1958.

Pittman, D. J. and Gordon, C. W. Criminal careers of the chronic drunkenness offender. *Quarterly Journal of Studies on Alcohol*, 1958, 19, 255–268.

Pittman, D. J. and Snyder, C. R. *Society, culture, and drinking patterns*. New York: Wiley, 1962.

Pollack, D. Experimental intoxication of alcoholics and normals: some psychological changes. Ph.D. Thesis, University of California at Los Angeles, 1965. Ann Arbor, Mich.: University Microfilms, Inc.

Quaranta, J. V. Alcoholism: a study of emotional maturity and homosexuality as related factors in compulsive drinking. Unpublished doctoral dissertation Fordham University, New York, 1947.

Remirez, S. *El Mexicano.* Mexico: Pat-Mexicano, 1960.

Research conference on problems of alcohol and alcoholism. *Quarterly Journal of Studies on Alcohol,* 1959, 20, 415–672.

Rosenthal, R. On the social psychology of the psychological experiment: The experimenter's hypothesis as unintended determinant of experimental results. *American Scientist,* 1963, 51, 268–283.

Sadoun, R., Lolli, G. and Silverman, M. *Drinking in French culture.* New Brunswick, N. J.: Rutgers Center of Alcohol Studies, 1965.

Sanford, N. Personality and patterns of alcohol consumption. *Journal of Consulting and Clinical Psychology,* 1968, 32, 13–17.

Sangree, W. H. The social functions of drinking in Bantu Tiriki. In D. Pittman and C. R. Snyder (Eds.), *Society, culture and drinking pattern.* New York: Wiley, 1962.

Schachtel, E. C. Projection and its relation to character attitudes and creativity in the kinaesthetic responses. *Psychiatry,* 1950, 13, 60–100.

Schafer, R. *Psychoanalytic interpretation in Rorschach testing.* New York: Grune and Stratton, 1954.

Seminario Latinoamericano Sobre Alcoholismo. Informe Final, Oficina Sanitaria Panamericana, Oficina Regional de la Organizacion Mundial de la Salud, con la colaboracion del Servicio Nacional de Salad y el auspicio de la Universidad de Chile y el Colegio Medico de Chile, 1961.

Shapiro, D. *Neurotic styles.* New York: Basic Books, 1965.

Shulman, A. J. Alcohol addiction. *University of Toronto Medical Journal,* 1951, 28, 219–229.

Siegman, A. A. Father absence during early childhood and anti-social behavior. *Journal of Abnormal Psychology,* 1966, 71, 71–74.

Skolnick, A. Motivational imagery and behavior over twenty years. *Journal of Consulting Psychology,* 1966, 39, 463–478.

Soustelle, J. *The daily life of the Aztecs.* London: Penguin Books, 1964.

Stone, P. S., Dunphy, D. C., Smith, M. S. and Ogilvie, D. M. *The general inquirer: a computer approach to content analysis.* Cambridge, Mass.: M.I.T. Press, 1966.

Straus, R. and Bacon, S. D. *Drinking in college.* New Haven: Yale University Press, 1953.

Strodtbeck, F. L. Family interaction, values, and achievement. In D. C. McClelland, *et al., Talent and society.* Princeton, N. J.: Van Nostrand, 1958, pp. 259–266.

Tähkä, V. *The alcoholic personality.* Helsinki, Finland: Finnish foundation for alcohol studies, 1966.

Takala, M., Pihkanen, T. A. and Markkanen, T. *The effects of distilled and brewed beverages.* Helsinki: Suomalaisen Kirjallisuden Kirjapaino, 1957.

Trentini, G., Spaltro, E. and Padovani, F. Analisi sperimentale di alcune modificazioni della personalità umana indotte dall'alcool. In *L'alcool al servizio del medico.* Torino, Italia: Edizioni Minerva Medica, 1963.

Uleman, J. A new TAT measure of the need for power. Unpublished doctoral dissertation, Harvard University, 1965.

Ullman, A. D. The psychological mechanism of alcohol addiction. *Quarterly Journal of Studies on Alcohol,* 1952, 13, 602–608.

Utley, R. M. *The last days of the Sioux nation.* New Haven: Yale University Press, 1963.

Veroff, J. Development and validation of a projective measure of power motivation. *Journal of Abnormal and Social Psychology,* 1957, 54, 1–8.

Veroff, J. and Feld, S. *Motives and roles: a nation wide interview study.* Princeton, N. J.: Van Nostrand, 1969.

Walker, H. M. and Lev, J. *Statistical inference.* New York: Holt, 1953.

Weber, M. *The theory of social and economic organization.* London and New York: Oxford University Press, 1947.

Weiss, M. Alcohol as a depressant in psychological conflict in rats. *Quarterly Journal of Studies on Alcohol,* 1958, 19, 226–237.

White, R. A. The urban adjustment of the Sioux Indians in Rapid City, South Dakota. Unpublished manuscript, Rapid City, 1964.

White, R. A. The crisis among the Sioux today. Unpublished manuscript, Rapid City, South Dakota, 1969.

Whiting, B. B. Sex identity conflict and physical violence: a comparative study. *American Anthropologist,* 1965, 67, 123–140.

Whiting, B. B. Unpublished data on cross-cultural sex difference in child behavior. Mimeograph, 1966, Harvard University.

Whiting, J. W. M. Effects of climate on certain cultural practices. In W. Goodenough (Ed.), *Cultural anthropology.* New York: McGraw-Hill, 1964, pp. 511–544.

Whiting, J. W. M. Unpublished ratings assembled in the Laboratory of Human Development, Harvard University, 1965.

Whiting, J. W. M., Kluckhohn, R. and Anthony, A. A. The function of male initiation ceremonies at puberty. In E. E. Maccoby, T. M. Newcomb and E. L. Harley (Eds.), *Readings in social psychology.* 3rd edition. New York: Wiley, 1960.

Whiting, M. A cross-cultural nutrition survey. Unpublished Ph.D. Thesis, School of Public Health, Harvard University, 1950.

Williams, A. F. Self-concept of college problem drinkers: II. Heilbrun Need Scales. *Quarterly Journal of Studies on Alcohol,* 1967, 28, 267–276.

Williams, A. F. Validation of a college problem-drinking scale. *Journal of Projective Techniques and Personality Assessment,* 1967, 31: 1, 33–40.

Winter, D. G. Power motivation in thought and action. Unpublished Ph.D. Thesis, Harvard University, 1967.

Winter, D. G. Need for power in thought and action. Unpublished paper. Department of Psychology, Wesleyan University, 1968.

Winter, D. G. A revised scoring system for the need for Power (*n* Power). Unpublished paper, Department of Psychology, Wesleyan University, 1968(a).

Winter, D. G. Studies in the need for power. Dittoed paper, Wesleyan University, 1968(b).

Winter, D. G., Alpert, R. A. and McClelland, D. C. The classic personal style. *Journal of Abnormal and Social Psychology,* 1963, 67, 254–265.

Witkin, H. A. Psychological differentiation and forms of pathology. *Journal of Abnormal Psychology,* 1965, 70, 317–336.

Wittenborn, J. R. The study of alternative responses by means of the correlation coefficient. *Psychological Review,* 1955, 62, 451–560.

Wolowitz, H. M. Food preferences as an index of orality. *Journal of Abnormal and Social Psychology,* 1964, 69, 650–654.

Wright, G. Projection and displacement: A cross-cultural study of folk-tale aggression. *Journal of Abnormal and Social Psychology,* 1954, 49, 523–528.

Young, F. *Initiation ceremonies.* Indianapolis: Bobbs-Merrill, 1965.

Young, F. W. The function of male initiation ceremonies: a cross-cultural test of an alternative hypothesis. *American Journal of Sociology,* 1962, 67, 379–396.

Zelditch, N., Jr. Role differentiation in the nuclear family. In T. Parsons and R. F. Bales, *Family, socialization and interaction process,* New York: The Free Press, 1955.

Zucker, R. A. and Fillmore, K. M. Motivational factors and problem drinking. East Lansing: Michigan State University, Department of Psychology, Mimeographed, 1968.

Zwerling, I. and Rosenbaum, M. Alcoholic addiction and personality. In S. Arieti (Ed.), *American handbook of psychiatry*. New York: Basic Books, 1959.

Index

A priori concept list, 53-55
Abstainers (*see* Dry subjects)
Acting-out syndrome, 188-191
Activity Change (masculine tag):
   correlation of Factor I and II with, 88
   correlation of male and female pronouns
     with, 78
Activity Inhibition (folk-tale tag), 83, 124
   correlations of drinking and community
     size with, 70
   correlations of Factor I and II with, 88
   covariance of Fear with, 81
   differing drinking histories and, 155-161
   effects of drinking on, 140-141
   high positive loading of, 80-81
   individual liquor consumption as joint
     function of n Power and, 153
   in motivational correlates of smoking
     pot, 372
   relation of socialized and personalized
     power categories to, 164-166
   relation of Time Concerns to, 138-139
   relative frequency in folk tales of, 58
   sober societies and, 60

Activity Inhibition Score, negative
   association of frequency and
   quantity drinking with, 151
Activity Questionnaire, 221-222
Adjective check list, ix
Adolescent Indians, drinking among,
   268-275
Aggression:
   acting out, 312
   in class of restraining thoughts (*see*
     Aggression restraints)
   defined, 9
   in discussion group experiment:
     frequency of sentient thoughts, 11
     general test results, 13, 21-22
     problems, 13-14
   effect of drinking on fantasies of, 128
   in fraternity cocktail party: average
     frequency of thoughts, 15
     discussion and results, 15, 17-18, 19,
     21-22
   increased by drinking, 279
   in Setting and Alcohol Experiments, 32
     conclusions, 39

data, 34-36
folksinger, 41-42
tests for, 7-8
  frequency of sentient thoughts, 11
  general results, 13
  problems, 13-14
  TAT samples, 150
Aggression Power, 125, 126
  coding of, 124
  increase by alcohol consumption, 124
  intercorrelations of other categories of
    power concerns with, 167-170
  restrained and unrestrained activities,
    176
  predictive of drinking in subtotals of, 133
  relation of Sex Power to, 167-169, 348-350
Aggression restraints:
  in class of restraining thoughts, 9
  in discussion group: average frequency,
    12
  general test results, 14
  in fraternity cocktail party: average
    frequency, 15
  discussion and results, 19
  in Setting and Alcohol Experiments:
    conclusions, 40, 43
  data, 36
Aggressive Implements (folk-tale tag):
  correlation of drinking with, 61
  entry words under, 56
  word counts for entries under, 55
Agricultural societies, 59
  correlation of drinking with themes in,
    60, 65
  food shortages in, 49
Agriculture:
  degree of dependence as prediction of
    drinking, 90
  detailed codes for, 368
  low Factor I loading of, 91
Alcohol:
  correlation of *n* Power with, 105
  physiological effects of, 282
  (*See also* Beer drinking; Liquor
    consumption)
Alcohol Experiment, 21-44
  effects of drinking on mean frequencies
    of Sex and Aggression imagery,
    128-129
  effects of drinking on Strong and Weak
    Power, 132
  general results and discussion of, 42-44
    inhibition, 43
    sentience, 42-43
    summary and conclusions, 43-44
  method in, 24-30
    coding of stories and intercoder
      reliability, 29-30
    data analysis, 30
    experimental conditions, 24-26
    procedure, 27-29
    selection and arrangement of TAT
      pictures, 26-27
    subjects, 27

preliminary observations on, 21-24
  design, 23
  factorial design, 24
  limitations of previous experiments,
    21-22
  new coding category, 23-24
  selection of subjects, 22-23
  in private apartment (*See* Private
    apartment experiment)
specific results and discussion of, 31-42
  effects of alcohol, female folksinger,
    and setting on fantasy, 33-40
  effects of female folksinger on fantasy,
    41-42
  effects of inhibition setting on fantasy,
    40-41
  effects of situational and personal
    sentience and inhibition on alcohol
    consumption, 31-33
  with folksinger: choice of folksinger, 24
    effect on fantasy, 41-42
    method, 24
  (*See also* Setting Experiment)
Alcoholics:
  adult characteristics of, 288-293
  developmental characteristics of, 286
  heavy drinkers compared with, 296-303
  socializing power needs of, 316-331
    data, 323-331
    treatment program, 317-323
  solving power needs of, 309-315
    acting out aggression, 312
    borrow strength, 310-312
    reducing need for personalized power,
      309-310
    socializing power drives, 313
    success at work, 313-314
    vicarious satisfaction of power drive,
      312-313
  summary reasons for, 333-334
Alcoholics Anonymous, 301
Alcoholism:
  college students with tendencies toward,
    217-231
    construction of personality scales,
      220-221
    cross validation of scales, 221-222
    discussion, 226-229
    heavy drinkers and alcoholics
      compared, 229-231
    personality characteristics, 217-219
    results, 222-226
    self-descriptive statements, 219-220
  in Mexican village, 232-262
    cultural vulnerability, 240-250
    economic vulnerability, 254-260
    features of village, 234-235
    importance of problem, 234
    method of study, 236-240
    origins of study, 233-234
    problems of accuracy, 235-236
    psychosocial vulnerability, 250-254
  patriarchal ideals and, 253
  psychodynamics of, 276-277, 302-303

research basis for alternate explanations of, 276-315
 adult characteristics of alcoholics, 288-293
 developmental sources of a personalized power concern, 305-309
 drinking among ethnic groups, 293-296
 evidence supporting dependency conflict hypothesis, 284-288
 points of view, 276-281
 psychological basis for power thoughts aroused by drinking, 281-282
 reasons for doubting dependency hypothesis, 282-284
 solutions to power needs, 309-315
 sources of need for personalized power, 303-305
 variations in rates of heavy drinking, 296-303
 review of studies on, 276-281
 among Teton Sioux, 265-266
 (*See also* Alcoholics; Heavy drinking)
"Alcoholism in a Mexican Village" (Maccoby), 232-262
Amphetamines, 370-378
 college men's characteristics correlated with using, 375
 correlations of normative and rebellious assertive activities in use of, 374
 motives for taking, by college men, 370-378
 procedure of study, 370-371
 results, 371-378
Anal Socialization Anxiety (folk-tale tag):
 correlation of drinking with, 59
 relative frequency in folk tales, 58
Anger (folk-tale tag), 70
 correlation of drinking with, 61, 71
 correlation of Factors I and II with, 88
 positive loading of, 80
 relative frequency in folk tales, 58
Anglo-Americans, drinking by Spanish-Americans and Indians compared with, 293-296
Anxiety (*See* Fear-anxiety)
Anxiety-arousing intravenous studies, limitations of, 5
Apartment cocktail party (*See* Private apartment experiment)
Assertive thoughts and acts, 162-197
 correlation of mind-altering substances with normative and rebellious, 374
 drinking and strong demands for, 303-304
 drinking in wider context of: drinking and personalized power syndrome, 185-192
 limits of partitioning and power-scoring systems, 162-163
 procedure, 163-164
 relations of power concern types to varieties of assertive activities, 170-185
 results, 164-170

values, power needs, and drinking, 193-197
Associative changes, invalid, 8
Attitude scales, ix
Authority impact in TAT samples, 150
Aztec society, drunkenness in, 251-252

Bar, home, correlation of *n* Power with, 105
Bar I study (*see* Working-class men)
Bar II study (*see* Working-class men)
Basuto tribe, 51
Beer drinking, 349
 n Power score and, 135-136
 power scores with, 134
Beer mug, correlation of *n* Power with, 105
Behavior scales:
 interaction of *n* Power Scoring System with, 110
 rotated factor loadings of *n* Power Scoring Systems and, 112
Black Americans, high drinking rates among, 305
Blind Man Game, 199-213
 procedure in, 199-203
 questionnaire in, 203
 results of, 203-213
Body-building equipment, correlation of *n* Power with, 105
Boisterousness, 84-85
 (*See also* Aggression)
Books for courses, correlation of *n* Power with, 105
Borrow strength, 310-312
Breton fishermen:
 alcoholism among, 298
 reducing need for personalized power among, 309-310
Bride service, correlation of drinking with, 67
Brule reservation, 266-267
Business administration students (*see* College men)

Capability (folk-tale tag):
 correlation of drinking with, 59
 correlation of Factors I and II with, 88
 correlation of male and female pronouns with, 78
 relationship of Power and Inhibitions to, 87
 relative frequency in folk tales, 58
Car accidents, correlation of Personalized Power scores with, 192
Cars, correlation of *n* Power with, 105
Change of State (folk-tale tag):
 as category, 62
 concern for potency indicated by, 75-76
 as neutral tag, 78
 relative frequency in folk tales, 58
 removal from empirical redefinition of magical potency, 79-80
Characteristic actions, ix

Child (folk-tale tag):
 as concern for others, 84
 correlation of drinking with, 69
 relationship of Factor II to, 83
 relative frequency in folk tales, 58
Childhood, obedience responses in, 67
Chinese, low drinking rates among, 300
Cigarettes, 349
 correlation of *n* Power with, 105
Classical music concerts, correlation of *n*
  Power with, 106
Classroom cocktail party:
 effects of drinking on mean frequencies
   of sex and aggression imagery,
   128-129
 effects of drinking on Strong and Weak
   Power, 132
 with folksinger: choice of folksinger, 24
  effects on fantasy, 41-42
  method, 24
 general results and discussion of, 42-44
  inhibition, 43
  sentience, 42-43
  summary and conclusions, 43-44
 method in, 24-30
  coding of stories and intercoder
    reliability, 29-30
  data analysis, 30
  experimental conditions, 24-26
  procedure, 27-29
  selection and arrangement of TAT
    pictures, 26-27
  subjects, 27
 preliminary observations on, 21-24
  design, 23
  factorial design, 24
  limitations of previous experiments,
    21-22
  new coding category, 23-24
  selection of subjects, 22-23
 specific results and discussion of, 31-42
  effects of alcohol, female folksinger,
    and setting on fantasy, 33-40
  effects of folksinger on fantasy, 41-42
  effects of inhibition setting on fantasy,
    40-41
  effects of situational and personal
    sentience and inhibition on alcohol
    consumption, 31-33
Cleaning equipment, correlation of *n*
  Power with, 105
Climate, 96
 as characteristic which predicts drinking,
   90
 correlation of drinking with, 65
 detailed codes for, 369
Clothing, correlation of *n* Power with, 105
Club memberships, correlation of *n* Power
  and assertive activities with, 176-177
Coding scheme:
 additions to, 23-24
 in Setting and Alcohol Experiments,
   29-30
 for Thematic Apperception Tests, 8-10

(*See also* Concepts in folk-tale analysis)
Collateral (folk-tale tag), relative
  frequency in folk tales of, 58
College men:
 alcoholic tendencies in, 217-231
  construction of personality scales,
    220-221
  cross validation of scales, 221-222
  discussion, 226-229
  heavy drinkers and alcoholics
    compared, 229-231
  personality characteristics, 217-219
  results, 222-226
  self-descriptive statements, 219-220
 motives for drug taking by, 370-378
  procedure, 370-371
  results, 371-378
 power and drinking in, 99-119
  action correlates of *n* Power
    system, 102-108
  arousal procedures and *n* Power
    scoring system, 100-102
  patterns of power motives and power
    behaviors, 114-116
  power-related behavior scales, 108-113
  summary, 117-119
Combined Drinking Score:
 correlation of masculine tags with, 84
 power and inhibition as joint function
   of, 86-87
 relationship between three components
   of Male Institution Scale and, 96
 variables correlated with, 89-90
Community size, correlation of drinking
  with, 64-65, 69
Competitive sports:
 correlation of *n* Power with, 103-104
 correlation of scoring system factors
   with, 116
 intercorrelation of other behavior scales
   and *n* Power with, 109-110
 power-related scales and, 108, 110-112,
   116
 rotated factor loadings and, 111-112
Concepts in folk-tale analysis:
 a priori, 53-55
 empirical, 55-58
Concerts of classical music, correlation of
  n Power with, 106
Conflict, tests for, 7-8
 (*See also* Aggression)
Consumption of drinks, 176, 349
 correlation of *n* Power and Activity
   Inhibition with, 153, 171, 176-177
 correlation of *n* Power and assertive
   activities with, 176-177
Conventionality, 88, 94, 96
 heavy drinking and, 91
Cook (folk-tale tag):
 correlation of drinking with, 61
 relative frequency in folk tales, 58
Cost of desired car, 349
 correlation of *n* Power and Activity
   Inhibition with, 171

Credit cards, correlation of Personalized
   and Socialized Power and
   Restrained Assertive activities with,
   179-180
Cross-cultural study of folk-tale content:
   alcohol's effects on, ix
   drinking and, 48-72
      conclusions, 70-72
      drinking ratings, 52-53
      inductive interpretation, 62-70
      method, 51-58
      mode of analysis, 53-58
      results of studies, 58-70
      selection of cultures, 51-52
      selection of folk tales, 52
   fantasy and, 46
   heavy-drinking factors in, 93
   individual activities and, 173-174
   limitations of, 45-46
   research value of, 50
   (*See also specific folk-tale tags*)
"Cross-Cultural Study of Folk-Tale
   Content and Drinking, A"
   (McClelland, Davis, Wanner, Kalin),
   48-72
Cultural analysis of folk tales (*see*
   Cross-cultural study of folk-tale
   content)
Cultural vulnerability to alcoholism,
   240-250
Cures for heavy drinkers, 336

Dances, correlation of *n* Power with, 106
Dating, correlation of *n* Power with, 105
Dating hours, correlation of *n* Power with,
   106
Davis, William N., xiii
   "A Cross-Cultural Study of Folk-Tale
      Content and Drinking," 48-72
   "The Influence of Unrestrained Power
      Concerns on Drinking in
      Working-Class Men," 142-161
   "A Pilot Attempt To Help Alcoholics
      by Socializing Their Power Needs,"
      310-313
Dead and Old (folk-tale tag):
   correlation of drinking with, 59, 71
   correlation of Factors I and II with, 88
   as powerful inhibition, 81
   relative frequency in folk tales of, 58
   sober societies and, 60
Deculturation of Indians, 261, 263-267
Deductive models, viii
Dependence on agriculture, predictability
   of drinking by, 90
Dependence on hunting, predictability of
   drinking by, 90, 91
Dependency:
   absence of relationship between
      drinking and, ix
   in alcoholics, 290
   as folk-tale tag: correlation of drinking
      with, 59, 60
      relative frequence in folk tales, 58

power concerns compared with, 198-213
   Blind Man Game, 199-203
   experimental issues, 198-199
   Game Questionnaire, 203
   results, 203-213
Dependency hypothesis:
   evidence for supporting, 284-288
   reasons for doubting, ix, 282-284
Discussion groups, 5-14
   tests on emotive responses of: coding
      scheme, 8-10
      procedure, 5-8
      results and discussion, 10-14, 21-22
Domestic (feminine tag):
   as concern for others, 84
   relationship to Factor II of, 83
Dreams:
   heavy drinking and, 93
   instrumental use of, 66
Drinking (folk-tale tag):
   correlation of alcoholic drinking with, 60
   relative frequency in folk tales of, 58
Drinking behavior:
   correlation of scoring system factors
      with, 116
   intercorrelation of other behavior scales
      and *n* Power with, 109-110
   rotated factor loadings and *n* Power,
      111-112
   (*See also* Liquor consumption)
Drinking ratings in cross-cultural study
   of folk tales, 52-53
"Drinking in the Wider Context of
   Restrained and Unrestrained
   Assertive Thoughts and Acts"
   (McClelland, Wanner,
   Vanneman), 162-197
Drinks consumed, 176, 349
   correlation of *n* Power and Activity
      Inhibition, 153, 171, 176-177
   correlation of *n* Power and assertive
      activities with, 176-177
Drug taking:
   by college men: procedure, 370-371
      results, 371-378
Dry subjects, 6, 249-250
   comparing "wet" with: general results,
      13-14
      inhibiting thoughts, 12, 38
      problems, 21-22
      sentient thoughts, 11, 33, 34, 36
   discriminating "wet" from, 9-10
   (*See also* Setting Experiment)
Dues, correlation of *n* Power with, 105

Eating (folk-tale tag):
   concern for potency indicated by, 76
   correlation of Combined Drinking score
      with, 84
   correlation of drinking with, 61, 65
   correlation of Factors I and II with, 88
   correlation of male and female pronouns
      with, 78
   high negative loading of, 79, 81

power-related concerns tapped by, 82
relative frequency in folk tales, 58
special concern for potency indicated
    by, 75
Eating Markers (folk-tale tag):
    correlation of drinking with, 61, 71
    correlation of Factors I and II with, 88
    relative frequency in folk tales, 58
Economic vulnerability to alcoholism,
    254-260
"Effect of Male Social Drinking on
    Fantasy, The" (Kalin, McClelland,
    Kahn), 3-44
Effective power, 88
"Effects of Drinking on Thoughts About
    Power and Restraint, The"
    (McClelland and Wilsnack), 123-141
Egalitarian kin terms, correlation of
    drinking with, 69
Ejiditarios and drinking, 256-260
Elation, tests for, 7-8
Empirical concept list, 55-58
Entering Implements (folk-tale tag):
    concern for potency indicated by, 76-78
    correlation of Combined Drinking Score
        with, 84
    correlation of drinking with, 61, 65,
        66, 283
    correlation of Factors I and II with, 88
    correlation of male and female pronouns
        with, 78
    high negative loading of, 79, 81
    power-related concerns tapped by, 82
    relative frequency in folk tales, 58
    special concern for potency indicated by,
        75
"Examining the Research Basis for
    Alternative Explanations of
    Alcoholism" (McClelland), 276-315
Excessive drinkers (*see* Heavy drinkers)
Exhibitionistic behavior, 84-85
Expanded consciousness, alcohol's role in,
    viii
Experimental procedure, general factors
    involved in, vii-ix
Exploitative Sex, 126-127
    as Personalized Power, 137
    in TAT samples, 150
Extreme Hostility, 84-85
Eysenck's Maudsley Personality Inventory,
    219

Factor I, 116
    assertive activities included in, 171-172
    characteristics with high loadings and,
        90-91
    characteristics with low loadings and, 90
    defining tags for, 88
    relationship of folk-tale and feminine
        tags to, 61, 65, 83, 88
    self-descriptive statements by college
        men grouped in, 223-224, 227
    variables loading on, 90
    Veroff scoring system and, 114

Factor II:
    activities loading on, 171-172
    criterion 2 of new system of power
        imagery in, 114
    defining tags for, 88
    high loadings on, 80-81, 86
    as power factor, 82-84
    relationship of folk-tale and feminine
        tags to, 61, 65, 83, 88
    as response to potency needs, 231
    self-descriptive statements by college
        students grouped in, 224, 227
    variables loading on, 81, 86, 90
Factor III, 116
    activities loading on, 171-172
    nature of, 114
    self-descriptive statements by college
        students grouped in, 225-227
    variables loading on, 115
Factor VI, 117
    nature of, 115-116
    variables loading on, 115
Families of pre-alcoholics, 286-288
Fantasy, 125
    alcohol's effects on, ix, 38-40
    effects of inhibition setting on, 40-41
    folk-tale material and, 46
    in Setting and Alcohol Experiments,
        38-42
        effects of alcohol, 38-40
        effects of folksinger, 41-42
Fastest speed driven, 348, 349
    correlation of *n* Power and Activity
        Inhibition with, 171
    relation of Personalized and Social
        Power scores with assertive activities,
        184
Father Distance, 95, 96
Fathers of pre-alcoholics, 286-288
Fear (folk-tale tag), 70, 124
    in class of restraining thoughts, 4
    covariance of Activity Inhibition with,
        81
    defined, 9
    relative frequency in folk tales, 58
    words classified under, 54
Fear-anxiety:
    in class of restraining thoughts, 9
    defined, 9
    in discussion group: average frequency,
        12
    general test results, 14
    in fraternity cocktail party: average
        frequency of thoughts, 15
    discussion and results, 18
    in Setting and Alcohol Experiments:
        conclusions, 40
        data, 38
Female pronouns, correlation of masculine
    tags with, 78
Feminine Adjective (feminine tag),
    relationship of Factor II to, 83
Feminine tags:
    as concern for others, 84

correlation of drinking with, 63-64
relationship of Factor II to, 83
Finnish alcoholics, 278, 299
First Order Generation (folk-tale tag):
as concern for others, 84
relationship of Factor II to, 83
relative frequency in folk tales, 58
Fish (folk-tale tag):
correlation of drinking with, 70, 71
correlation of Factors I and II with, 88
relative frequency in folk tales, 58
Fist fights, correlation of Personalized and
Socialized Power Scores and
Unrestrained Assertive activities
with, 181-182
Folksinger:
as factor in situational sentience, 24, 41
in Setting Experiment: alcohol
consumption, 31
correlations in alcohol consumption, 32
data analysis, 30
effects on fantasy, 41-42
general effects, 44
introduction to group, 28
mean frequencies of thematic fear, 38
mean frequencies of thematic physical
sex, 33
mean frequencies of thematic Time
Concern, 38
variation of situations, 25
Folk-tale data:
alcohol's effects on, ix
drinking and, 48-72
conclusions, 70-72
drinking ratings, 52-53
inductive interpretation, 62-70
method, 51-58
mode of analysis, 53-58
results of studies, 58-70
selection of cultures, 51-52
selection of folk tales, 52
fantasy and, 46
heavy-drinking factors in, 93
individual activities compared with,
173-174
limitations of, 45-46
research value of, 50
Food gatherers, 59
correlation of drinking with themes of,
60
food shortages among, 49
Formal organization, correlation of
drinking and folk-tale themes with,
59
France, drinking patterns in, 298
Fraternity cocktail party:
drinking at, 7
tests on emotive responses at, 14-20
average frequency of thoughts, 15
discussion and results, 15, 17-19, 21-22
prevailing conditions, 14-15
procedural flaws, 16-17
results and discussion, 15-20
Fromm, Erich, 239

Gambling:
correlation of *n* Power with, 105
correlation of Personalized and
Socialized Power scores with
Unrestrained assertive activities,
181-182
Ganda tribe, 51
Gather and Travel (folk-tale tag):
correlation of drinking with, 59
relative frequency in folk tales of, 58
Give (folk-tale tag):
correlation of drinking with, 59, 60
relative frequency in folk tales of, 58

Harvard beer mug, correlation of *n* Power
with, 103
Hat, correlation of *n* Power with, 105
Having (masculine tag)
correlation of Factor I and II with, 88
correlation of male and female pronouns
with, 78
highest loading on Factor II of, 81, 86
as measure of power concerns, 84
Heavy drinking, ix
accentuated needs for Personalized
Power among, 335-336
among Anglo-Americans, Spanish-
Americans, and Indians, 265-266,
293-296
behavior scales of, 157
among college men, 217-231
construction of personality scales,
220-221
cross validation of scales, 221-222
discussion, 226-229
heavy drinkers and alcoholics
compared, 229-231
personality characteristics, 217-219
results, 222-226
self-descriptive statements, 219-220
cure for, 336
drinking behavior and impulsive power
associated with, 84-85
high scoring on concerns, 185
intercorrelation of Personalized Power
and acting out with, 188
in Mexican village, 232-262
cultural vulnerability, 240-250
economic vulnerability, 254-262
features of village, 234-235
importance of problem, 234
method of study, 236-240
origins of study, 236-240
problems of accuracy, 235-236
psychosocial vulnerability, 250-254
power concerns as influence in, 296-303,
333-334
social variables and folk-tale themes
associated with, 92-93
summary reasons for, 333-334
types of, 334-335
variations in rates of, 296-303
Hierarchy:
correlation of drinking with, 64, 71

sober societies and, 60
Home bar, correlation of *n* Power with, 105
Housemaster interaction and power-related
    scales, 108, 112, 116
Hunt (folk-tale tag):
    correlation of drinking with, 59, 65, 66
    correlation of Factors I and II with, 88
    correlation of male and female pronouns
        with, 78
    highest loading on Factor II, 81, 86
    as measure of power concerns, 76-78, 84
    relative frequency in folk tales, 58
    special concern for potency indicated
        by, 75
Hunting:
    correlation of drinking and dependence
        on, 90, 91
    detailed codes for, 368
Hunting societies:
    correlation of drinking with themes of,
        60, 65
        childhood achievement, 66
    economic stability of, 91-92
    food shortages among, 49
    high-risk and low-probability character
        of, 92
    modern societies compared with, 97

Id Power Score, Other Power Score
    compared with, 175
Ifaluk tribe, 51
Imagination tests, 6-14
    for male social drinkers, 6-8
        coding scheme, 8-10
        results and discussion, 10-14
    See also Thematic Apperception Test
        (TAT)
Impermanence of settlement pattern, as
    characteristic which predicts
    drinking, 90
Impulsive Power, 88
    heavy drinking and, 93
    social situation which leads to, 95
Impulsive Power Score, correlation of
    heavy drinking with, 84-85
Indians:
    drinking by Spanish-Americans and
        Anglo-Americans compared with,
        293-296
    Teton Sioux (*see* Teton Sioux)
Individual activities, folk-tale activities
    compared with, 173-74
"Influence of Unrestrained Power Concerns
    on Drinking in Working-Class Men,
    The" (McClelland and Davis),
    142-161
Inhibiting thoughts (*see specific emotive
    restraints*)
Inhibition:
    correlation of drinking with, 73
    power and, 84-89
Inhibition Factor I (*see* Factor I)
Inhibition scale and heavy drinking, 93

Inhibition tags:
    correlation of drinking with, 71
    positive loading of, 80
Initiation impact:
    as characteristic predicting drinking, 90
    detailed codes for, 368
Instrumental dependence in adulthood
    and heavy drinking, 91
Interaction with housemaster:
    correlation of scoring system factors
        with, 116
    intercorrelation of other behavior scales
        and *n* Power with, 109-110
    rotated factor loadings and *n* Power,
        111-112
Intercoder reliability in Setting and
    Alcohol Experiments, 29-30
Interpretations, general factors involved
    in, vii-ix
Intravenous administration of alcohol,
    inhibiting effects of, 41
Irish, high drinking rates among, 299-300
Italy, drinking patterns in, 298

Jews, low drinking rates among, 298-300
Jurisdictional hierarchy, low degree of: as
    characteristic which predicts
    drinking, 90
    detailed codes for, 368

Kahn, Michael, xiii
    "The Effect of Male Social Drinking on
        Fantasy," 3-44
Kalin, Rudolf, xi, xiii
    "A Cross-Cultural Study of Folk-Tale
        Content and Drinking," 48-72
    "The Effect of Male Social Drinking on
        Fantasy," 3-44
    "Self-Description of College Problem
        Drinkers," 217-231
    "Social Drinking in Different Settings,"
        21-44
Khasis tribe, 51
Kikuyu tribe, 51
Kill (folk-tale tag):
    correlation of drinking with, 61
    relative frequency in folk tales, 58
Kung Bushmen, 91

Lack of inhibition in alcoholics, 289
Lakota (*see* Sioux Indians)
Landownership in Mexican village and
    drinking, 255-258
Laundry, correlation of *n* Power with, 105
Light drinkers:
    behavior scales of, 156-157
    cross-cultural folk-themes associated
        with, 71
    high scoring on Power Concerns of, 185
        intercorrelation of Personalized Power
            and acting out, 188
Liquor consumption, 349
    correlation of *n* Power and Activity
        Inhibition with, 153, 171, 176-177

correlation of *n* Power and assertive
    activities with, 176-177
n Power score and, 135-136
power scores with, 134
Liquor industry, economic interests of, 255
Local community, detailed codes for, 368
Love-making, correlation of *n* Power with,
    106
Low hierarchy:
as characteristic which predicts drinking,
    90
as folk-tale theme associated with light
    drinking, 71
Low inhibition, 88
Low power, 88
LSD, 370-378
college men's characteristics correlated
    with, 375
correlation of normative and rebellious
    assertive activities in use of, 374
motives for taking by college men:
    procedure, 370-371
    results, 371-378

McClelland, David:
"A Cross-Cultural Study of Folk-Tale
    Content and Drinking," 48-72
"Drinking in the Wider Context of
    Restrained and Unrestrained
    Assertive Thoughts and Acts,"
    162-197
"The Effects of Drinking on Thoughts
    About Power and Restraint,"
    123-141
"The Effects of Male Social Drinking on
    Fantasy," 3-44
"Examining the Research Bases for
    Alternative Explanations of
    Alcoholism," 276-315
"The Influence of Unrestrained Power
    Concerns on Drinking in
    Working-Class Men," 142-161
"Motion for Drug Taking Among
    College Men," 370-378
"Summary," 332-336
Maccoby, Michael, xi, xiv
"Alcoholism in a Mexican Village,"
    232-260
Magical potency, 73-98
empirical redefinition of, 76-82
problems in theory of, 73-76
(*See also* Power; Power concerns)
Male assertiveness (*see* Assertive thoughts
    and acts)
Male initiation, as characteristic predictive
    of drinking, 90
Male Institutions Scale, 90, 94
Combined Drinking Score and
    components of, 96
heavy drinking and, 93
subscales of, 95
Male pronouns, correlation of masculine
    tags with, 78

Male role, drinking and low support for,
    304
Male solidarity:
as characteristic which predicts
    drinking, 90
correlation of drinking with, 64, 65, 67, 71
detailed codes for, 369
Man-feminine tags, correlation of drinking
    with, 64
Marijuana, 370-378
college men's characteristics correlated
    with, 375
correlation of normative and rebellious
    assertive activities in use of, 374
as mode of expressing Personalized
    Power, 377-378
motives for taking by college men:
    procedure, 370-371
    results, 371-378
Marital problems, 349
correlations of drinking and Power
    Concerns with, 357
Masculine tags, correlation of female tags
    with, 78
Massachusetts Achievement Trainers, 318,
    321
Matriarchal communities, 252-253
high male drinking levels in, 305
Meaning Contrasts, 125
coding of, 124-125
defined, 7-9
in discussion group: difficulties of
    interpretation, 10, 13
frequency of sentient thoughts, 11
increase in wet condition, 10
effects of alcohol on, 42
in fraternity cocktail party: average
    frequency of thoughts, 15
results and discussion, 15-19
increase by alcohol consumption, 124
integration into more general theory, 135
power and, 130-132, 137
Socialized Power concern, 137
reinterpreting, 127
in Setting and Alcohol Experiments,
    36-37
Mental effects of alcohol, 1-44
effects of male social drinking on fantasy
    and, 3-20
on fantasy of males (*see* Fantasy)
social drinking in different settings and
    (*see* Alcohol Experiment; Setting
    Experiment)
Methodology:
deductive models, viii
factors involved in, vii-ix
Mexican village, 232-262
alcoholism in: cultural vulnerability,
    240-250
economic vulnerability, 254-260
features of village, 234-235
importance of problem, 234
method of study, 236-240
origins of study, 233-234

problems of accuracy, 235-236
psychosocial vulnerability, 250-254
macho values in, 304-305, 397
Middle-aged men, heavier drinking by,
296-297
Minnesota Multiphasic Inventory,
comparative response by alcoholics
to, 291-292
Mohatt, Gerald, xiv
"Sacred Water: The Quest for Personal
Power Through Drinking Among
the Teton Sioux," 261-275
Money for travel:
correlation of *n* Power and assertive
activities with, 176-177
correlation of Personalized and
Socialized Power scores and
unrestrained assertiveness with,
181-182
Money spending, correlation of *n* Power
with, 105-106
Mood themes for power/nurturance
study, 202
Mother-baby sleeping arrangements:
as characteristic which predicts
drinking, 90
detailed codes for, 369
Mother fixation, 233, 247-248
Mothers of pre-alcoholics, 286-288
"Motives for Drug Taking Among College
Men" (McClelland and Steele),
370-378
Motorcycles, correlation of *n* Power with,
105
Motorscooters, correlation of *n* Power
with, 105
Movies, correlation of *n* Power with, 106
Music concerts, classical, correlation of *n*
Power with, 106
Musical instrument, correlation of *n*
Power with, 105
Mysteries of life (*see* Meaning Contrasts)

n Achievement, 114
n Power, 124-125, 132-133
behavior scales intercorrelated with,
103-110, 171-177
individual liquor consumption as a joint
function of Activity Inhibition and,
153, 171, 176-177
intercorrelations with other categories
of power concerns, 167-171
restrained and unrestrained
activities, 176
money spending correlated with, 105-106
office-holding correlated with, 103-104
rotated factor loadings of behavior
scale and, 109-112
n Power categories:
partitioning of, 125-126
sources and classification of, 339-341
n Power Scores:
action correlates of, 102-108

arousal procedures and development of,
100-102
correlation with quantity/frequency
index for drinking, 151
effect of drinking history on, 135-136,
155, 158-161
features of, 117-119
improved, 99
interaction of behavior scales and, 110
loading on Factor II, 111
in motivational correlates of smoking
pot, 372
partitioning, 163
rotating factor loadings of behavior
scales and, 112
Narcissism, 246-247
National Institute of Mental Health, xi
"Need for Power in College Men, The:
Action Correlates and Relationship
to Drinking" (Winter), 99-119
Negation (folk-tale tag), relative frequency
in folk tales of, 58
Non-lineal descent, correlation of drinking
with, 64-65
Non-physical aggression (*see* Aggression)
Non-physical sex (*see* Sex)
Noun game, 75
Nurturance in drinking, 198-213
power concerns compared with: Blind
Man Game, 199-203
experimental issues, 198-199
Game Questionnaire, 203
results, 203-213
(*See also* Dependency; Dependency
hypothesis)

Office-holding, 103-104, 348
correlation of *n* Power and Activity
Inhibition with, 171
correlation of *n* Power and assertive
activities with, 176-177
correlation of Personalized and
Socialized Power with restrained
assertiveness, 179-180
correlation of scoring system factors
with, 116
intercorrelation of other behavior and *n*
Power with, 109-110
power-related scales and, 108, 110-112,
116
rotated factor loadings and *n* Power
with, 111-112
Officerships, 349
Old and Dead (folk-tale tag):
correlation of drinking with, 59, 71
correlation of Factors I and II with, 88
as powerful inhibition, 81
relative frequency in folk tales of, 58
sober societies and, 60
Omnibus Personality Inventory, 219
Open Class System:
as characteristic which predicts drinking,
90
detailed codes for, 368

Oral Body Parts (folk-tale tag):
close correlation of drinking with, 60, 283
correlation of male and female pronouns with, 78
relative frequency in folk tales of, 58
Other Power score, Id Power Score compared with, 175

p Power (*see* Personalized Power)
Palaung tribe, 51
Parent-child hierarchy, correlation of drinking with, 69
Parents
as characteristic which predicts drinking, 90
of pre-alcoholics, 286-288
Partitioning, limits of, 162-163
Passive receptiveness, absence of direct evidence for, 232-233
Patriarchal ideals and alcoholism, 253
Peasantry (*see* Mexican village)
Permanency of settlement patterns, detailed codes for, 368
Personal Reaction Inventory, 221-222
Personality tests, 219
Personalized Power:
correlation in opposite direction of conscious expectation variables, 195-197
correlation of restrained assertiveness with, 178-181
correlation of unrestrained assertiveness with, 181-183
correlation of values and drinking with, 193-195
developmental sources of, 305-309
differing drinking histories and, 155-161
Exploitative Sex as, 137
function of, 197
influence of drinking on, 185-192
intercorrelation of alternative manifestations before drinking, 186-192
intercorrelations of other categories of Power Concerns with, 167-170, 175, 176
in motivational correlates of smoking pot, 372
pot-smoking as mode of expressing, 377-378
predictability of participation in assertive activities and, 175-177
promise of scoring, 167
reducing need for, 309-310
relation of Activity Inhibition to, 164-166
relation of miscellaneous assertive activities to, 184-185
scoring manual for, 351-356
sources of needs for, 303-305
among Teton Sioux, 261-275
adolescent cases, 268-275
destruction of old ways, 263-264
liquor in early days, 264-266

old ways, 262-263
twentieth-century developments, 266-268
Personalized Power scores:
frequencies after alcohol consumption, 133
high-level drinking and, 135
nature of, 134
type of alcoholic beverage and, 134
Phonograph records, correlation of *n* Power with, 105
Physical aggression (*see* Aggressive thoughts and acts)
Physical health, 347
Physical sex (*see* Sex)
Physiological effects of alcohol, 137
Picture reproductions, 360-367
"Pilot Attempt To Help Alcoholics by Socializing Their Power Needs, A" (Davis), 310-331
Possessions:
correlation of *n* Power with, 103-104
prestige (*see* Prestige possessions)
Pot (*see* Marijuana)
Potency, associations of, 76-77
(*See also* Power)
Poverty and drinking, 355-356
Power:
college men and, 99-119
action correlates of *n* Power system, 102-108
arousal procedures and *n* Power Scoring System, 100-102
patterns of power motives and power behavior, 114-116
power-related behavior scales, 108-113
conclusions on, 97-98
inhibition and, 84-89
magical, 73-98
empirical redefinition, 76-82
problems in theory, 73-76
personalized (*see* Personalized Power)
sex and (*see* Sex; Sex Power; Sex restraints; Sex taboos)
social environment and, 89-97
socialized (*see* Socialized Power)
Power Concerns, 292
in alcoholics, 289
correlation of marital problems and drinking with, 357
dependency concerns compared with, 198-213
Blind Man Game, 199-203
experimental issues, 198-199
Game Questionnaire, 203
results, 203-213
in drinking by working-class men, 142-161
experimental problems, 142-144
procedure, 144-151
results, 151-161
patterns of, 114-117
sex and aggression as, 348-356
summary reasons for, 332-334

variations in rates of heavy drinking
explained in terms of, 296-303
varieties of assertive activities and,
170-185
Power Factor II (*see* Factor II)
Power fantasies, correlation of drinking
variables among working-class men
with, 152
"Power and Inhibition: A Revision of the
Magical Potency Theory" (Wanner),
73-98
Power motivation theory:
development of, 45-119
cross-cultural study of folk-tale
content, 48-72
need for power in college men, 99-119
power and inhibition, 73-98
testing of, 131-213
drinking in wider context of restrained
and unrestrained assertive thoughts
and acts, 162-197
effects of drinking on thoughts about
power and restraint, 123-141
influence of Power Concerns on drinking in working-class men, 142-161
relationship of drinking to nurturance
and power, 198-213
Power needs:
patterns of, 114-117
socializing, 216-231, 313
data on alcoholics, 323-331
treatment program for alcoholics,
317-323
vicarious satisfaction of, 312-313
solutions to, 309-315
Power outlets, drinking and lack of
socialized, 304-305
Power-related behavior scales, 108-116
Power-related themes of working-class
men, 150
Power scale and heavy drinking, 93
Power-scoring systems:
descriptions of, 338-341
limits of, 162-163
Power thoughts:
effects of drinking on, 123-141
experimental goals, 123-126
procedure, 126-128
relation of two measures of inhibitory
tendencies to drinking, 138-141
results, 128-138
physiological basis for drinking-induced,
281-282
Pre-alcoholism:
in college students, 217-231
construction of personality scales,
220-221
cross-validation of scales, 221-222
discussion, 226-229
heavy drinkers and alcoholics
compared, 229-231
personality characteristics, 217-219
results, 222-226
self-descriptive statements, 219-220

developmental characteristics in, 286
Predictability of drinking by social
characteristics and practices, 90
Prestige possessions:
correlation of scoring system factors
with, 116
intercorrelation of other behavior scales
and *n* Power with, 109-110
power-related scales and, 108, 110-112,
116
rotated factor loadings and *n* Power,
109-110
Prestige supplies in TAT samples, 150
Primitive societies (*see* Agricultural
societies; Foodgatherers; Hunting
societies; Indians; Mexican village)
Private apartment experiment, 21-44
alcohol consumption in, 31
correlations between predrinking TAT
sentience and subsequent alcohol
consumption in, 32
method in, 24-30
results and discussion in, 30-44
(*See also* Setting Experiment)
Protest masculinity, 307
Psychological theorizing, x
Psychosocial vulnerability to alcoholism,
250-254
Puritanism and social drinking, 4

Quantity/frequency index for drinking,
151
Questionnaires, viii, ix
in Bar Study of working-class men,
342-347

Receptive character, 244-246
Reckless driving:
correlation of *n* Power and assertive
activities with, 176-177
correlation of Personalized and
Socialized Power scores and
unrestrained assertive activities
with, 181-182
Recreation, correlation of *n* Power with,
105
Refrigerator, correlation of *n* Power with,
105
Research literature on male social drinking,
3-5
Respect themes, correlation of drinking
with, 71, 73
Restrained assertiveness:
correlation of *n* Power sub-scores with,
175-177
correlation of Personalized and
Socialized Power with, 178-182
(*See also* Assertive thoughts and acts)
Restraints:
average frequency of, 12
defined, 9
effects of drinking on, 123-141
experimental goals, 123-126
procedure, 126-128

relation of two measures of inhibitory
tendencies to drinking, 138-141
results, 128-138
general results of tests on, 14
(*See also* Aggression restraints;
Fear-anxiety; Sex restraints; Time
Concern)
Rosebud reservation, 265

s Power (*see* Socialized Power)
"Sacred Water, The: The Quest for
Personal Power Through Drinking
Among the Teton Sioux" (Mohatt),
261-275
Sadism, 246-247
Scheduling (folk-tale tag), 124
correlation of drinking with, 59
correlation of Factors I and II with, 88
correlation of male and female pronouns
with, 78
relationship of Power and Inhibition to,
87
relative frequency in folk tales, 58
sober societies and, 60
Scientific writing, deductive model of, viii
"Self-Description of College Problem
Drinkers" (Kalin), 217-231
Self-descriptive statements:
of college students with tendencies
toward alcoholism, 219-220
correlation of drinking with, 358-359
Sensuous Physical Pleasure:
as addition to coding scheme, 23-24
defined, 29
effects of alcohol on, 43
in Setting and Alcohol Experiments,
37-38
Sentience:
alcohol-induced, viii
as Id-need, 42
in private apartment experiment, 32
problem of defining, 22
in Setting Experiment: conclusions, 42-44
effects on fantasy, 40
situational, 31-33
variation, 25
Setting Experiment, 21-44
aggression in (*see* Aggression, in Setting
and Alcohol Experiments)
alcohol consumption in, 31
correlation between predrinking TAT
sentience and subsequent alcohol
consumption in, 32
effects of drinking on mean frequencies
of Sex and Aggression imagery,
128-129
effects of drinking on Strong and Weak
Power, 132
fear-anxiety in, 38, 40
with folksinger (*see* Folksinger, in
Setting and Alcohol Experiments)
general results and discussion of, 42-44
inhibition, 43
sentience, 42-44

summary and conclusions, 43-44
Meaning Contrasts in, 36-37
method in, 24-30
coding of stories and intercoder
reliability, 29-30
data analysis, 30
experimental conditions, 24-26
procedure, 27-29
selection and arrangement of TAT
pictures, 26-27
subjects, 27
preliminary observations on, 21-24
design, 23
factorial design, 24
limitations of previous experiments,
21-22
new coding category, 23-24
selection of subjects, 22-23
Sensuous Physical Pleasure in, 37-38
sex in (*see* Sex, in Setting and Alcohol
Experiments)
situation inhibition in, 25, 40, 44
specific results and discussion of, 31-42
effects of alcohol, female folk singer
and setting on fantasy, 33-40
effects of inhibition setting on fantasy,
40-41
effects of situational and personal
sentience and inhibition on alcohol
consumption, 31-33
Thematic Apperception Test in (*see*
Thematic Apperception Test, in
Setting and Alcohol Experiments)
Time Concern in, 38, 40-43
Settlement patterns, detailed codes for, 368
Sex:
in class of restraining thoughts (*see* Sex
restraints)
correlation of scoring systems factors
with, 116
defined, 8-9
in discussion group: frequency of
sentient thoughts, 11
general test results, 13, 21-22
exploitative, 126-127
Personalized Power, 137
TAT samples, 150
in fraternity cocktail party: average
frequency of thoughts, 15
discussion and results, 18, 19, 21-22
intercorrelation of other behavior scales
and *n* Power with, 109-110
as nearly always Exploitative, 137
power-related scales and, 83-84, 109,
110-112, 116
rotated factor loadings and *n* Power,
111-112
in Setting and Alcohol Experiments:
conclusions, 41, 43
data, 33-34
presence of folksinger, 41
tests for, 7-8
Sex Power:
increase by alcohol consumption of, 124

intercorrelation with other categories of
Power Concerns, 167-170
restrained and unrestrained activities,
176
relation of Aggression Power to, 167-169,
348-350
subtotals predictive of drinking, 133
Sex restraints:
in class of restraining thoughts, 9
in discussion group: average frequency,
12
general test results, 14
in Setting and Alcohol Experiments:
conclusion, 34
data, 34
Sex taboos:
as characteristic predictive of drinking,
90
detailed codes for, 369
Sioux Indians, 261-275
myths about drinking among, 265-266
Personalized Power among: adolescent
cases, 268-275
destruction of old ways, 263-275
liquor in early days, 264-266
old ways, 262-263
twentieth-century developments,
266-268
Situation inhibition:
in classroom cocktail experiment, 31-33
in Setting Experiment: conclusions, 44
effects on fantasy, 40
variation, 25
Size of local community, as characteristic
predictive of drinking, 90
Sleeping distance of mother and father:
as characteristic predictive of drinking,
90
detailed codes for, 369
Sober societies and hierarchy, 60
Sobriety (see Dry subjects)
Social characteristics which predict
drinking, 90
Social control and sober societies, 60
"Social Drinking in Different Settings"
(Kalin), 21-44
Social interaction, 5-14
by business administration students:
coding schemes, 8-10
results and discussion, 10-14
test procedures, 5-8
Socialized Power:
correlation of restrained assertiveness
with, 178-181
correlation of unrestrained assertiveness
with, 181-183
intercorrelation of other categories of
Power Concerns with, 167-170, 175
Meaning Contrast as nearly always, 137
in motivational correlations of smoking
pot, 372
promise of scoring, 167
relation of Activity Inhibition to, 164-166

relation of miscellaneous assertive
activities to, 183-185
scoring manual for, 351-356
Socialized Power scores:
differing drinking histories and, 155-161
frequencies after alcohol consumption,
133
function of, 197
low-level drinking and, 135
nature of, 134
type of alcoholic beverage and, 134
Socio-economic simplicity scale, 90
Sorrow (feminine tag):
as concern for others, 84
relationship of Factor II to, 83
Spanish Americans, drinking by
Anglo-Americans and Indians
compared with, 293-296
Speed (see Amphetamines)
Speeding, 348-349
correlation of n Power and assertive
activities with, 176-177
correlation of Personalized Power scores
with, 192
Spending money correlated with n Power,
105-106
Sports, competitive, correlation of n Power
with, 103-104
Sports participation, 349
correlation of n Power and activities
inhibition with, 171
correlation of n Power and assertive
activities with, 176-177
correlation of Personalized and
Socialized Power and assertive
activities with, 179-180
"Sporty" magazines, 176
correlation of n Power and Activity
Inhibition with, 171
correlation of n Power and assertive
activities with, 176-177
correlation of Personalized Power
scores with, 192
relation of Personalized and Socialized
Power and assertive activities with,
184
Stag cocktail parties, qualification of term,
40
Stateless societies, correlation of drinking
with, 64-67
Steele, Robert, "Motives for Drug Taking
Among College Men," 370-378
Strong Power:
intercorrelations of other categories of
Power Concerns with, 167-170
restrained and unrestrained
activities, 176
as characteristic predictive of drinking,
132-133
Subsistence Anxiety:
correlation of folk-tale themes with, 59
insobriety and, 48, 49
"Summary" (McClelland), 332-336
Supplies, correlation of n Power with, 105

Taking (folk-tale tag):
   relative frequency in folk tales, 58
   correlation of drinking with, 59, 60
Taking walks, correlation of *n* Power with,
   106
Television set, correlation of *n* Power
   with, 105
Television viewing, 348, 349
   correlation of *n* Power and Activity
      Inhibition with, 171
Television "violence," 348
   correlation of *n* Power and assertive
      activities with, 176-177
   correlation of Peronalized and Socialized
      Power scores and unrestrained
      assertive activities with, 181-182
Temperature:
   as characteristic predictive of drinking,
      90
   detailed codes for, 369
Teton Sioux:
   myths about drinking among, 265-266
   Personalized Power among: adolescent
      cases, 268-275
   destruction of old ways, 263-275
   liquor in early days, 264-266
   old ways, 262-263
   twentieth century developments,
      266-268
Thematic Apperception Test (TAT):
   coding scheme for, 8-10
   differing drinking histories and power
      scores in, 155-161
   in fraternity cocktail party, 14-20
   general use of, 6-8
   in helping socializing alcoholics' power
      needs, 322, 328
   in Setting and Alcohol Experiments:
      data analysis, 30-40
      instructions for TAT, 28
      procedure, 24, 28-29
      selection and arrangement, 26-27
   in social discussion group, 5-14
   for working-class men, 145-151
Thinking, alcohol's role in, viii, ix
Thonga tribe, 51
Thought samples, ix
Time Concern, 125
   in class of restraining thoughts, 9
   defined, 9
   differing drinking histories and, 155-161
   in discussion group: average frequency,
      12
      general test results, 14
   effects of drinking on, 124, 139-140
   in fraternity cocktail party, 18, 19
   as lacking predictive value, 151-152
   relation of Activity Inhibition to,
      138-139
   in Setting and Alcohol Experiments:
      conclusions, 40, 43
      data, 38
      folksinger, 41-42

Time hanging around, correlation of *n*
   Power and Activity Inhibition with,
   171
Time with women, 176, 349
   correlation of *n* Power and Activity
      Inhibition with, 171
   correlation of *n* Power and assertive
      activities with, 176-177
   correlation of Personalized and
      Socialized Power and restrained
      assertive activities with, 179-180
Time working, 349
Title (folk-tale tag):
   correlation of drinking with, 59, 71
   correlation of Factors I and II with, 88
   positive loading of, 80
   relative frequency in folk tales, 58
   sober societies and, 60
Transportation, correlation of *n* Power
   with, 105
Travel and Gather (folk-tale tag):
   correlation of drinking with, 59
   relative frequency in folk tales, 58
Travel money, correlation of Personalized
   and Socialized Power scores and
   unrestrained assertive activities
   with, 181-182
Treatment of heavy drinkers, 336

Uleman system, 114-115
Ulithi tribe, 51
Unable (folk-tale tag), words classified
   under, 54
Unrestrained assertiveness:
   correlation of *n* Power sub-scores with,
      175-177
   correlation of Personalized and
      Socialized Power with, 178-182
   (*See also* Assertive thoughts and acts)
Unstructured societies:
   correlation of drinking with, 64
   factors involved, 67-68
   instrumental use of dreams in, 66

Value expectations, correlations of
   Personalized Power needs and
   drinking with, 193-195
Vanneman, Reeve, xiv
   "Drinking in the Wider Context of
      Restrained and Unrestrained
      Assertive Thoughts and Acts,"
      162-197
Veroff scoring system, 114-115
Vertical Space (folk-tale tag):
   correlation of drinking with, 59
   relative frequency in folk tales, 58
   sober societies and, 60
Vicarious experience:
   correlation of scoring system factors
      with, 116
   intercorrelation of other behavior scales
      and *n* Power with, 109-110
   power-related scales and, 108-112, 116

rotated factor loadings and *n* Power, 111-112
Vicarious magazines, reading, 349
Vigorous Activities (folk-tale tag):
  assertive factors loading on, 173
  correlation of Factors I and II with, 88
  correlation of male and female pronouns with, 78
  highest loading of Factor II on, 81, 86
  as measure of Power Concerns, 84
Violent Physical Manipulation (folk-tale tag):
  as additional masculine tag, 79
  correlation of Combined Drinking Score with, 84
  correlation of Factor I and II with, 88
  drinking closely correlated with, 283
  negative loading of, 81
  power-related concerns tapped by, 82
  relative frequency in folk tales, 58
"Violent" television:
  correlation of *n* Power and assertive activities with, 176-177
  correlation of Personalized and Socialized Power scores and unrestrained assertive activities with, 181-182

Wanner, Eric, xiv
  "Power and Inhibition: A Revision of the Magical Potency Theory," 73-98
  "A Cross-Cultural Study of Folk-Tale Content and Drinking," 48-72
  "Drinking in the Wider Context of Restrained and Unrestrained Assertive Thoughts and Acts," 162-197
Want (folk-tale tag):
  correlation of drinking with, 59, 60
  correlation of male and female pronouns with, 78
  relative frequency in folk tales, 58
War (folk-tale tag):
  correlation of drinking with, 61
  correlation of Factors I and II with, 88
  correlation of male and female pronouns with, 78
  highest loading on Factor II, 81, 86
  as measure of power coercion, 84
  relative frequency in folk tales, 58

Warm winter temperature, as characteristic predictive of drinking, 90
Weak Power:
  as characteristic predictive of drinking, 132-133
  intercorrelation of other categories of Power Concerns with, 167-170
  restrained and unrestrained activities, 176
Wet climate, as characteristic predictive of drinking, 90
Wilsnack, Sharon Carlson, xiv
  "The Effects of Drinking on Thoughts About Power and Restraint," 123-141
Wine consumed, 349
  correlation of *n* Power and assertive activities with, 176-177
  correlation of Personalized and Socialized Power and restrained assertive activities with, 179-180
Wine glasses, correlation of *n* Power with, 105
Winter, David G., xiv, 47
  "The Need for Power in College Men: Action Correlates and Relationship to Drinking," 99-119
Winter coding system, 114-115, 124, 126
Winter temperature, detailed codes for, 369
Work, success at, 313-314
Working-class men:
  activities' questions asked of, 342-347
  descriptive characteristics of, 148-149
  Power Concerns in drinking by, 142-161
    correlation of marital problems and drinking with Power Concerns, 357
    experimental problems, 142-144
    index of Power Concerns, 185-186
    intercorrelation of alternative manifestations of Personalized Power Concerns, 186-187
    Personalized Power score, 187-192
    procedure, 144-151
    results, 151-161
  relation of Socialized and Personalized Power categories to Activity Inhibition in, 164-166
  restrained and unrestrained assertiveness in, 175-181